MANAGEMENT OF
SPINAL CORD INJURIES

This volume is one of the series,
Rehabilitation Medicine Library,
edited by John V. Basmajian

* Originally published as part of the Physical Medicine Library, edited by
   Sidney Licht.

MANAGEMENT OF SPINAL CORD INJURIES

Edited by

Ralph F. Bloch, M.D., Ph.D., F.R.C.P.(C)

Associate Professor of Medicine
McMaster University
Faculty of Health Sciences
Director of Neurotrauma Program
Chedoke Rehabilitation Centre
Hamilton, Ontario, Canada

Mel Basbaum, M.S.W.

Social Work Department
Chedoke-McMaster Hospitals
Chedoke Rehabilitation Centre
Hamilton, Ontario, Canada

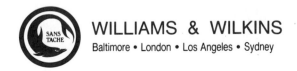

WILLIAMS & WILKINS
Baltimore • London • Los Angeles • Sydney

Editor: John Butler
Associate Editor: Carol Eckhart
Copy Editor: CRACOM Corporation
Design: Bob Och
Illustration Planning: Reginald Stanley
Production: Anne G. Seitz

Accurate indications, adverse reactions, and dosage schedules for drugs are
provided in this book, but it is possible that they may change. The reader is urged
to review the package information data of the manufacturers of the medications
mentioned.

Printed in the United States of America

Library of Congress Cataloging in Publication Data

Main entry under title:
Management of spinal cord injuries.
   (Rehabilitation medicine library)
   Includes index.
   1. Spinal cord—Wounds and injuries—Treatment. 2. Spinal cord—Wounds and
injuries—Complications and sequelae. I. Bloch, R. F. II. Basbaum, Mel. III. Series.
[DNLM: 1. Spinal Cord Injuries—therapy.
WL 400 M266]
RD595.M255   1986   617′.482044   85-17807
ISBN 0-683-00851-X
Composed and printed at the   86 87 88 89 90
Waverly Press, Inc.   10 9 8 7 6 5 4 3 2 1

Series Editor's Foreword

A wide spectrum of people have a deep interest in the various aspects of spinal cord injuries. They range from government and insurance officials at one end to the patients and their immediate relatives at the other. In between are many people who come in touch with the individual patient—sometimes only transiently as onlookers but sometimes for long periods either of cooperation or of conflict.

This book emphasizes the ways in which a compact can be arranged with the prime actor of each individual drama to bring about the best results possible under difficult circumstances. Shakespeare aptly compared our world to a stage and all of us mere players on it. Suddenly the patient with a spinal cord injury is thrust unwillingly and unrehearsed into the role of a "star." Little does either the patient or the immediate family realize that a large cast of well-trained supporting players stands by, ready to help. Increasingly their training and skills have been honed to the point today where it bears little resemblance to the uniformly tragic dramas I first saw enacted some 40 years ago.

Of course tragedy still holds center stage in many cases. But with ideal management combined with the buoyant will of most human beings in times of duress, many patients with spinal cord injuries bounce back with a vigor that never fails to thrill me. The tragedy is turned into high drama and the professional members of the management team are proud to have had their important moments on the stage with a real star.

This book illuminates that stage. Each chapter is like a light. Some chapters provide back lighting, some are floodlights, and some are brilliant spotlights. All are essential for achieving total success. That some of the stars can and do achieve brilliant successes comes as no surprise for those who read and implement the lessons of this book. Ralph Bloch and Mel Basbaum, along with all our authors, have performed a great service in the writing of this important volume in the *Rehabilitation Medicine Library* series. And I am happy to have been silent "producer" behind the scenes.

JOHN V. BASMAJIAN

Preface

Injuries to the spinal cord are among the most devastating physical insults an individual may suffer. They spare the mind, leaving intact all desires and aspirations, while rendering the body unable to obey many, if not most, of the commands necessary to achieve these goals.

Medical science and technology have made great progress in the field of spinal cord injury care over the past 50 years. Life expectancy, even for patients with high quadriplegia, is starting to approach that of the healthy population. Quality of life, on the other hand, is lagging behind physical homeostasis. Only a small number of paraplegics and even fewer quadriplegics return to gainful employment. Access to avocational activities is limited by physical and attitudinal barriers. Many patients feel discriminated against, even during their rehabilitation phase. They perceive themselves as being subject to excessive control by physicians and hospital staff, and this accentuates their own sense of lost control.

Professionals who care for patients with spinal cord injuries require specific knowledge and skills, and also an appropriate attitude. This book focuses on transmitting information, thus increasing knowledge. Skills are most effectively developed by demonstration and practice; we do not fully understand how attitudes are shaped. However we would feel remiss, simply providing information without pointing out the importance of the simultaneous development of technical skills and healthy attitudes.

RALPH BLOCH
MEL BASBAUM

January 1986

vii

Contributors

Michael R. Achong, M.D., F.R.C.P.(C), F.A.C.P.
Associate Professor
Department of Medicine
St. Joseph's Hospital
Hamilton, Ontario, Canada

Natalie Bahry, B.Sc. (O.T.), O.T.(C)
Hamilton-Wentworth Home Care Program
Hamilton, Ontario, Canada

Mel Basbaum, M.S.W.
Chedoke-McMaster Hospitals
Social Work Department
Chedoke Rehabilitation Centre
Hamilton, Ontario, Canada

Ralph F. Bloch, M.D., Ph.D., F.R.C.P.(C)
Associate Professor of Medicine
McMaster University
Faculty of Health Sciences
Director of Neurotrauma Program
Chedoke Rehabilitation Centre
Hamilton, Ontario, Canada

Pamela J. Cluff, F.R.A.I.C., F.R.I.B.A.
Associated Planning Consultants, Inc.
Toronto, Ontario, Canada

M. Decker, Dip.P.T., M.C.P.A.
Chedoke-McMaster Hospitals
Physiotherapy Department
Chedoke Division-Holbrook Pavilion
Hamilton, Ontario, Canada

Ronald Gerridzen, F.R.C.S.(C)
Assistant Professor of Surgery (Urology)
University of Ottawa
Ottawa, Canada

Stanley D. Gertzbein, M.D., F.R.C.S.(C)
Associate Professor
Department of Surgery
University of Toronto
Consultant Orthopaedic Surgeon
Acute Spinal Injuries Units
Sunnybrook Medical Centre
Toronto, Ontario, Canada

A. Hall
Graduate Student
Design Measurement & Evaluation Program
Department of Clinical Epidemiology & Biostatistics
Faculty of Health Sciences
McMaster University
Hamilton, Ontario, Canada

Robert R. Hansebout, M.D., F.R.C.S.(C), F.A.C.S.
Head of Neurosurgery
St. Joseph's Hospital
Professor of Surgery
McMaster University
Hamilton, Ontario, Canada

S. Herschorn, B.Sc., M.D., C.M., F.R.C.S.(C)
Assistant Professor of Surgery
Chief of Urology
Sunnybrook Medical Centre
Toronto, Ontario, Canada

R. Hollingworth, M.D., F.R.C.P.(C)
McMaster Clinic
Hamilton General Hospital
Hamilton, Ontario, Canada

Jeanette Keenan
Associated Planning Consultants, Inc.
Toronto, Ontario, Canada

M. D. L. Morgan, M.D., (Cantab), M.R.C.P.(U.K)
Department of Chest Medicine
East Birmingham Hospital
Bordesley Green
Birmingham, England

T. Seaton, M.B., F.R.C.P.(C)
Head, Service of Gastroenterology
Hamilton Civic Hospitals
Associate Clinical Professor
McMaster University
Hamilton, Ontario, Canada

Bhagwan T. Shahani, M.D., D.Phil.(Oxon)
Clinical Neurophysiology Laboratory
Department of Neurology
Massachusetts General Hospital
Harvard Medical School
Boston, Massachusetts

J. R. Silver, M.D., B.S., F.R.C.P.(Ed. & Lond.)
Consultant in Spinal Injuries
Stoke Mandeville Hospital
Aylesbury, Bucks, England

Samuel L. Stover, M.D.
Professor and Chairman
Department of Rehabilitation Medicine
The University of Alabama at Birmingham
Birmingham, Alabama

George Szasz, M.D.
Professor and Director of In-Patient Services
Sexual Medicine Unit
Faculty of Medicine
University of British Columbia
Shaughnessy Hospital
Vancouver, British Columbia, Canada

Roberta B. Trieschmann, Ph.D.
Consulting Psychologist
Scottsdale, Arizona

Eldon Tunks, M.D., F.R.C.P.(C)
Director of Chedoke-McMaster Pain Programs
Professor of Psychiatry
McMaster University
Hamilton, Ontario, Canada

A. G. G. Turpie, M.B., F.R.C.P.(Glas. & Lon.), F.A.C.P., F.R.C.P.C.
Professor of Medicine
Hamilton General Hospital
McMaster Clinic
Hamilton, Ontario, Canada

A. Vaugeois
Chedoke-McMaster Hospitals
Chedoke Division
Hamilton, Ontario, Canada

S. J. Williams
Lung Function Unit
Bromptom Hospital
London, England

Robert R. Young, M.D.
Movement Disorder Clinic
Clinical Neurophysiology Laboratory
Department of Neurology
Massachusetts General Hospital
Harvard Medical School
Boston, Massachusetts

Contents

Introduction

The purpose of this book is to give an inventory of the state of the art of rehabilitating individuals with spinal cord injuries in the 1980s. Rather than attempting to put together a "How to" book, we had asked the contributors for a critical appraisal of the literature they review. It is difficult to steer a safe course between the uncritical empiricism of the clinical craftsman and the therapeutic nihilism of the methodologist sitting at his desk. Various contributors have succeeded to different degrees.

This book does not quite have the breadth originally intended because there were some areas for which we were unable to find experts who were both able and willing to meet the deadlines necessary to publish a multi-authored book. Specifically, we lack chapters on the epidemiology of spinal injuries, on clinical assessment, on spinal cord nursing care, on prevention and treatment of pressure sores, on wheelchairs and bracing, and on fertility in spinal cord patients. This book puts its emphasis on those areas that have seen new developments and insights over the past ten years.

The first chapter reviews current neurosurgical management of cord injuries, surgical and conservative. Experimental treatments currently being evaluated are discussed together with more time-hallowed procedures. Whether established or experimental, the various interventions are largely based on face evidence and animal experiments. Most are justified on the basis of case reports and case series. Case control studies are few; analytical cohort and randomized controlled studies are not available. Many methods in current clinical use remain to be supported or refuted by properly controlled studies. Even though the efficacy of various methods of cord resuscitation has not been well established, these methods are widely practiced. Cord regeneration has not yet reached the state where it can be used clinically.

Chapter 2, dealing with the orthopedic management of the fractured spine, describes various surgical techniques in current use. The fundamental questions of conservative management versus surgical stabilization and the exact role of decompression are still subjects for debate.

The third chapter deals with the altered physiology of breathing in patients with quadriplegia. Therapeutic interventions are discussed based on their role in current practice and the fact that they make clinical sense. The various suggested techniques have not been subjected to critical evaluation.

Chapter 4 deals with the pathophysiology of the neurogenic bladder, basing therapeutic suggestions on an understanding of physiology and various case studies. Historic controls are of some help since the dire complications of chronic reflux and urinary tract infections are well known. Manometric and videourodynamics have greatly contributed to our understanding of the altered function of the urinary tract. Whether their use affects outcome in the majority of patients is, at present, conjectural. Use of parasympatholytic drugs and their side effects are presented.

The fifth chapter discusses function and management of the neurogenic bowel. The chapter is largely based on nonspinal cord data, extrapolating general principles. The use of high fiber diets, stool softeners, and laxatives is discussed.

Chapter 6 reviews the various syndromes associated with autonomic de-efferentation and automatism. Most of the data come from physiological animal and human experiments and case studies. From a clinical point of view, elucidation of prevalence and natural history, as well as prevention and treatment of the apneic bradyarrhythmia syndrome in quadriplegics might offer a significant impact on quality of care.

In Chapter 7 we return to the urinary tract, focusing on the management of infections. The two major issues are the effects of antibacterial prophylaxis and the treatment of asymptomatic bacteruria on long-term health and on patient survival.

Chapter 8 deals with the problem of pain in spinal cord injured patients. Diagnosis of the cause of pain and its treatment is no easier in these patients than in pain sufferers without damage to the spinal cord.

Prevention and treatment of venous thrombosis and pulmonary embolism are discussed in Chapter 9. This clinical entity has been well studied in other patient groups with the effectiveness of various interventions carefully evaluated.

Spasticity, a major cause of discomfort for individuals with spinal cord damage is addressed in Chapter 10. Most of the effort has been directed at elucidating the pathophysiology of spasticity. Conservative interventions against spasticity have limited efficacy. There is a need for comparative studies of the various pharmacological antispasticity agents. Similarly, there is a need for case series that evaluate the long-term effects of different operative procedures for the reduction of spasticity.

Chapter 11 discusses a less common complication of spinal cord injury, heterotopic ossification. While the exact role of spasticity, associated injuries, and aggressive range of movement exercises in the pathogenesis of heterotopic ossification is still somewhat speculative, it appears that disodium edetate is effective in preventing the progression of ossification.

Chapter 12 examines the literature on the psychosocial adjustment to spinal cord injury. By necessity, this chapter is very descriptive. This descriptive chapter reveals the difficulty of conducting controlled trials of various interventions in the psychosocial field.

In Chapter 13, efficacy of physical therapy is carefully reviewed in light of current literature. A useful conceptual framework in the approach to therapy is provided.

Occupational therapy is addressed in Chapter 14. In contrast to physical therapy, the current approach in occupational therapy is very strongly focused on the needs of individual patients. There are fewer physiologically generalizable principles and clinical trials are practically nonexistent.

Chapter 15 addresses possible solutions to the functional problems encountered in the living environment. While emphasis is placed on the many pragmatic issues of architectural design, and accessibility, the authors remain cognizant of individual differences that exist in terms of physical disability, life-style, and personal goals.

If we have been slow to validate the results of physiologically based treatment modalities, this is even more true of the social and psychological success or failure following spinal cord rehabilitation. Chapter 16 identifies the many complex treatment, personality, family, and community variables that influence outcomes in the years following spinal cord injury. Again, by necessity, many hypotheses are proposed but few empirical data are presented. It is apparent from the information, however, that as life expectancy of the spinal cord injured patient improves, quality of life issues have become increasingly relevant. Rehabilitation professionals must begin to look beyond the walls of the institution for the answers they require.

Finally, in Chapter 17, adaptation to the physiological, functional, psychological, and social consequences of spinal cord injury are addressed in respect to sexuality. While practical assessment and treatment approaches are provided, the scope of the issue and the need for multidisciplinary cooperation in addition to the specialist in "sexual health care" are emphasized.

From a methodological point of view, most of the therapeutic interventions in current clinical use are poorly validated. This is not necessarily due to lack of intention. Spinal cord injuries have a low incidence and are fairly variable in their presentation, depending on level and completeness. This makes it difficult for all but the largest centers to collect sufficient subjects for a proper evaluation of any intervention. We lack generally accepted and validated clinical and paraclinical descriptive tools, which are necessary to allow for valid multicenter studies. Above all, for patients, families, and professionals alike, spinal cord injury constitutes such a major and irreversible threat to homeostasis and function that it is psychologically, if not ethically, difficult to withhold any therapy that could possibly be of benefit.

If we want to become more confident that our treatments do more good than harm, we must move toward more rigid evaluation of therapeutic efficacy and effectiveness. Given the practical barriers, we have to start by developing mechanisms that will make large multicenter trials possible.

1

The Neurosurgical Management of Cord Injuries

ROBERT R. HANSEBOUT

For at least 4500 years, the treatment of spinal cord injuries has been cloaked in an aura of pessimism. It was written in the Edwin Smith Surgical Papyrus that such injuries were hopeless (178). Unfortunately, this attitude has persisted through the centuries.

Attempts at the reduction of fracture dislocations of the spine have been described since the mid-17th century. Sporadic operative attempts at decompression of the fractured spine are noted in the mid-18th century. With the advent of anesthesia in 1846, surgery of the spine became more common. During the latter part of the 19th century, some attempts where made at anastomosing the severed spinal cord. In 1905 Cushing formulated the indications and contraindications for surgery in spinal injuries (178). Since that time the pendulum has swung to and fro from those who believe surgical therapy is of no avail to those who advocate surgery in almost every case. Thus even today the surgical treatment of spinal injuries remains controversial.

Some of the issues remain unresolved for a number of reasons. First, the spinal cord is a relatively small structure. In the past, diagnostic methods did not adequately reveal the cord pathology. Moreover, the surgeon rarely explores the inside of the spinal cord during surgery. The basic mechanisms of spinal cord injury dysfunction have been poorly understood. In addition, there has been conflicting evidence in the literature concerning spinal cord injury pathophysiology. Second, there is no uniform universal classification of spinal cord injury. In many papers it is difficult to know whether the patients have sustained complete or incomplete functional cord syndromes. Third, there is a lack of controlled clinical studies in man comparing the results of one treatment with another. This is compounded by the fact that few centers treat enough patients on a yearly basis to obtain statistically

1

significant information. Lastly, if a properly conducted study is ever carried out amongst a number of centers, it will take several years to obtain significant information. For these reasons the present management of patients with spinal injuries is somewhat based on anecdotal evidence, the experience of the treating physician, and regional practices.

During the past 15 years, a great deal of research has been done to delineate some of the alterations in spinal cord injury pathophysiology. Moreover, there have been broad advances in diagnostic capabilities. The use of somatosensory evoked responses and computed tomography (CT) is becoming more commonplace. With the advent of nuclear magnetic resonance (NMR), hopefully it may become easier to categorize spinal injuries on an individual patient basis in the future.

The following outline is based on the current management of patients with spinal injuries at the Hamilton General Hospital. The author's personal bias of timely aggressive treatment will undoubtedly be reflected.

Pathophysiology

After being subjected to a sudden force, the spinal cord may not function for a variable period of time. Then function may gradually return. This altered state has been termed *spinal shock*, although its exact mechanism is not known. After cord injury, there may be a gradual loss of potassium from the injured cord tissues (112). It is possible that this potassium gathers in excess concentrations in the extracellular fluid to cause spinal shock (54). As the potassium level subsequently normalizes, spinal shock may wear off.

Even after severe injury, the spinal cord is rarely completely transected either in animals (181) or in man (15, 157). The cord may look fairly normal for a few minutes after such an injury, although it may be rendered nonfunctional due to a direct force to the axons (100). Within a few minutes, small hemorrhages develop within the central gray matter (8), and these hemorrhages progressively increase (49) until, by 4 hours after injury, there is central hemorrhagic necrosis of the gray matter and adjacent white matter. By 24 hours, the central gray and white matters are necrotic with only a rim of white matter remaining (175).

Cord injury is followed by the development of edema that becomes maximal between the third and sixth day after the injury (112) and persists until the 15th day (179). It had been postulated that such edema expands the cord, causing pressure therein and thus reducing blood flow, resulting in necrosis (5). However, other evidence suggested that structural damage rather than edema is the main culprit (111) in spinal cord dysfunction.

Vascular damage (50) has been singled out as a major problem after severe spinal cord injury with hypoxia (63) and severe ischemia (10) beginning immediately after trauma and persisting for at least 24 hours (165), leading to a reduction in the cord's oxygen tension (113). Some researchers do not believe ischemia is the main deleterious factor following cord injury

(12, 16, 73, 74, 101, 103). Two investigators found a global decrease in blood flow both in the white and gray matters of the cord following injury (135, 150). However, other investigators found that after severe cord injury there was decreased blood flow in the gray matter but increased flow in the white matter (16, 102, 154). Thus there are some contradictions concerning the role of decreased blood flow following spinal cord injury.

One report suggests that a mitochondrial lesion is responsible for cord dysfunction after injury (92), while another implicates the release of lysosomes (98). Further work indicates that toxic free-radicals may be responsible (33). An interesting theory is that norepinephrine is released from the gray matter following injury, temporarily halting functions in the white matter and later causing vasospasm with cord autodestruction and permanent loss of function (127). However, there was much criticism of the norepinephrine theory by a number of investigators (17, 85, 121, 131).

Regardless of the ultimate mechanism of cord dysfunction following injury, necrosis of the gray matter and a large amount of the inner white matter occurs after severe cord injury, typically leaving only the shell of the outer rim of the cord by 2 months following the injury.

There is still a lot of debate about the pathogenesis of cord injury but not the final pathology. There is general agreement that the cord is usually not initially destroyed, but in order to preserve the white matter, something extraordinary has to be accomplished within the first few hours following the injury. After that, cord preservation is out of the question, and one is left with consideration of regeneration.

Emergency Management

The first principle is to try and prevent further harm to the cord in any patient with a suspected spinal fracture or cord injury. It is well known that cord injuries can be accentuated by improper first aid care (67, 71). Therefore, unless there is danger of burning or drowning, the patient should be moved only when adequate help is present, after bleeding and respiratory distress are under control. The patient should be moved with the spine held as straight as possible, exerting traction on the head and countertraction on the lower extremities. However, we advise the transferring physician to immediately give a loading dose of intramuscular steroid on notification that a patient with a potential spinal cord injury has been diagnosed. The easiest position for transport is the supine position, allowing access to the airway; an indwelling urinary catheter should be used if the transportation period is going to be lengthy.

In the emergency room, a complete neurological examination is performed to determine the level of injury and whether the patient has a complete cord injury with absence of any sensorimotor, bowel, or bladder function below the injury, or an incomplete spinal cord syndrome. A multiple system examination is also carried out to determine any bony, chest, or adominal injuries. In addition, treatment of shock is undertaken when necessary. Attention is directed to respiratory care, especially with a high cervical cord injury. Blood samples are drawn for various studies, and blood is cross-matched in anticipation of possible surgery. It is to be noted that patients with cervical cord injury often have hypotension, bradycardia, and decreased body temperature, and that this does not necessarily indicate hemorrhagic shock (178). It is important to obtain blood gas measurements. I feel there is rarely an indication for "diagnostic" lumbar puncture in spinal injury cases.

Diagnostic Procedures

The main diagnostic procedure is the patient's medical history, if obtainable, and good neurological and physical examinations. Unless the patient is exposed to a life-threatening situation, plain x-rays should be taken immediately while providing that there is no spinal movement, especially in the cervical region. Films should be made in at least two planes. An open-mouth view should be made to visualize the C1–2 region. Especially in muscular males, the C6–7-T1 region may be difficult to visualize. Sometimes clarification is obtained by pulling the shoulders down, obtaining oblique views, or getting a "swimmer's view" (165). A prevertebral soft tissue thickness of greater than 5 mm is indirect evidence of a cervical vertebral injury (172).

Special Radiography

If a fracture is suspected but cannot be seen on plain x-rays, tomograms are indicated, especially in the C1–2 area and the lower cervical region (94). Facet displacement may sometimes be better appreciated using tomography than plain x-rays. Tomography may also obviate the need for oblique views or excess manipulation of the head and neck. The above investigation is often ample in patients without any neurological deficit. It may give sufficient information to determine whether external stabilization is adequate or whether operative fusion is required. In patients with complete or incomplete lesions, further diagnostic evaluation may be required.

High resolution computed tomography of the vertebral column gives an accurate cross-sectional view of the spinal canal (65). It can also reveal the presence of small pieces of bone compressing the cord from within or without and may also disclose disc protrusion in the thoracic and thoraco-lumbar regions. Even intramedullary hematomas can sometimes be shown (130).

Whether more than the above examinations will be performed in any particular patient depends on that patient's neurological and general clinical condition. For example, intra-abdominal hemorrhage, shock, or respiratory complications may preclude further investigation prior to lifesaving surgery. In addition, some of the newer treatment methods require rapid exposure of the dura or cord, in which case information that would have been gained by diagnostic radiographic procedures may be obtained during surgery. In patients with complete cord lesions of longer than 24 hours duration, there is no good evidence that conventional treatment helps in the acute stage and perhaps no further investigation is indicated except in a few exceptional cases. Patients with a complete neurological deficit of the cauda equina region will require further investigation especially if no cause is seen in the preceding investigation (165) since these have a greater propensity for recovery than cord lesions. Patients with incomplete neurological deficits for which there is no obvious cause on the plain x-rays or who show progressive deterioration also require further investigation. In such cases myelography should be considered (165).

The use of oil (iophendylate) for myelography in acute cases has been controversial since it has been said that arachnoiditis may be initiated in combination with a bloody cerebrospinal fluid (148). Oil has been injected by the C1–2 lateral puncture in cervical injuries to demonstrate persistent cord compression after spinal alignment by skeletal traction (142) or by the lumbar route (165) for thoracic and lumbar injury. However, the use of oil myelography in acute trauma may be of little diagnostic value (144).

Myelography using gas by a C1–2 puncture has been advocated (138) in cervical spinal injuries. This may be performed with the patient in a supine position and is said to give excellent visualization of the entire subarachnoid space and spinal cord (165), although one usually does not see much detail (178). It is not being used in our unit.

Water-soluble contrast material (metrizamide) gives good quality myelograms (153). This does not require removal, causes few complications, but may rapidly become diluted. For cervical studies it is given by the C1–2 lateral spinal puncture. This may reveal cord compression and pathology. This material may be used to enhance computed tomography of the spine. In this way, sometimes cord swelling can be differentiated from extrinsic cord pressure demonstrating the need for medical or surgical therapy (130). It may also show radicular compression (28). In the cervical region this technique is said to offer advantages over oil or gas myelography (110).

Computed tomography and/or myelography may demonstrate the need for surgical decompression and in addition may allow more precise planning of an anterior or posterior approach to the spine.

During the last two years the technique of imaging (MRI) magnetic resonance has been developed in medicine. The advantage of this technique is that apparently no radiation is imparted to the patient while giving extremely clear images of the central nervous system, including the spinal cord and nerve roots (76). Whether or not this technique will prove useful in the diagnostic management of acute spinal cord trauma remains to be seen. It is highly likely that this type of study will prove useful in the evaluation of cases of chronic spinal cord injury.

Evoked Potentials

There has been a great deal of interest in the use of evoked responses, first described in 1947 (42), to study patients with disorders of the central nervous system. In spinal cord injury the most applicable is the somatosensory evoked response or potential. An electrode is placed externally over a major nerve in the body, such as the posterior tibial or the median nerve. Electrodes are applied to the scalp in the same fashion as for an electroencephalogram. A volley of stimuli is applied to a peripheral nerve, causing minute potentials to appear over the brain when the spinal cord is intact. When a number of such potentials are averaged in a computer, a characteristic evoked response is obtained. However, when the spinal cord is severely damaged, the impulses are not conducted across the point of injury and the evoked response is absent. This then corroborates the findings of a complete cord injury during the clinical examination. Of course incomplete cord injury causes variations in the wave form and often a delay in conduction of the evoked response.

It has been found that the prognosis for recovery in dogs with spinal injuries is poor if the somatosensory cortical evoked potential (SSEP) cannot be recorded within 4 hours following injury (45). It was also shown that cord compression can obliterate the SSEP (38). It is thought that the evoked response is carried mainly in the posterior column, based on a study conducted on seven patients with lesions involving these tracts (69). The author has noted also that evoked responses are not altered in patients who have undergone lateral spinothalamic tractotomies to alleviate pain, further substantiating that conclusion.

In experimental animals the evoked response may disappear within 20–90 sec after injury (152). Complete cord transection in animals can change the EEG with an increase in fusiform spindle bursts and the addition of long, symmetrical runs of regular fast and low amplitude activity (109). Other studies showed that severe, irreversible neurological deficits could occur in cats in which the SSEP disappeared following cord injury. In animals with cord injury in which the SSEP did not disappear, only mild neurological loss was evident 6 weeks after injury (115).

The SSEP has been said to be of great assistance in the early distinction of patients with complete or incomplete spinal cord injuries (129). The SSEP has also been used in the treatment of some spinal condition such as scoliosis, with intraoperative monitoring during changes in angulation of the spine. Diminution of the evoked response signifies incipient injury to the cord and a change in operative strategy (159). Progressive normalization of the somatosensory evoked potential antedates the appearance of clinical improvement, and therefore the test can be of prognostic value in man (140). Moreover, this test may confirm completeness of an injury in unconscious patients and also determine the response to treatment in humans (165).

Although the SSEP is becoming more widely used for various spinal cord conditions, we have found some disadvantages to its use during acute trauma. The test is time-consuming, especially in a critically ill patient, the results are sometimes difficult to interpret, and it is questionable whether it adds a great deal to the conclusions obtained from a good neurological examination.

The "H" reflex has also been used following spinal cord trauma. Its absence may indicate damage to the central gray matter of the cord both in animals (40) and humans (168).

Other Investigations

Arteriography of the spinal cord has been used especially in cervical and high thoracic spinal injuries (66). However, in monkeys it was found that changes in the spinal artery were inconsistent following trauma (46). One study in humans found little usefulness for arteriography in cervical cord injury (174). In addition, spinal cord damage has been noted following angiography (52, 178). However, spinal angiography is time-consuming and difficult to perform. Moreover, the information obtained is indirect. It has not been used much in the past for investigation of spinal cord trauma, and with the newer techniques now available, it is likely that its use will decline even further in the investigation of spinal cord injury.

It is often desirable to investigate patients with complete chronic spinal cord injuries to see if there is persistant pressure on cervical nerve roots with a view toward regaining one or two root levels by decompression. Moreover, some patients with incomplete lesions and some remaining cord function may have substantial residual cord compression, especially if they have never undergone any decompressive operation. There may also be a few patients who are initially deemed to have complete lesions but who recover significant function that might be improved by surgery.

In such cases the plain x-rays may give an indication of narrowing of the spinal canal. The SSEP is also of interest in chronic cases, although we have seen quite normal-appearing evoked responses in cases with an anterior cord syndrome. We feel that one of the best current procedures is the metrizamide myelogram, done by the lateral cervical route in cervical injuries or the lumbar route for thoracic or lumbar spinal injuries, to determine the degree of myelographic block and other abnormalities. In conjunction with the CT scan, the size of the cord can be determined and the degree of compression at the site of the bony abnormality. It is also possible to detect posttraumatic syrinxes and sometimes determine the cause of myelographic defects even in total block (125, 130). Radicular compression can sometimes be noted (28).

The value of nuclear magnetic resonance in chronic spinal injuries remains to be determined.

Timeliness of Intervention

Studies of the pathological changes after cord injury indicate a progressive process (49) with major cord damage occurring between the fourth and eighth hour after injury (8). Several studies in the literature indicate that the longer the spinal cord is compressed, the worse is the neurological recovery (136, 160, 162). In the experimental lab, cooling was found to be of value when applied early (4) while its application 8 hours after injury was not of value (7). Two clinical notations indicated that early decompression (within 2 hours) was better than late treatment in humans (70, 158). On the other hand, a large study in human cervical spinal injury indicates that early spinal surgery does not influence the outcome of neurological function (83).

The Surgery of Spinal Injuries

Spinal cord function can be compromised by compression due to a tumor. Following acute spinal injury, there is often cord compression. It appears therefore logical for the surgeon to remove this compression in order to try and restore cord function. However, in cord injury there are factors at work other than physical compression. There is considerable controversy as to the role of surgery in the treatment of spinal injuries. Traditional surgical decompression with dural opening appears ineffective in restoring cord function (21, 141). However, early decompression may be of some value (44).

In man, the main neurosurgical treatment of spinal injuries has been laminectomy. Guttmann campaigned against laminectomy for many years (75). Some (14, 35) were guarded in their enthusiasm for laminectomy while others (114, 119) suggested that it was of no benefit to patients with complete or incomplete cervical cord lesions. The same is true for patients with complete thoracic cord injury (87). In patients with complete or incomplete cervical cord injury, one series (35) indicated that no operation at all was better than laminectomy. Moreover, in such cases, no operation also appeared superior to posterior fusion without laminectomy (124). A more recent study suggested that early spinal operation does not influence the outcome of neurological function in patients with severe cervical cord injury (83). In 185 patients with gunshot wounds of the spine, there was no apparent difference in neurological outcome in either complete or incomplete cord injuries (155) whether laminectomy was done or not.

In complete cervical cord injury treated mostly without operation (75, 87) or by various means (116), no patient with a complete injury of greater than 24 hours duration ever walked again. Others have indicated that laminectomy carries a low mortality and morbidity rate (36) while resulting in neurological improvement (11, 61). It should be performed as soon as possible even in patients with complete lesions to give them at least a chance of recovery (162). There are cases of cord injury deemed complete who then improved neurologically either spontaneously or following surgical decompression (48, 59, 138, 139, 157, 182). There are also reports that immediate decompression within a couple of hours may improve cord recovery (70, 158).

In most cases traumatic cord compression occurs at the anterior aspect of the cord (132, 169). Laminectomy gives only partial decompression of such an anteriorly situated compression (47). In 1962 Cloward (34) reported a return to ambulation in 33% of complete cervical cord injured patients following anterior decompression and fusion. However, when several other series were added to that of Cloward, the ambulation rate attained by patients with complete injuries was only about 3% (78). Seventy-three percent of patients with incomplete cord injuries showed neurological improvements in that combined series (78). These figures are better than those seen following cervical laminectomy. Another study (23) of cervical injury also suggested that the anterior approach gives better results than laminectomy.

Anterior decompression and fusion can be done virtually anywhere in the spine but the C1-2 region is difficult to approach (178). Operations in the thoracic and lumbar regions usually involve a team approach with thoracic and general surgeons rather than neurosurgeons and orthopaedic surgeons alone. For this reason, the posterior approach has been used most often in the thoracic and lumbar regions in the past.

There are therefore no absolute criteria for operation, especially in the case of complete cord injury. Nevertheless, in view of recent developments, there may be some reasons to proceed with surgery with a minimum of delay in selected acute cases.

There is no properly controlled clinical study in the literature of early decompression either by laminectomy and fusion or anterior decompression and fusion to indicate whether early surgical intervention is of benefit. Most of the surgeries reported have been performed after extensive cord damage has already occurred. Most of the traditional literature concerns laminectomy rather than the anterior approach, which is now becoming more popular. Some of the newer methods of treatment require rapid access to the cord. Despite the controversies, I believe that in any patient with an acute spinal cord injury, attention must be directed toward decompression of the spinal cord itself and stabilization of the spine to prevent further cord damage.

With respect to complete chronic cord injuries, there is no convincing evidence that late decompression is of value in restoring cord function. However, even in patients with complete injury, sometimes relief of pressure on a single nerve root may add one level of function that can be of tremendous importance to a quadriplegic. Moreover, late anterior decompression in patients with incomplete cord injury can result in significant functional improvement (24). Occasionally, drainage of a posttraumatic central cord cyst can promote some functional neurological improvement (51) and pain relief (151).

Conservative Management

In a patient with an acute cervical injury, initial stabilization is often accomplished using sandbags. However, to provide immobilization (and possibly to realign the spine and decrease pain) cranial tongs are often used (39). These come in a number of varieties (178). The point of insertion is usually in a line along the posterior aspect of the ear and 2 cm superior to the upper margin of the ear. This area of parietal scalp is shaven, the patient mildly sedated, and a local anesthetic agent infiltrated down to the periosteum. A tiny incision is made, and the pins are inserted into drill holes in the outer margin of the parietal bone. With the patient supine, traction can be applied using a rope, pulley, and some weights. With increasing weight, realignment of the spine may be accomplished with a decompression of the spinal contents (1). Therefore, increments of weight are added periodically with control radiography until reduction is accomplished. There is controversy as to the maximum amount of weight that should be used. Crutchfield began with 18 pounds and then gradually went up to double this weight (39). Others apply no greater than 50 pounds (88), while some go up to 75 pounds (178). I have seen up to 100 pounds used with locked facets. Occasionally, to help achieve reduction, a sandbag is placed behind the shoulders to slightly extend the neck while moving the chin gently from side to side to cause slight rotation of the spine. If reduction is accomplished, the patient may report considerable pain relief, and there may be rapid improvement in neurological function in those with incomplete cord injury. The patient can then be placed in a bed with the traction pulley raised so that the back of the head rests lightly against the mattress. The maintenance weight in pounds is approximately the sum of the numerical levels of cervical vertebrae involved, i.e. 3 pounds for C2, but 28 pounds for C7. The patient is moved from side to back to side every 2 hours for a period of up to 12 weeks when maintained in tong traction.

In acute thoracic and lumbar injuries immobilization can be accomplished using positioning in bed and padded supports (59, 75). Recently halo devices have been used more in cervical spine injury (165). The halo takes longer to apply than tongs, but a body jacket can subsequently be added for stabilization while the patient is being mobilized. A number of experts indicate that long-term treatment using the above measures usually results in good bony stability (13, 30, 59, 120).

Conventional Surgical Approach

Although most studies indicate that patients with immediate complete cord injury do not improve with decompression (41, 157), such operations have traditionally been carried out after some delay. There is therefore no absolute indication for decompression operations in patients with complete cord injuries. However, there are relative indications to consider surgery in those cases.

If the patient's dislocation remains substantial (e.g. 3 mm) in the cervical region, an open reduction should be considered. This is especially true if the patient has severe pain on the basis of stretching and compression of nerve roots, even in the thoracic region. A lesion involving the cauda equina should be decompressed even if complete since there is a greater potential for recovery than in cord injury (35). In cases of cervical injury, especially with radiological evidence of nerve root compression, an anterior decompression of the cervical roots and fusion may give one level of recovery and allow earlier mobilization (89, 123, 132, 139). However, owing to the dangers of respiratory complications in cervical patients, it is sometimes wise to wait several days prior to undertaking such surgery (165).

In patients with acute incomplete lesions the absolute indication for decompression surgery is progressive deterioration of neurological function (145, 147). There are some relative indications for surgery such as cord compression due to bone fragments in the spinal canal or a ruptured disc compressing the anterior part of the cord (25). The presence of a complete block on the myelogram is usually taken to indicate that decompression should be undertaken (178). Open or compound wounds leading down to the spine or spinal cord should be debrided (25, 178). Patients with a stable neurological deficit but persistent cord compression may improve significantly from early decompression, especially through an anterior approach (108, 128, 139, 173). Occasionally patients without neurological deficits are seen with unstable fractures that may benefit from internal stabilization alone.

There is no indication for a decompression operation for an incomplete injury in a patient who is showing progressive improvement in neurological function (165). Furthermore, there is no indication for immediate surgery in patients with central cord injury syndromes since these often improve spontaneously (146). Contraindications to surgery include the presence of hemorrhagic shock, certain blood dyscrasias, or another injury, more life threatening than the spinal cord injury.

If there is no neurological involvement, fusion alone may be required if surgery is indicated. When decompression is indicated, a decision for the anterior or posterior approach will depend on the clinical findings and the site of cord compression. If the lamina and spines are fractured, a posterior approach may be indicated. If there is anterior compression of the cervical cord by disc or bone fragments, an anterior approach is better. The same is true in the thoracic and lumbar regions, although with the excellent stabilization afforded by Harrington rods, the posterior approach is more commonly used. With marked anterior compression in the thoracic region, a posterolateral transthoracic approach is sometimes used.

Great care must be undertaken to prevent movement of the spine during transport of the patient to the operating room and during anesthetic induction. In patients with a cervical injury, skull traction is continued throughout the operation, including anesthetic induction. Blind nasotracheal intubation is preferred in the awake patient while avoiding neck movement (68). However, transoral intubation can sometimes be accomplished using a fiberoptic laryngoscope. Care should be taken to inspect the skin and pad it well to prevent pressures sores, since the patient may have been in the same position for a number of hours prior to surgery. Urinary catheterization may also be necessary.

When surgery is indicated via a posterior approach, the patient is usually placed in the prone position in order to avoid orthostatic hypotension. For the cervical region, the patient is left in traction with the forehead and sides of the face resting against a well padded head rest. The spine is kept as straight as possible. In the cervical region, a neutral position is preferred, although slight flexion of the neck may be preferred for the posterior approach as long as it does not redislocate the spine. For the thoracic and lumbar regions, slight flexion or extension may be preferred to better align the spine.

After meticulous prepping and draping, a midline incision is made. Bleeding is controlled using electrocautery. After retraction, we prefer to use a cutting cautery down to the level of the spinous processes to minimize bleeding. The muscles are separated from the spinous processes and laminae of the vertebrae subperiostially. Great care should be taken to avoid damage to the spinal cord, which may be unprotected owing to extensive fracturing of the laminae. Bilateral hemilaminectomies may be carried out to inspect the dura, but most often a laminectomy is done at one level. The surgeon should avoid removing more than the mesial one third of the facet joints to ensure as much stability as possible later on. Pieces of bone compressing the dura are removed. Palpation can locate anteriorly displaced disc fragments that can often be removed through a posterior approach, but care must be taken to avoid damage to the cord when extracting them. There may be retropulsion of bone fragments due to an anteriorly compressed vertebral body; these cannot be removed via the posterior route. Hemostasis can be a problem, and small epidural veins may be coagulated using biopolar coagulating forceps while venous bleeding can be stopped using small pieces of gelfoam. Sometimes the dura is widely torn so that the cord or nerve roots can easily be seen. If possible, the dura is repaired. If torn too extensively, it is left open and gelfoam is placed over the cord and nerve roots. If the dura remains intact, we do not open it since durotomy appears ineffective in promoting functional improvement (21, 141). Opening the dura does not give a clear indication of prognosis unless the cord is transected (35) and may create a danger of herniation of the cord structures.

Once decompression has been accomplished, it is important to assure spinal stability by fusion to prevent any further cord damage.

We believe autogenous bone is the best material for fusion in the cervical region. The orthopaedic surgeon places wires under the laminae or through the base of the spinous processes followed by onlay bone grafts to incorporate vertebrae one level above and two levels below the injury. The bone grafts are then wired firmly into place.

In the thoracic and lumbar regions, posterior fusion is commonly employed (178). Harrington rods are often used for posterior immobilization in conjunction with bone chips (43, 77). Of course, bone onlay grafts can also be used. A fusion can be carried out laterally involving only facets and transverse processes (178).

More recently, the anterior approach has been advocated (165). For the cervical spine, the approach is usually from the right side. The patient remains supine in traction, with the back of the head on a head rest. The neck in slight extension is preferred. Although less cosmetic than a horizontal incision, an oblique incision affords better exposure along the anterior border of the sternomastoid muscle. Even the upper cervical vertebrae can be reached using this approach (178). However, it is most commonly used in fractures of the mid- and lower cervical regions.

The platysma is divided longitudinally. Dissection proceeds along the mesial border of the sternomastoid. The carotid sheath is retracted laterally to expose the longus colli muscles, which are divided along the anterior border of the vertebral bodies. Retraction is facilitated using Cloward instruments (178). Great care must be taken during retraction of the longus colli muscles not to compress the carotid artery on the right side or the esophagus and trachea on the left side. Bleeding from the vertebral bodies can be controlled using bone wax. A fracture may be obvious although it may be necessary to obtain x-rays after inserting a needle into a disc space to confirm the level. Pieces of bone may be removed using rongeurs or a laminectomy punch. Quite often a high speed air drill removes a vertebral body more easily in an atraumatic fashion.

If myelography has shown a localized disc protrusion without significant bone damage, a drill hole may be made as for discectomy using the Cloward instruments. In this way compressive elements of bone and disc material are removed from the dura. It is important to palpate under the edges of the vertebral bodies between the dura and bone to ensure that no further compressive pieces of tissue are present. When decompression is completed, a bone dowel can be inserted into the drill hole, distracting the vertebrae with a bone spreader.

If a complete vertebral body has been removed, the adjacent discs must also be removed using curettes. Then a piece of iliac crest or other suitable bone can be placed tightly between the remaining adjacent vertebral bodies.

Notches should be made in the upper and lower intact vertebral bodies with a high speed air drill so that the graft can be countersunk and fit tightly.

The thoracic cord can also be decompressed using a transthoracic route after removal of the pedicle (128). In our hands a transthoracic extrapleural approach has been used occasionally in the thoracic region with partial removal of the anterolateral body and adjacent pedicle for access to the cord. Anterior transperitoneal lumbar fusion is also advocated (60). Such an approach may present a problem because of the diaphragm. The hypogastric nerve plexus should be protected as well (178).

Whether an anterior or posterior approach is used, external stabilization is usually required following decompression and fusion. The halo apparatus is ideal for cervical fractures. The halo can also be used for an upper thoracic fracture. However, an external vest is usually used for immobilization in thoracic and lumbar fractures. External stabilization is maintained until clinical and radiological evidence shows union.

Of course, the same surgical techniques apply to cord decompression in chronic cases. The Russians have been advocating late decompression to improve cord function even years after the injury (107), especially by laminectomy. More recent attempts in North America to improve patients with incomplete chronic injuries have used the anterior approach (24). Depending on whether spine stability is intact after surgery, internal stabilization may or may not be necessary.

Newer Treatments of Acute Cord Injuries

Since the realization that the cord is rarely transected after cord injury, but rather undergoes progressive pathological changes leading to irreversible cord destruction, investigators have during the last 15 years tried various means of stopping these processes with a view towards preservation of tissues to enhance later rehabilitation. A number of drugs and physical agents have been tried in experimental animals, sometimes without any success and at other times with rather encouraging results. A few treatments have been used in humans with acute and sometimes even chronic cord injury. After human application, the results are often not so spectacular as those seen in controlled animal experiments. Nevertheless, a few treatments are still being administered, and some of these will be briefly dealt with below.

Osmotic Diuretics

Because increased water content in the spinal cord following injury causes increased volume, various agents have been administered to try and reduce the cord volume and presumably increase blood flow. Mannitol given to animals after cord injury decreased astrocyte swelling, but the effects were thought to be transient (133). However, its use in humans was thought not to improve neurological recovery (83). Intravenous urea was used in animals (96) while 50% glucose and water was given to humans to decrease edema (143). There is no controlled study of the effects of diuretics in human cord injury. In many centers the use of such agents is usually not considered a definitive form of treatment.

Steroids

Neurosurgeons are generally enthusiastic about giving steroids to patients with cord injury (29), but orthopaedic surgeons do not all agree (23). Steroids may stabilize membranes, preserve lysosome integrity after trauma, prevent the release of proteolytic enzymes, and thereby prevent edema (78). However, this author's work indicates that steroids do not reduce edema significantly (81) but do prevent tissue potassium depletion (106, 111, 112). This may be due to preservation of cellular elements resulting in a better functional motor state (81). However, the exact mechanism of action of steroids is unclear.

Ten series of experimental animals with cord injuries were treated with steroids in order to determine any beneficial effect on motor recovery following acute injuries (19, 27, 31, 50, 53, 72, 80, 86, 97, 112). Sixty-five percent of the treated animals improved neurologically. Eighty percent of the investigators favored steroid utilization. Another series (23) indicated that recovery in humans was no better with steroids than without but the incidence of gastrointestinal bleeding was greater. In another study the incidence of bleeding with patients on steroids was not increased (55). On the other hand, other case reports of patients with incomplete (37) and complete cord injury (70) are quoted to suggest that treatments using steroids helped patients regain useful functions. A search of the literature to date does not disclose the results of controlled studies on the effects of steroids in humans with complete and incomplete cord injury.

This author feels that some of the cord injuries sustained by humans are more severe than those seen in experimental animals. There are degrees of injury which no form of treatment will help, including steroids. On the other hand, since steroids appear to help in animal experimental series, I feel that a controlled series of steroid administration in humans with incomplete injury will probably show some beneficial effects.

Thus, no one really knows if steroids are of value in humans with complete cord injuries. However, there is a rationale for their use in all cases of cord injury since there may be decreased endogenous steroid production in the cord-injured patient (72). Until a clear-cut answer becomes available, we are giving steroids according to the following regime: a loading dose of 20 mg of dexamethasone is given as soon as possible following the injury. The patient is then given 10 mg every 6 hours for the first 11 days after the injury. The dose is then tapered off to discontinuation on the 18th day after the injury.

Hypothermia

For many years hypothermia has been thought to exert a protective influence on central nervous system tissues during surgical procedures. This may be due to a reduced demand for oxygen and decreased metabolic activity in the tissues (137). Hypothermia may also decrease edema and the inflammatory response (5). One study postulated that in perfusion cooling, the irrigation itself washed toxic substances from the cord (164). However, studies in our laboratory (80, 105) and others (166) showed that extradural cooling without perfusion was effective as well. The exact reasons for the beneficial effects of hypothermia are not known.

Seventeen studies were conducted in animals that received hypothermia locally at the site of cord injury (4, 6, 7, 18–20, 31, 50, 53, 90, 99, 105, 106, 164, 166, 167, 171). Cooling the cord locally caused beneficial functional results in 87% of the studies. Even when cooling was delayed up to 5 hours, it still significantly helped promote motor function in 80% of the studies (78). However, one study in animals showed there was no functional improvement when local cooling was applied 8 hours after injury (7). Another study (171) showed that prolonged cooling was not as effective as delayed short-term cooling. In the 17 series, 77% of the treated animals improved and many became ambulatory. Eight-two percent of the investigators found that cooling gave favorable results (78).

In human cases the cord injury has usually been treated using local cord cooling, most often with the addition of parenteral steroids. In the literature there were 43 cervical and 27 thoracic patients, all with complete cord injuries (2, 3, 22, 26, 79, 104, 117, 122, 149, 163, 176). Cooling was usually done for 1 to 4 hours, although in one study it was continued for several days (26). Of a total of about 70 patients, 54% improved neurologically, ranging from return of some useful function all the way up to ambulation (78). Those cases receiving steroids fared about the same, although it is not known whether steroids were given in some series. An astonishing 14% of the patients with complete cord injuries became ambulatory; this is several times the expected ambulation rate using conventional treatment. Moreover, only 13% of the patients in the 11 studies died, which is about one-third of the expected mortality rate for comparable injuries in other series. Six of the investigators commented favorably on cooling, four were against it, and one said it was ineffective (78).

Disadvantages of cooling are that a lot of equipment is needed, and the procedure requires surgery providing access to the dura via an anterior or posterior approach. Most of the patients arrive at the hospital too late to undergo cooling, which should be administered within the first 4 to 8 hours following the injury to be effective. This then may prove to be a factor in reducing the usefulness and applicability of cooling.

In humans there is no controlled series of comparable patients undergoing cooling versus no cooling. Historical controls have been used for the studies hitherto. Perhaps cooling will prove to be most effective in severe incomplete cord injury. Of course such patients do not have standardized injuries, and therefore it will always be difficult to prove the efficacy of cooling. The author has used this procedure in 20 patients, the results of which will be the subject of a future publication.

Myelotomy

Myelotomy was first performed by Cushing in 1905 (15). It may remove pressure from within the cord (8) and is said to decrease cavitation (62). It may release vasoactive substance from the cord (134). The removal of blood may diminish free radical formation (31) or decrease the neurotransmitter response, thus reducing hemorrhage within the cord (126).

Seven series of animal experiments were done in which myelotomy was performed for treatment of experimental cord injury (9, 27, 32, 62, 93, 134, 167). Sixty-seven percent of the animals showed a significant neurological improvement. Five of the seven investigators were impressed with myelotomy.

Myelotomy has been performed by three groups in humans (8, 15, 170). In a total of 24 patients half the patients improved, with 17% becoming ambulatory. However, it is not certain if all the patients subjected to myelotomy had complete injuries. Two authors were in favor of myelotomy. The ambulation result is truly striking compared with conventional therapy. On the other hand, there was a 42% mortality rate associated with the procedure, which is somewhat above the expected mortality rate using conventional procedures (78). Several surgeons (118, 143, 161) considered that the procedure could cause additional damage. We have not been using it in our patients.

Hyperbaric Oxygenation

It seems logical to improve the oxygen supply to the injured spinal cord if ischemia is truly a factor. In the laboratory, administration of hyperbaric oxygen increases the pO_2 of the injured cord (99). Improvement in one of five baboons with spinal cord injury treated with hyperbaric oxygen was also observed (84). There is also a report that exposure to high pressure using hyperbaric oxygenation may increase hemorrhage in the central gray matter of the cord (12). There are reports of hyperbaric oxygenation being utilized in humans following spinal cord injury (64, 95, 156, 180). There are some encouraging indications, but futher controlled studies will have to be done. A major difficulty with hyperbaric oxygenation is that facilities are not available everywhere to perform this type of treatment.

Other New Methods

In view of the proposed ischemia following cord injury, one study used hypertension and hypercarbia in experimental spinal cord injury (91) without improving the clinical outcome.

Oxygenated fluorocarbon perfusion has also been used in order to deliver oxygen to the injured segment of the spinal cord (82) with demonstration of some functional improvement. However, this substance is not yet generally available in the clinical setting.

Preliminary reports on the use of naloxone look encouraging in the treatment of spinal cord injury in animals (56, 57). Clinical trials are under way at this time with utilization of the substance in man.

Thus, a number of physical agents and drugs have been used in the treatment of acute spinal cord injury in attempts to preserve the cord from ongoing self-destruction shortly after injury. In many instances these treatments look encouraging in animal studies. However, most often the results in humans are not as striking. Those criticizing such new treatments quote the lack of controlled studies following their application in humans. Of the above treatments, studies are still being conducted concerning the efficacy of steroids, naloxone, hypothermia, and hyperbaric oxygen.

Regeneration Studies

For chronic cord injury there have been attempts at regeneration of the cord or attempts to bypass the injured area of the cord. It has been shown that there can be regeneration of cut axons in the adult rat brain (58). Moreover, delayed nerve grafting of the injured area of the cord can result in reinnervation of the nerve graft by axons (177). Thus far, there has been no indication that these axons, which may regenerate, are successful in making connections with target cells. Thus, attempts at regeneration at this time have not caused functional improvement in animals. Further trials in the laboratory are indicated to determine whether spinal cord reconstruction in the human will ever be feasible.

Summary

During trauma both the spine and spinal cord may be injured. The cord is rarely transected in such an injury but is often subjected to a sudden mechanical force followed by compression and additional poorly understood factors, possibly of a chemical or vascular nature. The end result is a progressive hemorrhagic necrosis beginning within the center of the cord and spreading in a few hours to damage the white matter with variable loss of function. Over the years clinicians and researchers have tried to minimize these destructive changes using various forms of treatment ranging from conservative to very aggressive modalities.

The most universally agreed upon treatments involve immobilization of the spine to prevent further cord injury and early reduction of dislocations to reduce pressure on the cord. Attention is also directed toward the effects of other bodily injuries and maintenance of homeostatic functions.

A preponderance of clinical studies indicates that surgical intervention in patients with functionally complete cord injuries rarely results in clinical improvement. On the other hand, progressive deterioration of function is an indication for early decompressive surgery in patients with functionally incomplete cord injuries. A few selected cases of patients with incomplete injuries may also benefit from a late decompression, especially by the anterior approach, which is gaining in popularity. Internal stabilization is usually indicated after decompression. Most of the literature concerns the effects of treatment undertaken after cord necrosis has occurred. There is no carefully controlled series concerning the effects of early (within 4 hours) aggressive decompression and stabilization, a task which remains to be undertaken.

A great deal of effort has been directed toward arrest of the autodestructive secondary forces tending to further damage the cord after injury using drugs and physical agents. A few of these treatments have been encouraging in the animal laboratory; however, the results have been less spectacular in man, possibly because such forms of therapy in the clinical setting have usually been used only in the most hopeless cases. The value of newer forms of treatment in the patient with an incomplete injury remains to be proven.

The surgical treatment of the patient with a chronic complete cord injury remains an uncharted area. Much current research is directed toward attempts at regeneration of cord elements. Thus far restoration of function has not occurred in animals, and therefore, at the present time, there is little clinical applicability to man.

Nevertheless, developments in modern medicine have led to a significant reduction in morbidity and mortality in the victims of spinal injury during the last decade. In addition, advances in diagnostic capabilities have enhanced both the treatment and understanding of spinal injuries.

The problem of spinal cord injury and the tremendous physical and psychological effects in man have proven to be formidable challenges to clinician and researcher alike. It is fervently hoped that ongoing efforts will ultimately provide a breakthrough to lessen the suffering of the millions of people throughout the world whose lives have been so dramatically altered following a serious spinal cord injury.

REFERENCES

1. Abbott, K. H., and Hale, N. Cervical trapeze. *J. Neurosurg., 10:*436–437, 1953.
2. Acosta-Rua, G. J. Treatment of traumatic paraplegic patients by localized cooling of the spinal cord. *J. Iowa Med. Soc., 60:*326–328, 1970.
3. Albin, M. S., Hung, T., and Babinski, M. The patient with spinal cord injury. Epidemiology, emergency and acute care: Advances in physiopathology and treatment. *Curr. Probl. Surg., 17:*190–204, 1980.
4. Albin, M. S., White, R. J., Acosta-Rua, G., et al. Study of functional recovery produced by delayed localized cooling after spinal cord injury in primates. *J. Neurosurg., 29:*113–120, 1968.
5. Albin, M. S., White, R. J., Locke, C. S., et al. Localized spinal cord hypothermia—anesthetic effects and application to spinal cord injury. *Anesth. Analg., 46:*8–16, 1967.
6. Albin, M. S., White, R. J., and Locke, G. E. Treatment of spinal cord trauma by selective hypothermic perfusion. *Surg. Forum., 16:*423–424, 1965.

7. Albin, M. S., White, R. J., Yashon, D., et al. Effects of localized cooling on spinal cord trauma. *J. Trauma, 9:*1000–1008, 1969.

8. Allen, A. R. Remarks on the histopathological changes in the spinal cord due to impact: An experimental study. *J. Nerv. Ment. Dis., 41:*141–147, 1914.

9. Allen, A. R. Surgery of experimental lesion of spinal cord equivalent to crush injury or fracture dislocation of spinal column: A preliminary report. *J.A.M.A., 57:*878–880, 1911.

10. Anderson, D. K., Means, E. D., Waters, T. R., et al. Spinal cord energy metabolism following compression trauma to the feline spinal cord. *J. Neurosurg., 53:*375–380, 1980.

11. Aufranc, O. E., Jones, W. N., and Harris, W. H. Thoracic spine fracture with paralysis. *J.A.M.A., 189:*1018–1021, 1964.

12. Balentine, J. D. Central necrosis of the spinal cord induced by hyperbaric oxygen exposure. *J. Neurosurg., 43:*150–155, 1975.

13. Bedbrook, G. M. Spinal injuries with paralysis. *Surg. Neurol., 5:*185–186, 1976.

14. Benassy, J., Blanchard, J., and Lecoq, A. Neurological recovery rate in para- and tetraplegia. *Paraplegia, 4:*259–263, 1967.

15. Benes, V. *Spinal Cord Injury.* Balliere, London, 1968, pp. 94–96.

16. Bingham, W. G., Goldman, H., Friedman, S. J., et al. Blood flow in normal and injured monkey spinal cord. *J. Neurosurg., 43:*162–171, 1975.

17. Bingham, W. G., Ruffolo, R., and Friedman, S. J. Catecholamine levels in the injured spinal cord of monkeys *J. Neurosurg., 42:*174–178, 1975.

18. Black, P. Recovery of spinal cord trauma: Comparison of hypothermic and normothermic perfusion with and without durotomy. *Proceedings of the 26th Annual Meeting of the Congress of Neurological Surgeons,* New Orleans, 1976.

19. Black, P., and Markowitz, R. S. Experimental spinal cord injury in monkeys: Comparison of steroids and local hypothermia. *Surg. Forum, 22:*409–411, 1971.

20. Black, P., Shepard, R. H., and Markowitz, R. S. Experimental spinal cord injury in monkeys: Comparison of normothermic and hypothermic perfusion. *Proceedings of the 25th Annual Meeting of the Congress of Neurological Surgeons,* Atlanta, 1975.

21. Black, T. M., Markowitz, R. S., Cianci, S. M., et al. Recovery of function after spinal cord injury in monkeys. Comparison of various experimental treatments. Presented at the Annual Meeting of the American Association of Neurological Surgeons, Saint Louis, 1974.

22. Blume, H. G. Surgical management of the cervical fracture dislocation with neurological deficit in conjunction with hypothermia of the spinal cord. *Proceedings of the 4th European Congress of Neurosurgery,* Prague, 1971, pp. 605–609.

23. Bohlman, H. H. Acute fractures and dislocations of the cervical spine. An analysis of three hundred hospitalized patients and review of the literature. *J. Bone Joint Surg., 61A:*1119–1142, 1979.

24. Bohlman, H., and Eismont, F. J. Surgical techniques of anterior decompression and fusion for spinal cord injuries. *Clin. Orthop., 154:*57–67, 1981.

25. Branch, C. L. The definitive treatment and late management of spinal cord injuries with neurological involvement. In Moseley, H. F. (ed): *Accident Surgery.* Appleton-Century-Crofts, New York, 1964, pp. 213–221.

26. Bricolo, A., Ore, G. D., Da Pian, R., et al. Local cooling in spinal cord injury. *Surg. Neurol., 6:*101–106, 1976.

27. Brodner, R. A., Van Gilder, J. C., Collins, W. F., Jr., et al. Experimental spinal cord trauma: The efficacy of treatment. *Proceedings of the Annual Meeting of the American Association of Neurological Surgeons,* San Francisco, 1976.

28. Brown, B. M., Brant-Zawadzki, M., and Cann, C E. Dynamic C.T. scanning of spinal column trauma. *A.J.R., 139:*1177–1181, March, 1982.

29. Bucy, P. C. Emergency treatment of spinal cord injury. Editorial. *Surg. Neurol., 1:*216, 1973.

30. Burke, D. C., and Tiong, T. S. Stability of the cervical spine after conservative treatment. *Paraplegia, 13:*191–202, 1975.

31. Campbell, J. B., Decrescito, V., Tomasula, J. J., et al. Experimental treatment of spinal cord contusion in the cat. *Surg. Neurol.,* 1:102–106, 1973.
32. Campbell, J. B., Decrescito, V., Tomasula, J. J., et al. Experimental treatment of acute spinal cord contusion. Proceedings of the Annual Meeting of the American Association of Neurological Surgeons, Boston, 1972.
33. Clendenon, N. R., Allen, N., Gordon, W. A., et al. Inhibition of Na+-K+-activated ATPase activity following experimental spinal cord trauma. *J. Neurosurg.,* 49:563–568, 1978.
34. Cloward, R. B. Treatment of acute fractures and fracture dislocations of the cervical spine by vertebral-body fusion: A report of eleven cases. *J. Neurosurg.,* 18:201–209, 1961.
35. Comarr, A. E., and Kaufman, A. A. A survey of the neurological results of 858 spinal cord injuries. A comparison of patients treated with and without laminectomy. *J. Neurosurg.,* 13:95–106, 1956.
36. Covalt, D. A., Cooper, I. S., and Hoen, T. I. et al. Early management of patients with spinal cord injury. *J.A.M.A., 151:*89–94, 1953.
37. Cranston, R. W. Dexamethasone in spinal cord injury. Letter to the Editor. *Surg. Neurol.,* 1:290, 1973.
38. Croft, T. J., Brodkey, J. S., and Nulsen, F. P. Reversible spinal cord trauma: A model for electrical monitoring of spinal cord function. *J. Neurosurg., 36:*402–406, 1972.
39. Crutchfield, W. G. Skeletal traction in treatment of injuries to the cervical spine. *J.A.M.A., 155:*29–32, 1954.
40. D'Angelo, C M. The H-reflex in experimental spinal cord trauma. *J. Neurosurg., 39:*209–213, 1973.
41. Davidoff, L. M. Spinal cord injuries. *Surg, Clin. North Am., 21:*433–441, 1941.
42. Dawson, G. D. Cerebral responses to electrical stimulation of peripheral nerve in man. *J. Neurol. Neurosurg. Psychiatry, 10:*137–140, 1947.
43. Dickson, J. H., Harrington, P. R., and Erwin, W. D. Harrington instrumentation in the fractured, unstable thoracic and lumbar spine. *Tex. Med., 69:*91, 1969.
44. Dolan, E. J., Tator, C. H., and Endrenyi, L. The value of decompression for acute experimental spinal cord compression injury. *J. Neurosurg., 53:*749–755, 1980.
45. Donaghy, R. M. P., and Numoto, M. Prognostic significance of sensory evoked potentials in spinal cord injury. *Proceedings of the 17th Veterans' Administration Spinal Cord Injury Conference,* Bronx, 1969, pp. 251–257.
46. Doppman, J. L. Angiographic changes following acute spinal cord compression: An experimental study in monkeys. *Br. J. Radiol., 49:*398–406, 1976.
47. Doppman, J. L., and Girton, M. Angiographic study of the effect of laminectomy in the presence of acute anterior epidural masses. *J. Neurosurg., 45:*195–202, 1976.
48. Drake, C. G. Cervical spinal-cord injury. *J. Neurosurg., 19:*487–494, 1962.
49. Ducker, T. B., Assenmacher, D. R. Microvascular response to experimental spinal cord trauma. *Surg. Forum, 20:*42–430, 1969.
50. Ducker, T. B., and Hamit, H. G. Experimental treatments of acute spinal cord injury. *J. Neurosurg., 30:*693–697, 1969.
51. Edgar, R. E. Surgical management of spinal cord cysts. *Paraplegia, 14:*21–27, 1976.
52. Editorial: Spinal cord damage after angiography. *Lancet, 2:*1067–1068, 1973.
53. Eidelberg, E., Staten, E., Watkins, L. J., et al. Treatment of experimental spinal cord injury in ferrets. *Surg. Neurol., 6:*243–246, 1976.
54. Eidelberg, E., Sullivan, J., and Bringham, A. Immediate consequences of spinal cord injury: Possible role of potassium in axonal conduction block. *Surg Neurol., 3:*317, 1975.
55. Epstein, N., Hood, A. C., and Ransohoff, J. Gastrointestinal bleeding in patients with spinal cord trauma. Effects of steroids, cimetidine, and mini-dose heparin. *J. Neurosurg., 54:*16–20, 1981.
56. Faden, A. Pharmacological agents for treatment of spinal cord injury. Presented at Spinal Cord Injury Cure Workshop. Paralysis Cure Research Foundation, Airlie, Va., September 12, 1981.

57. Flamm, E. S., Young, W., Demopoulos, H. B., et al. Experimental spinal cord injury: Treatment with naloxone. *Neurosurg., 10:* 227–231, 1982.
58. Foerster, A. P. Spontaneous regeneration of cut axons in adult rat brain. *J. Comp. Neurol., 210:*335–356, 1982.
59. Frankel, H. L., Hancock, D. O., Hyslop, G., et al. The value of postural reduction in the initial management of closed injuries of the spine with paraplegia and tetraplegia. Part I. *Paraplegia, 7:*179–192, 1969.
60. Freebody, D., Bendall, R., and Taylor, R. D. Anterior transperitoneal lumbar fusion. *J. Bone Joint Surg., 53B:*617–627, 1971.
61. Freeman, L. W. Treatment of paraplegia resulting from trauma to the spinal cord. *J.A.M.A., 140:*949–958, 1949.
62. Freeman, L. W. and Wright, T. Experimental observations of concussion and contusion of the spinal cord. *Ann. Surg., 137:*433–443, 1953.
63. Fried, L. C., and Goodkin, R. Microangiographic observations of the experimentally traumatized spinal cord. *J. Neurosurg., 35:*709–714, 1971.
64. Gamache, F. W., Jr., Myers, R. A. M., Ducker, T. B., et al. The clinical application of hyperbaric oxygen therapy in spinal cord injury: A preliminary report. *Surg. Neurol., 15:*85–87, 1981.
65. Gargano, F. P., Meyer, J., Houdek, P. B., et al. Transverse axial tomography of the cervical spine. *Radiology, 113:*363–367, 1974.
66. Gargour, G. W., Wener, L., and DiChiro, G. Selective arteriography of the spinal cord in post-traumatic paraplegia. *Neurol. (Minn.), 22:*131–134, 1972.
67. Geisler, W. O., Wynne-Jones, M., and Jousse, A. T. Early management of the patient with trauma to the spinal cord. *Med. Serv. J. Can., 22:*512–523, 1966.
68. Gilbert, R. G. D., Brindle, G. F., and Galindo, A. *Anesthesia for Neurosurgery.* Little Brown, Boston, 1966.
69. Gilbin, D. R. Somatosensory evoked potentials in healthy subjects and in patients with lesions in the nervous system. *Ann. N.Y. Acad. Sci., 112:*93–142, 1964.
70. Gillingham, J. Early management of spinal cord trauma. Letter to the Editor (C). *J. Neurosurg., 44:*766–767, 1976.
71. Gillingham, J. The problem of head and spinal injuries: Prevention of the second accident. *Med. Sci. Law, 10:*104–109, 1970.
72. Green, B. A., Kahn, T., and Klose, K. J. A comparative study of steroid therapy in acute experimental spinal cord injury. *Surg. Neurol., 13:*91–97, 1980.
73. Griffiths, I. R. Ultrastructural changes in spinal gray matter microvasculature after impact injury. *Adv. Neurol., 20:*415–422, 1978.
74. Griffiths, I. R., Trench, J. G., and Crawford, R. A. Spinal cord blood flow and conduction during experimental cord compression in normotensive and hypotensive dogs. *J. Neurosurg., 50:*353–360, 1979.
75. Guttman, L. *Spinal Cord Injuries: Comprehensive Management and Research.* Blackwell, Oxford, 1973.
76. Hall, L. Basic principles of NMR. Paper presented at the XVIII Can. Cong. Neurol. Sci., St. John's Nfld. June 23, 1983.
77. Hannon, K. M. Harrington instrumentation in fractures and dislocations of the thoracic and lumbar spine. *South. Med. J., 69:*1269–1273, 1976.
78. Hansebout, R. R. A comprehensive review of methods of improving cord recovery after acute spinal cord injury. In Tator, C. H. (ed): *Early Management of Acute Spinal Cord Injury.* Raven Press, New York, 1982, pp. 181–196.
79. Hansebout, R. R. (unpublished data), 1980.
80. Hansebout, R. R., Kuchner, E. F., and Romero-Sierra, C. Effects of local hypothermia and of steroids upon recovery from experimental spinal cord compression injury. *Surg. Neurol., 4:*531–536, 1975.

81. Hansebout, R. R., Lewin, M. G., and Pappius, H. M. Evidence regarding the action of steroids in injured spinal cord. In Reulen, H. J., and Schurmann, K. (eds): *Steroids and Brain Edema.* Springer-Verlag, Berlin, 1972, pp. 153–155.

82. Hansebout, R. R., van der Jagt, R. H., Sohal, S. S., et al. Oxygenated fluorocarbon perfusion as treatment of acute spinal cord compression injury in dogs. *J. Neurosurg., 55:*725–732, 1981.

83. Harris, P., Karmi, M. Z., McClemont, E., et al. The prognosis of patients sustaining severe cervical spinal injury (C2–C7 inclusive). *Paraplegia, 18:*324–330, 1980.

84. Hartzog, J. T., Risher, R. G. and Snow, C. Spinal cord trauma: Effect of hyperbaric oxygen therapy. *Proceedings of the 17th Veterans' Administration Spinal Cord Injury Conference.* Bronx, 1969, pp. 70–71.

85. Hedeman, L. S., Shellenberger, M. K., and Gordon, J. H. Studies in experimental spinal cord trauma. Part 1: Alterations in catecholamine levels. *J. Neurosurg., 40:*37–43, 1974.

86. Hedeman, L. S., and Sil, R. Studies in experimental cord trauma. Part 2: Comparison of treatment with steroids, low molecular weight dextan, and catecholamine blockades. *J. Neurosurg., 40:*44–51, 1974.

87. Holdsworth, F. W. Fractures, dislocations, and fracture-dislocations of the spine. *J. Bone Joint Surg., 52A:*1534, 1970.

88. Hollin, S. A., Hayashi, H., and Gross, S. W. Management of cervical spine dislocations with locked facets. *Surg. Gynecol. Obstet., 124:*521–524, 1967.

89. Horsey, W J., Tucker, W. S., Hudson, A. R., et al. Experience with early anterior operation in acute injuries of the cervical spine. *Paraplegia, 15:*110–122, 1977.

90. Howitt, W. M., and Turnbull, I. M. Effects of hypothermia and methysergide on recovery from experimental paraplegia. *Can. J. Surg., 15:*179–186, 1972.

91. Hukuda, S., Mochizudi, T., and Ogata, M. Therapeutic trial of combined hypertension and hypercarbia on experimental acute spinal cord injury. *Neurosurg., 6:*644–648, 1980.

92. Ito, T., Allen, N., and Yashon, D. A mitochondrial lesion in experimental spinal cord trauma. *J. Neurosurg., 48:*434–442, 1978.

93. Iwasaki, Y., Isu, T., Ito, T., et al. Effect of longitudianl myelotomy on experimental spinal cord injury. *No Shinkei Geka, 8:*65–72, 1980.

94. Janda, W. E., Kelly, P. J., Rhoton, A. L., et al. Fracture-dislocation of the cervical part of the spinal column in patients with ankylosing spondylitis. *Mayo Clin. Proc., 43:*714–721, 1968.

95. Jones, R. F., Unsworth, I. P., and Marosszeky, J. E. Hyperbaric oxygen and acute spinal cord injuries in humans. *Med. J. Aust., 2:*573–575, 1978.

96. Joyner, J., and Freeman, L. W. Urea and spinal cord trauma. *Neurol. (Minn.), 13:*69–72, 1963.

97. Kajihara, K., Kawanaga, H., Dela Torre, J. C., et al. Dimethyl sulfoxide in the treatment of experimental acute spinal cord injury. *Surg. Neurol., 1:*16–22, 1973.

98. Kao, C. C., and Chang, L. W. The mechanism of spinal cord cavitation following spinal cord transection. Part 1: A correlated histochemical study. *J. Neurosurg., 46:*197–209, 1977.

99. Kelly, D., Lassiter, K., Calogero, J., et al. Effects of local hypothermia and tissue oxygen studies in experimental paraplegia. *J. Neurosurg., 33:*554–563, 1970.

100. Kobrine, A. The neuronal theory of experimental traumatic spinal cord dysfunction. *Surg. Neurol., 3:*261–264, 1975.

101. Kobrine, A. I., and Doyle, T. F. Role of histamine in post-traumatic spinal cord hyperemia and the luxury perfusion syndrome. *J. Neurosurg., 44:*16–20, 1976.

102. Kobrine, A. I., Doyle, T. F., and Martin, A. N. Local spinal cord blood flow in experimental myelopathy. Presented at the Annual Meeting of the American Association of Neurological Surgeons, Saint Louis, 1974.

103. Kobrine, A. I., Evans, D. E., and Rizzoli, H. V. The effects of ischemia on long-tract

neural conduction in the spinal cord. *J. Neurosurg., 50:*639–644, 1979.

104. Koons, D. D., Gildenberg, P. L., Dohn, D. F., et al. Local hypothermia in the treatment of spinal cord injuries: Report of seven cases. *Cleve. Clin. Q., 39:*109–117, 1972.

105. Kuchner, E. F., and Hansebout, R. R. Combined steroid and hypothermia treatment of experimental spinal cord injury. *Surg. Neurol., 6:*371–376, 1976.

106. Kuchner, E. F., Mercer, I. D., Pappius, H. M., et al. Experimental spinal cord injury: Effects of steroids and/or cooling on edema, electrolytes and motor recovery. In Pappius, H. M., and Feindel, W. (eds): *Dynamics of Brain Edema.* Springer-Verlag, Berlin, 1976, pp. 315–322.

107. Landeau, B., Campbell, J. D., and Ransohoff, J. Surgical reversal of the effects of long-standing traumatic lesions of the conus medullaris and cauda equina. *Proceedings of the Annual Clinics on Spinal Cord Injury Conference, 17:*23–27, 1967.

108. Larson, S. J., Holst, R. A., Hemmy, D. C., et al. Lateral extracavitary approach to traumatic lesions of the thoracic and lumbar spine. *J. Neurosurg., 45:*628–637, 1976.

109. Lavy, S., and Herishanu, Y. The effect of complete transection of thoracic spinal cord on cat's electrocorticogram. *Epilepsia, 12:*117–122, 1971.

110. Leo, J. S., Bergeron, R. T., Kricheff, I. I., et al. Metrizamide myelography for cervical spinal cord injuries. *Radiology, 129:*707–711, 1978.

111. Lewin, M. G., Hansebout, R. R., and Pappius, H. M. Chemical characteristics of traumatic spinal cord edema in cats. *J. Neurosurg., 40:*65–75, 1974.

112. Lewin, M. G., Pappius, H. M., and Hansebout, R. R. Effects of steroids on edema associated with injury of the spinal cord. In Reulen, H. G., and Schurmann, K. (eds): *Steroids and Brain Edema.* Springer-Verlag, Berlin, 1972, pp. 101–112.

113. Locke, G. E., Yashon, D., Feldman, R. A. et al. Ischemia in primate spinal cord injury. *J. Neurosurg., 34:*614–617, 1971.

114. Lucas, J. T., and Ducker, T. B. Laminectomies in acute spinal cord injury. Presented at the Annual Meeting of the American Association of Neurological Surgeons, New York, 1980.

115. Martin, S. H., and Bloedel, J. R. Evaluation of experimental spinal cord injury using cortical evoked potentials. *J. Neurosurg., 39:*75–81, 1973.

116. Maynard, F. M., Reynolds, G. G., Fountain, S., et al. Neurological prognosis after traumatic quadriplegia. Three-year experience of California Regional Spinal Cord Injury Care System. *J. Neurosurg., 50:*611–616, 1979.

117. Meacham, W. F., and McPherson, W. F. Local hyperthermia in the treatment of acute injuries of the spinal cord. *South. Med. J., 66:*95–97, 1973.

118. McVeigh, J. F. Experimental cord crushes with special reference to the mechanical factors involved and subsequent changes in the areas of the cord affected. *Arch. Surg., 7:*573–600, 1923.

119. Morgan, T. H., Wharton, G. W., and Austin, G. N. The results of laminectomy in patients with incomplete spinal cord injuries. *Paraplegia, 9:*14–23, 1971.

120. Munro, D. Treatment of fractures and dislocations of the cervical spine, complicated by cervical cord and root injuries: A comparative study of fusion vs nonfusion therapy. *N. Engl. J. Med., 264:*573–582, 1961.

121. Naftchi, N. E., Demeny, M., Decrescito, V., et al. Biogenic amine concentrations in traumatized spinal cord of cats. Effect of drug therapy. *J. Neurosurg., 40:* 52–57, 1974.

122. Negrin, J. Spinal cord hypothermia. Neurosurgical management of immediate and delayed post-traumatic neurologic sequelae. *N.Y. State J. Med., 75:*2387–2392, 1975.

123. Norrell, H., and Wilson, C. B. Early anterior fusion for injuries of the cervical portion of the spine. *J.A.M.A., 214:*525–530, 1970.

124. Norton, W. L. Fractures and dislocations of the cervical spine. *J. Bone Joint Surg., 44(A):*115–139, 1962.

125. Osborne, D. R., Vavoulis, G., Nashold, B. S., Jr., et al. Late sequelae of spinal cord

trauma. Myelographic and surgical correlations. *J. Neurosurg., 57:*18–23, 1982.
126. Osterholm, J. L. The pathophysiological response to spinal injury. The current status of related research. *J. Neurosurg., 40:*5–33, 1974.
127. Osterholm, J. L., and Mathews, G. J. Altered norepinephrine metabolism following experimental spinal cord injury. Part 1: Relationship to hemorrhagic necrosis and post-wounding neurological deficits. *J. Neurosurg., 36:*386–394, 1972.
128. Paul, R. L., Michael, R. H., Dunn, J. E., et al. Anterior transthoracic surgical decompression of acute spinal cord injuries. *J. Neurosurg., 43:*299–307, 1975.
129. Perot, P. L., Jr. The clinical use of somatosensory evoked potentials in spinal cord injury. *Clin. Neurosurg., 20:*367–381, 1973.
130. Post, M. J., Green, D. A., Quencer, R. M., et al. The value of computed tomography in a spinal trauma. *Spine, 7:*417–431, 1982.
131. Rawe, S. E., Roth, R. H., Boadle-Biber, M., et al. Norepinephrine levels in experimental spinal cord trauma. Part 1: Biochemical study of hemorrhagic necrosis. *J. Neurosurg., 46:*342–349, 1977.
132. Rayner, R. B. Severe injuries of the cervical spine treated by early anterior interbody fusion and ambulation. *J. Neurosurg., 28:*311–316, 1968.
133. Richardson, H. D., and Nakamura, S. Electron microscopic study of spinal cord edema and the effects of treatment with steroids, mannitol and hypothermia. Presented at the Annual Meeting of the American Association of Neurological Surgeons, Houston, 1971.
134. Rivlin, A. S., and Tator, C. H. Effect of vasodilators and myelotomy on recovery after acute spinal cord injury in rats. *J. Neurosurg., 50:*349–352, 1979.
135. Rivlin, A. S., and Tator, C. H. Regional spinal cord blood flow in rats after severe cord trauma. *J. Neurosurg., 49:*844–853, 1978.
136. Rivlin, A. S., and Tator, C. H. Effect of duration of acute spinal cord compression in a new acute cord injury model in the rat. *Surg. Neurol., 10:*38–43, 1978.
137. Rosomoff, H. L. Experimental brain injury during hypothermia. *J. Neurosurg., 16:*177–187, 1959.
138. Rossier, A. B., Berney, J., Rosenbaum, A. E., et al., Value of gas myelography in early management of acute cervical spinal cord injuries. *J. Neurosurg., 42:*330–337, 1975.
139. Rossier, A. B., Hussey, R. W., Kenzora, J. E. Anterior fibular interbody fusion in the treatment of cervical spinal cord injuries. *Surg. Neurol., 7:*55–60, 1977.
140. Rowed, D. W., McLean, J. A. G., and Tator, C. H. Somatosensory evoked potentials in acute spinal cord injury: Prognostic value *Surg. Neurol., 9:*203–210, 1978.
141. Sandler, A. N., and Tator, C. H. Pathological effect and therapeutic value of durotomy in acute experimental spinal cord injury. Presented at the Annual Meeting of the American Association of Neurological Surgeons, Saint Louis, 1974.
142. Saul, T. G., Carol, M., and Ducker, T. B. Immediate mini-myelography in acute cervical cord injuries. *Am. Surg., 48:*463–468, 1982.
143. Scarff, J. E. Injuries of the vertebral column and spinal cord. In Brock, S. (ed): *Injuries of the Brain and Spinal Cord and Their Coverings,* ed. 4. Springer-Verlag, New York, 1960, pp. 530–589.
144. Scher, A. T. Is positive-contrast myelography of value in acute cervical spinal cord injury? *Paraplegia, 15:*215–220, 1977.
145. Schneider, R. C. A syndrome in acute cervical spine injuries for which early operation is indicated. *J. Neurosurg., 8:*360–367, 1951.
146. Scneider, R. C., Cherry, G., and Pantek, H. The syndrome of acute central cervical spinal cord injury. *J. Neurosurg., 11:*546–577, 1954.
147. Schneider, R. C., Crosby, E. C., Russo, R. H., et al. Traumatic spinal cord syndromes and their management. *Clin. Neurosurg., 20:*424–492, 1973.
148. Sehgal, A. D., Gardner, W. J., and Dohn, D. F. Pantoppaque "arachnoiditis": Treatment with subarachnoid injections of corticosteroids. *Clev. Clin. Q., 29:*177–188, 1962.

149. Selker, R. G. Icewater irrigation of the spinal cord. *Surg. Forum, 22:*411–413, 1971.
150. Senter, H. J., and Venes, J. L. Altered blood flow and secondary injury in experimental spinal cord trauma. *J. Neurosurg., 49:* 569–578, 1978.
151. Shannon, N., Symon, L., Logue, V., et al. Clinical features, investigation and treatment of post-traumatic syringomyelia. *J. Neurol. Neurosurg. Psychiatry, 44:*35–42, 1981.
152. Singer, J. M., Russell, G. V., and Coe, J. E. Changes in evoked potentials after experimental cervical spinal cord injury in the monkey. *Exp. Neurol., 29:*449–461, 1970.
153. Skalpe, I. O., and Amundsen, P. Thoracic and cervical myelography with metrizamide. *Radiology, 116:*101–106, 1975.
154. Smith, A. J. K., McCareery, D. B., Bloedel, J. R., et al. Hyperemia, vasoparalysis and loss of autoregulation in the white matter following spinal cord injury. *Proceedings of the 26th Annual Meeting of the Congress on Neurological Surgery,* San Francisco, 1976.
155. Stauffer, E. S., Wood, R. W., and Kelly, A. T. Gunshot wounds of the spine: The effects of laminectomy. *J. Bone Joint Surg., 61A:*389–392, 1979.
156. Sukoff, M. H. Central nervous system: Review and update cerebral edema and spinal cord injuries. *HBO Review, 1:*189–195, 1980.
157. Suwanwela, C., Alexander, E., Jr., and Davis, C. H., Jr. Prognosis in spinal cord injury, with special reference to patients with motor paralysis and sensory preservation. *J. Neurosurg., 19:*220–227, 1962.
158. Sussman, B. J. Early management of spinal cord trauma. Letter to the Editor (C). *J. Neurosurg., 44:*766, 1976.
159. Tanner, J. A. Personal communication, 1982.
160. Tarlov, I. M. Acute spinal cord compression paralysis. *J. Neurosurg., 36:*10–20, 1972.
161. Tarlov, I. M. *Spinal cord compression. Mechanisms of Paralysis and Treatment.* Charles C. Thomas, Publisher, Springfield, Illinois, 1957.
162. Tarlov, I. M. Spinal cord injuries—early treatment. *Surg. Clin. North Am.,* April:591–607, 1955.
163. Tator, C. H. Spinal cord cooling and irrigation for treatment of acute cord injury. In Popp, J. A., Bourke, R. S., Nelson, L. R., Kimelberg, H. K., (eds): *Neural Trauma.* Raven Press, New York, 1979, pp. 363–370.
164. Tator, C. H., and Deecke, L. Value of normothermic perfusion, hypothermic perfusion, and durotomy in the treatment of experimental acute spinal cord trauma. *J. Neurosurg., 39:*52–64, 1973.
165. Tator, C. H., and Rowed, D. W. Current concepts in the immediate management of acute spinal cord injuries. *C.M.A.J., 121:*1453–1464, 1979.
166. Thienprasit, P., Bantli, H., Bloedel, J. R., et al. Effect of delayed local cooling on experimental spinal cord injury. *J. Neurosurg., 42:*150–154, 1975.
167. Tomasula, J. J., Decrescito, V., Goodkin, R., et al. A survey of the management of experimental spinal cord trauma. *Proceedings of the 17th Veterans' Administration Spinal Cord Injury Conference, 17:*12–16, 1969.
168. Van Gilder, J. Data presented to the National Paraplegia Foundation, Milwaukee, June 1972.
169. Verbiest H. Anterolateral operations for fractures or dislocations of the cervical spine due to injuries or previous surgical interventions. *Clin. Neurosurg., 20:*334–366, 1973.
170. Wagner, F. C., and Rawe, S. E. Microsurgical anterior cervical myelotomy. *Surg. Neurol., 5:*229–231, 1976.
171. Wells, J. D., and Hansebout, R. R. Local hypothermia in experimental spinal cord trauma. *Surg. Neurol., 10:*200–204, 1978.
172. Weir, D. C. Roentgenographic signs of cervical injury. *Clin. Orthop., 109:*9–17, 1975.
173. Weiss, M. H., Heiden, J. S., Apuzzo, M. L. J., et al. Anterior decompression of the thoracic and thoraco-lumbar spine. *Bull. Los Angeles Neurol. Soc., 40:*112–115, 1975.

174. Wener, L., DiChiro, G., and Gargour, G. W. Angiography of cervical cord injuries. *Radiology, 112:*597–604, 1974.
175. White, R. J. Pathology of spinal cord injury in experimental lesions. *Clin. Orthop., 112:*16–26, 1975.
176. White, R. J., Yashon, D., Albin, M. S., et al. The acute management of cervical cord trauma with quadriplegia. *Proceedings of the Annual Meeting of the American Association for Neurological Surgery,* Boston, 1972.
177. Wrathall, J. R., Rigamont, D. D., Braford, N. R., et al. Reconstruction of the contused cat spinal cord by the delayed nerve graft technique and cultured peripheral non-neuronal cells. *Acta Neuropathol. (Berl.), 57:*59–69, 1982.
178. Yashon, D. *Spinal Injury.* Appleton-Century-Crofts, New York, 1978.
179. Yashon, D., Bingham, W. G., Faddoul, E. M., et al. Edema of the spinal cord following experimental impact trauma. *J. Neurosurg., 38:* 693–697, 1973.
180. Yeo, J. D., Lowry, C., and McKenzie, B. Preliminary report on 10 patients with spinal cord injuries treated with hyperbaric oxygenation. *Med. J. Aust., 2:*572–573, 1978.
181. Yeo, J. D., Payne, W., Hinwood, B. et al. The experimental contusion injury of the spinal cord in sheep. *Paraplegia, 12:*279–298, 1975.
182. Young, J. S., and Dexter, W. R. Neurological recovery distal to the zone of injury in 172 cases of closed, traumatic spinal cord injury. *Paraplegia, 16:*39–49, 1978.

2

Orthopaedic Management of the Injured Spine[1]

STANLEY D. GERTZBEIN

The management of injuries to the spinal column continues to be a controversial issue (7, 9, 12, 14–16, 29, 30, 32, 34, 36, 42, 47, 48, 53, 57, 61, 74, 76, 77). The conservative approach practiced in many centers appears to provide satisfactory results (7, 8, 12, 24, 32, 34, 48, 66, 78), yet a significant number of patients are left with serious deformity, pain, and disability because of inadequate correction of the bony injury (28, 50, 54, 73). Improved medical facilities, such as regional trauma centers and acute spinal injury units, have dramatically improved the quality of care for spinal injury patients in the past decade (70). Furthermore, a better understanding of the pathology, biomechanics, and pathophysiology has led to a more rational approach to the management of patients with spinal injuries (10, 60, 61).

The goals of treatment are: (a) to prevent further neurological damage; (b) to improve neurological function where possible; (c) to restore stability and alignment; and (d) to rehabilitate the patient to the maximum potential of his disability.

Neurosurgical indications for decompression are presented elsewhere in this text. This chapter will focus on the management of the spinal column with particular emphasis on the determination of spinal instability. A rational approach to treatment will be developed based on whether the spine is stable or unstable.

Spinal Instability

The spinal column consists of an anterior column and a posterior complex. (36). The former includes the vertebral bodies, the intervertebral disc, and

---

[1] The author wishes to thank Miss R. Verman for the preparation of this chapter and the Medical Art and Photography Department, Sunnybrook Medical Centre, for the figures.

the anterior and posterior longitudinal ligaments. The latter is composed of the supraspinous ligament, the interspinous ligaments, the capsular ligaments, the ligamentum flavum, the facets and articular processes, the pedicles, and the spinous and transverse processes (Fig. 2.1). More recently, a middle vertebral segment has been identified which includes portions of the anterior column and the posterior complex (15, 62) (Fig. 2.2). This entity consists of the posterior half of the vertebral body, the posterior longitudinal ligament, the articular facets, and the pedicles. It appears that the middle segment plays a major role in maintaining spinal stability.

Spinal instability may be described as the inability to resist physiological forces. Although imprecise, this definition allows one to place an injury along a spectrum ranging from minor to major degrees of instability. At one end of the scale, relatively little instability exists, obviating the need for intensive treatment. At the opposite end of the scale, more definitive methods of management are indicated. Injuries in the midspectrum require accurate diagnosis since it is these that create the greatest controversy.

Factors Leading to Instability

Various anatomical structures have been described which provide spinal stability (75). Damage to these structures and, therefore, to the anterior and posterior columns can be determined by assessing: (a) the pattern of fractures; (b) the amount of displacement; and (c) the forces involved.

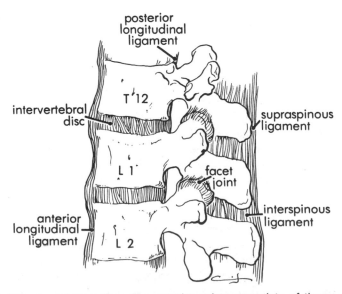

Figure 2.1. Diagram of the spine. The anterior column consists of those structures anterior to and including the posterior longitudinal ligament. The posterior complex includes the remaining posterior structures.

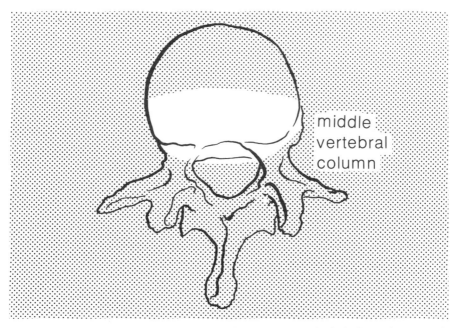

Figure 2.2. The middle vertebral column. The structures included are the posterior vertebral body and the posterior longitudinal ligament.

Fracture Patterns

Holdsworth was one of the first to appreciate the importance of studying fracture patterns in order to evaluate the stability of spinal injuries (36). Such lesions as the wedge compression fracture (Fig. 2.3), the burst injury (Fig. 2.4), and most extension injuries were felt to be stable. Unstable fractures included slice fractures (Fig. 2.5) and dislocations (Fig. 2.6). Some of the fractures described as stable by Holdsworth are now considered relatively unstable because of other factors, such as trauma to the middle vertebral segment (15, 62). Most burst injuries do in fact involve the middle segment and should be considered relatively unstable (Fig. 2.4).

Displacement

In their list of factors that play a role in spinal instability, White and Panjabi (76) have included various degrees of displacement such as sagittal translation, increased sagittal rotation (kyphosis), and distraction. By attaching a numerical value to these parameters (along with other factors), they were able to determine if a significant degree of instability was present. Five or more points indicated an unstable spine.

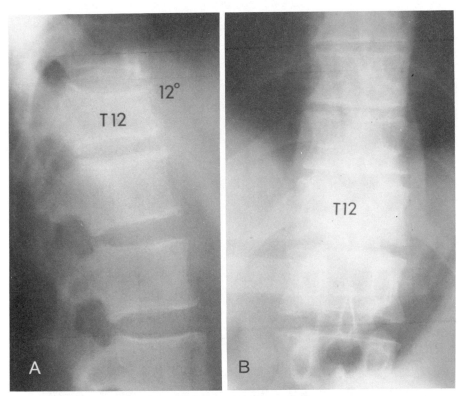

Figure 2.3. Wedge compression fracture. (*A*) Lateral. The body of T12 is wedged with a crush anteriorly, relatively sparing the posterior cortex and posterior complex. (*B*) AP. The alignment of the spine is maintained and the distance between the pedicles is not widened.

Force Vectors

The forces that create spinal injury also play an important role in determining the degree of instability (11, 51). The most important forces include flexion and vertical compression, flexion and rotation, and vertical compression and extension. Specific force vectors create predictable fracture patterns. For example, a vertical compression force will lead to a burst fracture, whereas a flexion and rotation injury may result in the slice fracture described by Holdsworth.

Late Instability

All of the factors mentioned above may lead to late instability with progressive deformity associated with pain and, in some cases, neurological deficit. In addition, the loss of vertebral height of greater than 30% to 50%

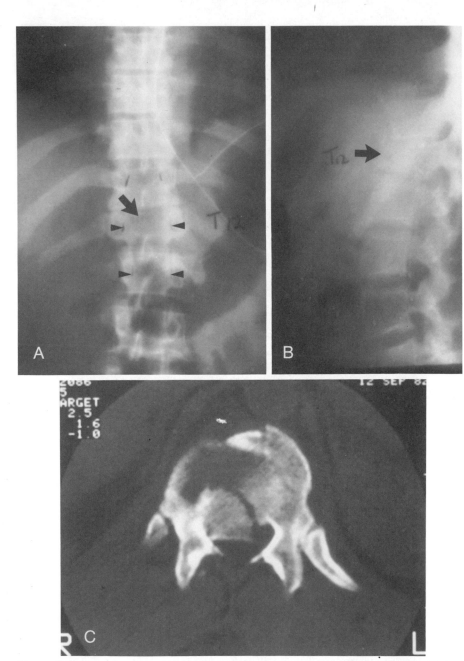

Figure 2.4. Burst fracture. (*A*) AP. The body of T12 is crushed with loss of vertebral height. The pedicles are widened relative to the pedicles of the vertebrae above (arrowheads). (*B*) Lateral radiograph demonstrating loss of height both anteriorly and posteriorly (arrow). (*C*) Bony fragment extruded into the spinal canal. Note the disruption of the posterior half of the vertebral body indicating significant disruption of the middle vertebral segment.

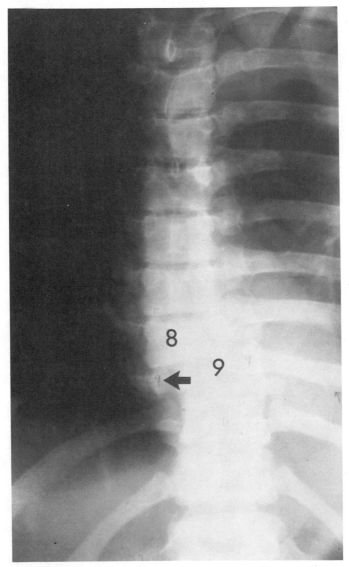

Figure 2.5. Slice fracture. This flexion and rotation injury has resulted in a fracture dislocation with the superior portion of the body of T9 displacing with the upper vertebral column (arrow).

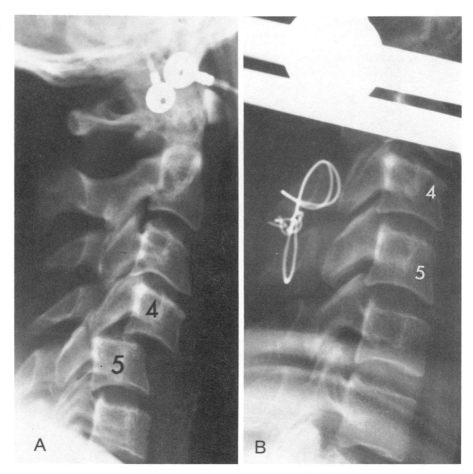

Figure 2.6. Dislocation of C4 on C5. (*A*) Note the displacement of C4 is greater than 50% of the width of the body of C5. The articular facets of C4 are anterior to those of C5 and are locked anteriorly. (*B*) The dislocation is reduced and held by wires. Note the normal relationship of the facets.

or angular deformity greater than 30° are factors that may lead to these complications (51, 75, 76) (Fig. 2.7). Lateral angulation of greater than 10° may also cause late pain. We and others (28, 71) have come to recognize the potential for deformity when adjacent vertebrae have been damaged (Fig. 2.8).

Clinical Assessment of Instability

Several conditions have led to delays in the diagnosis of a spinal injury (10). These include head injury with loss of consciousness, alcoholic intoxication, and associated fractures or multiple injuries. Greater care in as-

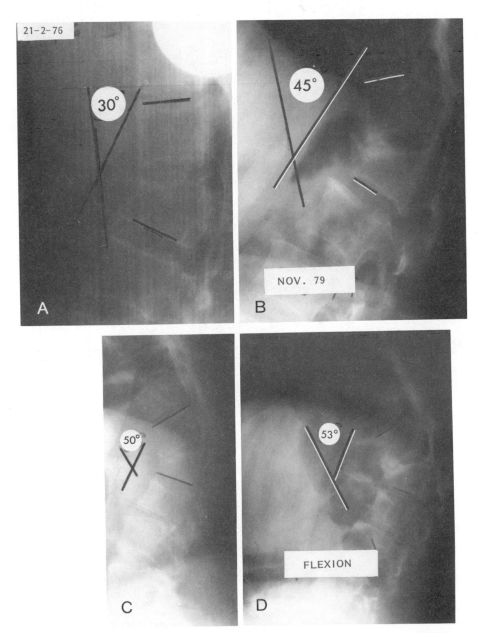

Figure 2.7. Fracture L1 with 30° angulation. (A) Lateral on date of injury. (B) After 3½ years, the angle has increased to 45°. (C) At 4 years the kyphosis is 50°, and (D) with forward flexion the angle is 53°.

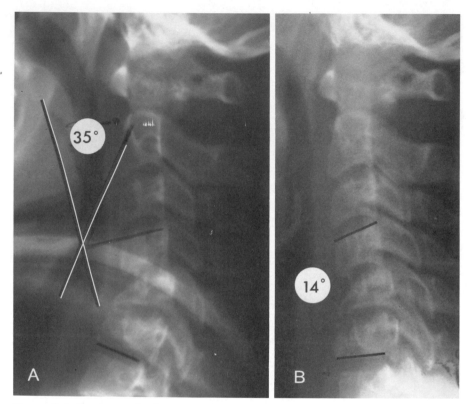

Figure 2.8. Fractures of adjacent vertebrae. (*A*) Lateral of fracture of C5 and C6 with 14° angulation. (*B*) At 2 months the deformity has increased to 35° in spite of halo vest immobilization.

sessing spinal injuries must be taken under these conditions to avoid delays in diagnosis.

From the patient's history, one can determine the mechanism of injury and the violence of the forces involved. Neurological symptoms are usually manifestations of significant instability, although some burst fractures with neurological deficits may be relatively stable. A history of progressive neurological deficit is another indication that the spine is unstable.

On physical examination, abrasions, contusions, and hematomas about the skull or back may indicate rotational forces, especially if these findings are unilateral. The presence or absence of intercostal breathing may be a clue to the level of injury. Palpation of a posterior gap or a gibbus as well as malalignment of the spinous processes is a sign of significant disruption (Fig. 2.9).

An accurate neurological examination will reveal the presence or absence of neurological involvement and will provide a baseline for subsequent

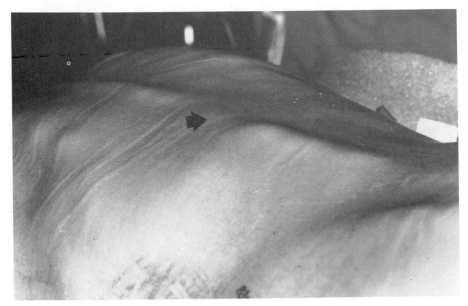

Figure 2.9. Clinical instability can be determined by a gap or malalignment of the spinous processes (arrow).

improvement or deterioration. Determination of the extent of neurological injury is extremely important, particularly if the lesion is incomplete. Anterior, lateral, and central cord syndromes should be well documented. A rectal examination is a necessary part of the physical examination since it assists in determining whether there is involvement of the sacral segments and whether the patient is in spinal shock. A neurological lesion is usually indicative of a significant spinal column injury, and, therefore, instability should be suspected.

Radiographic Assessment of Instability

Anteroposterior and lateral x-ray views are most helpful in delineating spinal injuries (Fig. 2.10). In the cervical spine, oblique views, pillar views, and cone down projections may also be beneficial in defining less obvious fractures. Because of the risk of neurological damage, flexion and extension views in the early stage are not indicated unless there is no obvious bony trauma. If required, they should be performed with a physician in attendance. Anteroposterior and lateral tomograms are routinely performed in this center to delineate fracture patterns, especially of the posterior elements (Fig. 2.11). Angular deformities are also accurately defined by this study.

The CT scan has become an invaluable tool in the diagnosis and management of spinal injury, often revealing lesions which may be missed by other techniques (35, 52, 58). The most important feature of the CT scan

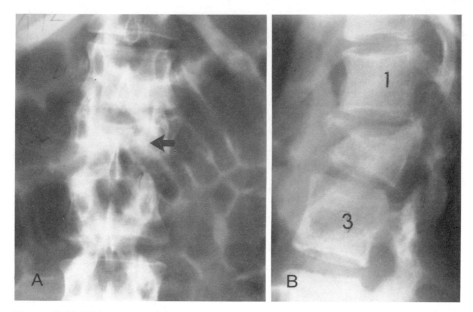

Figure 2.10. Plain x-rays of the spine. (*A and B*) AP and lateral of L2 demonstrating a burst fracture with loss of vertebral height, widening of the pedicles (arrow), and widening of the interspinous distance.

is an evaluation of the size of the spinal canal and the encroachment of bony fragments. Additional unsuspected fractures, particularly in the posterior elements, can be identified (Fig. 2.12). For these reasons, the CT scan has been extremely useful in determining whether anterior spinal surgery for decompression of the spinal cord is indicated.

Metrizamide myelography has been used independently or in combination with CT scans in this and other centers (10, 52). We have found it useful in evaluating spinal cord compression, particularly in incomplete spinal cord lesions that have plateaued.

Diagnosis of Instability

In summary, the following features are important in establishing a diagnosis of spinal instability:

1. the history of violent forces affecting the spinal column with associated neurological symptoms or progressive neurological deficit;
2. physical findings indicative of rotational forces as well as local features in the spine representing posterior element disruption;
3. presence of neurological signs;
4. radiographic evidence of anterior, middle, and posterior spinal column disruption as evidenced by fracture patterns and displacements (angular and translational); and
5. presence of two or more adjacent fractures.

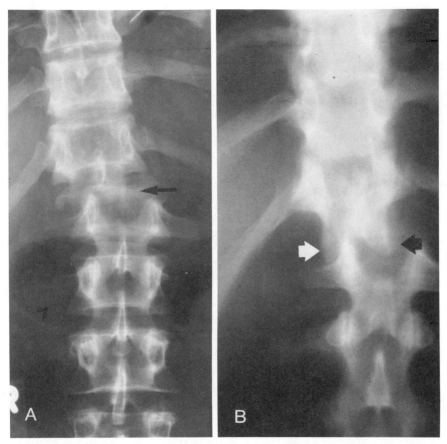

Figure 2.11. Value of tomography. (*A*) Plain film demonstrating fracture dislocation with malalignment (arrow). (*B*) Tomogram demonstrates lateral dislocation of the articular facets (arrows).

Management of Stable Spinal Injuries

Our approach to most stable spinal injuries is nonoperative. If, after careful assessment of the injury, the fracture is deemed relatively stable and the spinal column well-aligned (less than 30° kyphosis, less than 30% loss of vertebral height or less than 10° scoliosis), the patient is kept on bed rest until pain decreases. He is ambulated with a collar or brace for a period of 6 to 12 weeks. Most patients in this group have no neurological impairments, but occasionally, patients present with complete quadra- or paraplegia and stable spinal injuries. They may be treated in a similar fashion. Regular radiographic assessment should be undertaken to ensure that progressive deformity does not develop. Should this occur, operative intervention will be necessary.

If a partial spinal cord lesion shows substantial improvement in the first

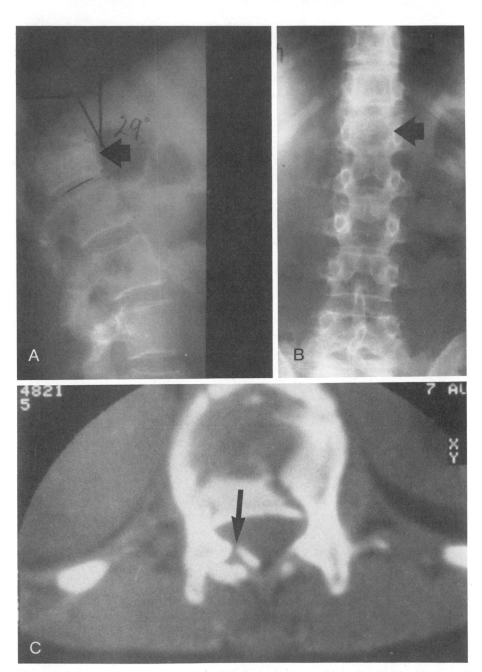

Figure 2.12. Value of CT scan. (*A and B*) Burst fracture of L1 with slight widening of the interpedicular distance (arrows). The posterior elements are poorly visualized. (*C*) Fracture of the laminae is well demonstrated (arrow) by the CT scan.

few days of injury, no further surgical intervention is performed. If, however, there is no improvement after a few days, decompression surgery is recommended, provided that significant encroachment on the spinal cord can be demonstrated radiographically.

Management of Unstable Spinal Injuries

In general, surgical stabilization is recommended for unstable spinal injuries. The anterior approach is reserved for those patients requiring decompression surgery. There is no place for posterior laminectomy in the treatment of spinal cord decompression since it does not relieve pressure on the cord and may in fact cause late complications (11, 13).

In a study undertaken at our center between January 1974 and June 1979, the results of conservative treatment for lumbar and thoracic fractures caused by major trauma were reviewed. Of the 45 patients who were treated conservatively, 22 had either angular deformities of greater than 30°, loss of height of greater than 30%, or a combination of both. Follow-up averaged 15 months with an average patient age of 34 years. There were 5 burst fractures, 38 wedge fractures, and 2 fracture dislocations. Of the 19 patients who had loss of height greater than 30%, 7 (37%) had mild to moderate pain. Angular deformities greater than 30° were seen in 9 of the 22 patients. Of these, 8 (89%) had mild to moderate discomfort. Because of these findings, we have elected to treat patients with spinal deformities greater than 30° or loss of height greater than 30% (whether stable or unstable) by means of an open reduction and internal fixation. In addition to these indications, we recommend surgery for the following specific injuries to the spinal colum.

Cervical Spine

Fractures of C1 (Jefferson fractures)

Fractures to the first cervical vertebra are secondary to bursting of the ring caused by axial loading and resulting in two or more fractures with spreading fragments. If 7 mm or more of transverse displacement of the lateral masses is noted, a rupture of the transverse ligament is likely (63). This injury is not usually associated with a neurological deficit and is relatively stable. The identification of these injuries is best seen with the CT scan (Fig. 2.13). A firm cervical orthosis is the treatment recommended for this fracture. Protection of the cervical cord is best achieved with a halo vest used for 6 to 12 weeks if the fracture is felt to be more unstable, as in the case of odontoid fractures (19). If the fracture fails to heal (a very rare occurrence), an occiput to C2 fusion is recommended (57).

Fractures of C2

Fractures of the Odontoid. Odontoid fractures are found in 10% to 15% of all cervical fractures (1). The injury may be divided into three types

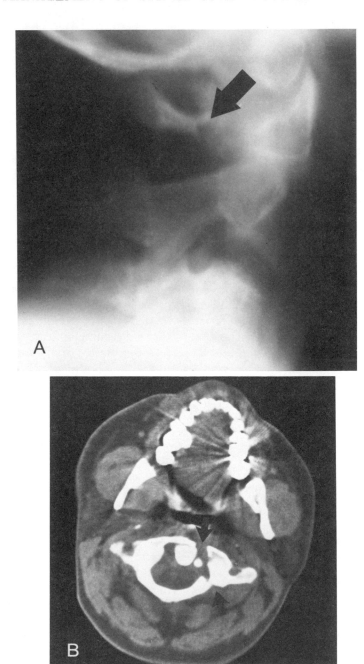

Figure 2.13. Jefferson fracture. (*A*) Fracture of the ring posteriorly (arrow). (*B*) CT scan demonstrating a fracture of both anterior and posterior portions of the ring (arrows).

according to the classification of Anderson and D'Alonzo (2). Type I is an oblique fracture through the upper odontoid process, representing an avulsion fracture of the attachments of the alar ligaments. Type II is a fracture at the junction of the odontoid process and the body of the axis. Type III extends into the cancellous bone of the axis body and represents a fracture of the body of C2. The fracture line often extends into the superior articular facet of C2 (Fig. 2.14).

The nonunion rate of fractures of the odontoid varies from 5% to 64% (5, 19, 63). The higher rate of nonunion has been associated with lack of treatment or conservative treatment other than the use of the halo vest. More recently, however, the halo vest has been applied to this injury because of its ability to provide relative rigidity. Variable results have been reported (17, 19, 69). Some have claimed that there is no significant improvement in the union rate (2, 5, 63). Sweigil (69) showed that 21 out of 22 patients

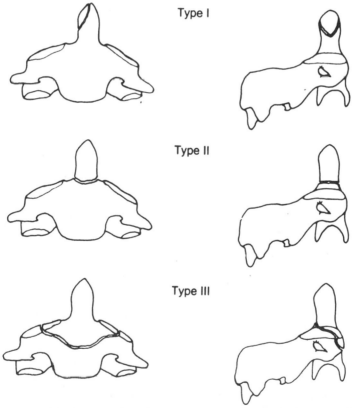

Type I

Type II

Type III

Figure 2.14. Classification of odontoid fractures according to Anderson and D'Alonzo (2). (From Anderson, L. D., D'Alonzo, R. T. Fractures of the odontoid process of the axis. *J. Bone Joint Surg., 56A:*1663–1674, 1974.)

experienced union using the halo vest. Donovan (17) noted a 75% union rate, although the Type II fractures had a higher rate of nonunion. Ekong and associates noted an increased nonunion rate in patients over 55 as well as those with posterior displacement (19). Southwick indicated that there was no satisfactory conservative treatment for Type II injuries (65).

Because of the possibility of late myelopathy associated with nonunions (10, 56), it is important to ensure that union of the odontoid occurs. Our routine, comparable to that described by Fried (25), is to apply traction for several days followed by the application of a halo vest. If the fracture is undisplaced or reduced by traction and the reduction is maintained with a halo vest as determined by frequent serial radiographs, then no surgical intervention is undertaken. A C1–2 fusion is performed at the end of 2 to 3 months if union has not occurred. If, however, the patient is over the age of 55 or 60 and had a posteriorly displaced type 2 fracture, we tend to operate primarily.

If a reduction cannot be obtained or maintained, particularly if the lesion is displaced posteriorly, a C1–2 interlaminar wiring and bone block is applied according to the Gallie technique (53) (Fig. 2.15).

The success rate with this operation is extremely high, ranging from 79% to 100% (3, 30, 56, 72). We have noted only one failure of primary arthrodesis at our center. (19). The Brooks fusion described by Griswald (30) has also enjoyed a high rate of success. The neck should be supported by a halo vest for 6 to 8 weeks postoperatively.

If a fracture of the atlas is associated with an odontoid fracture, we recommend that a halo vest be applied until the atlas has healed. If a nonunion of the odontoid persists, surgery is recommended.

Traumatic Spondylolisthesis of the Axis (Hangman's Fracture). This unique injury results from a hyperextension force coupled with axial loading, causing a fracture through the pedicle of the axis (Fig. 2.16). The initial injury may be undisplaced, but as loading continues, the disruption of the anterior and posterior longitudinal ligaments may occur with further displacement of the fracture. With sufficient extension force, disruption of the C2–3 disc may cause further displacement and instability. A major disruption may displace the anterior elements anteriorly (18, 23, 27).

Because the posterior elements separate from the anterior, the spinal canal becomes more capacious. This accounts for the relative sparing of the spinal cord. The stability of this injury must be assessed by appropriate radiographs. If there is any suspicion of instability, flexion and extension x-rays may be undertaken with care under the direction of a physician.

Stable injuries may be treated by a cervicothoracic brace and early ambulation in reliable patients. All other injuries should be treated by means of initial traction in slight extension in order to reduce the injury. A halo vest is applied within 1 to 2 days and early ambulation is initiated. The brace is worn for a period of 3 months. Two patterns of healing have

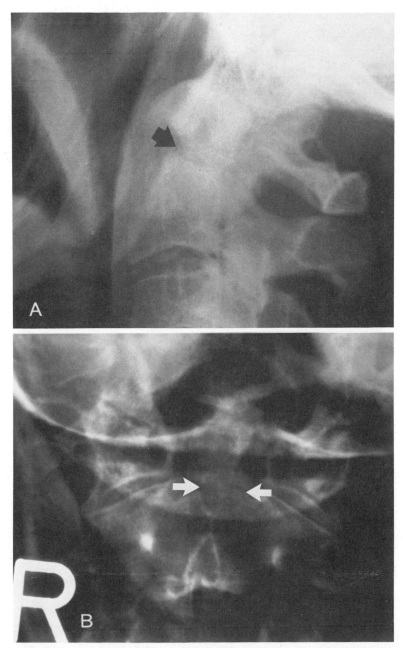

Figure 2.15. Odontoid fracture. (*A and B*) Fracture through the base (arrows) of the odontoid (Type II). (*C and D*) AP and lateral tomograms demonstrating the fracture more clearly (arrows). (*E*) Lateral tomogram at 5 months demonstrating nonunion (arrow). (*F and G*) AP and lateral radiographs demonstrating wiring technique of C1 to C2 with union occurring through the graft site at 9 months following the injury.

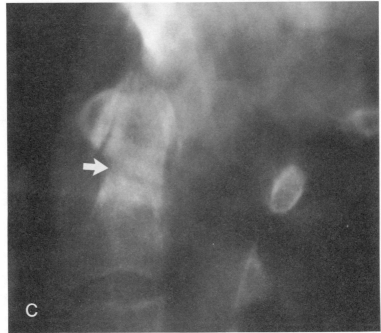

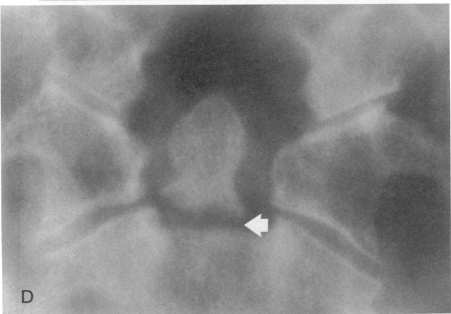

Figure 2.15 C and D

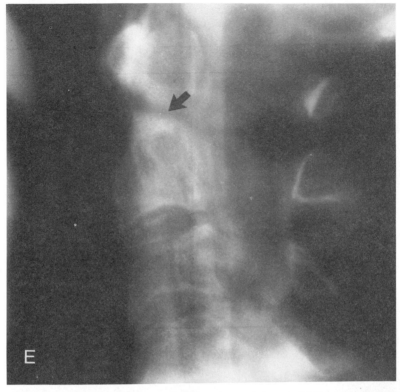

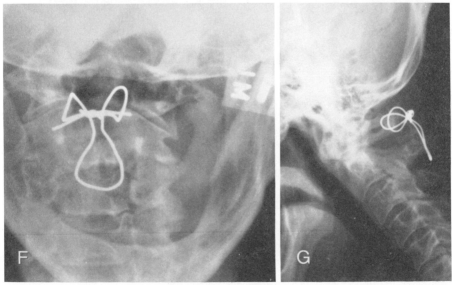

Figure 2.15 E–G

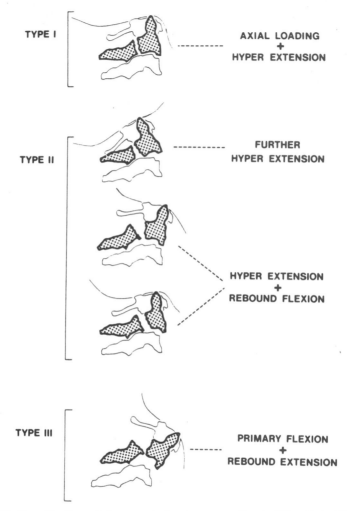

Figure 2.16. Classification of Hangman's fracture according to Effendi et al (18). (From Effendi, B., Roy, D., Cornish, B., Dussault, R. G., Laurin, C. A. Fractures of the ring of the axis. *J. Bone Joint Surg., 63B:*319–327, 1981.)

been noted with this injury (27). In the first case, the fracture heals by bony union (Fig. 2.17). Mild residual displacement is not an important concern because nonunion is rare and displacement results in a wider spinal canal. Spontaneous anterior fusion of C2–3 may also occur, stabilizing the injury.

Rarely, the injury requires stabilization because of marked displacement or late pain. A C2–3 anterior body fusion is recommended (27).

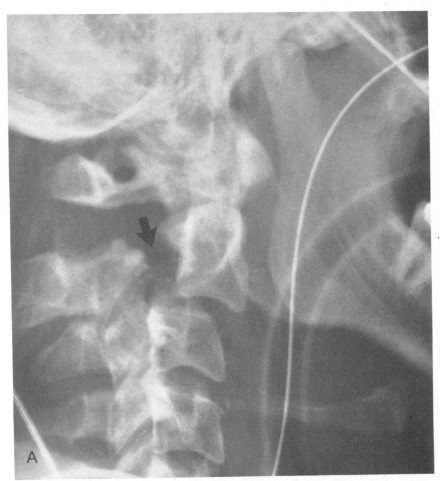

Figure 2.17. Hangman's fracture. (*A*) Fracture through the pedicles with anterior displacement of the body of C2 on C3 (arrow). (*B*) Healed fracture at 4 months. Note anterior displacement of the body of C2 on C3.

Fractures and Dislocations of the Lower Cervical Spine.

Adequate radiographic visualization of the lower cervical spine is mandatory since more than one fracture may be present. Furthermore, occult injuries at the C7-T1 level can be easily missed (21) (Fig. 2.18). Radiographs at the lowest levels of the cervical spine can be obtained by various views as noted elsewhere in this text. Since the advent of the halo vest, many unstable injuries have been treated by this technique. This method of management is satisfactory as long as the reduction of the fracture can be maintained.

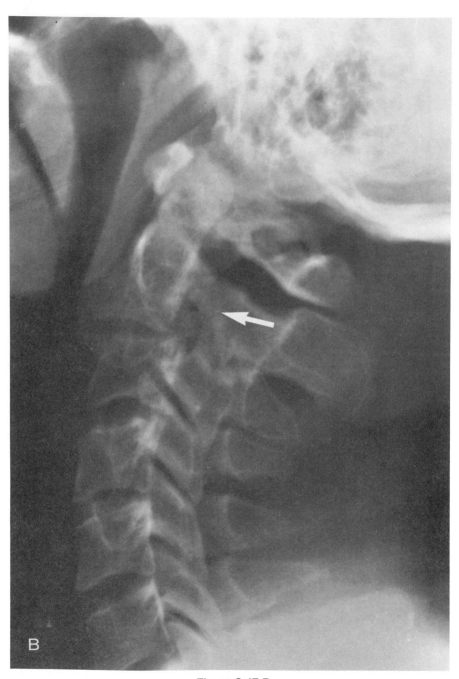

Figure 2.17 B

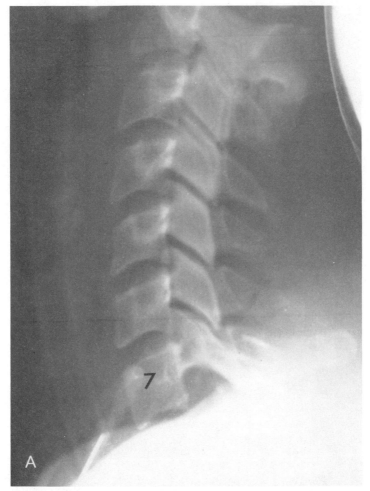

Figure 2.18. Occult injury of the cervicothoracic junction. (*A*) Lateral of the cervical spine down to C7 with no apparent abnormality. (*B*) Swimmer's view demonstrating anterior subluxation of C7 on T1 (arrows). (*C*) Tomogram demonstrating anterior subluxation of C7 on T1 (small arrows) with an avulsion fracture of the superior end plate of T1 (large arrow).

The immediate management of patients with cervical injuries must include initial immobilization by paramedical and medical personnel. Patients have developed increasing neural deficit from unintentional movement of the injured spinal cord (10). Appropriate resuscitative measures, such as the institution of an airway and the maintenance of adequate circulation, are not only important in resuscitating the patient but may also improve

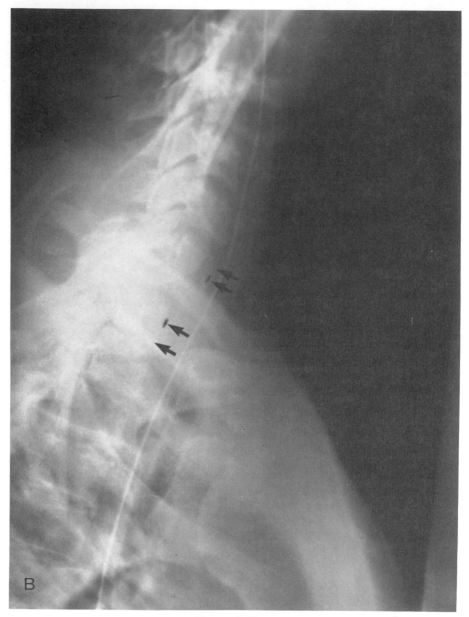

Figure 2.18 B

spinal cord perfusion. Such conditions as multiple trauma, hypovolemic shock, and water inhalation may contribute to poor respiratory function and thus, inadequate oxygenation of the cord.

The importance of restoring spinal alignment cannot be overstressed

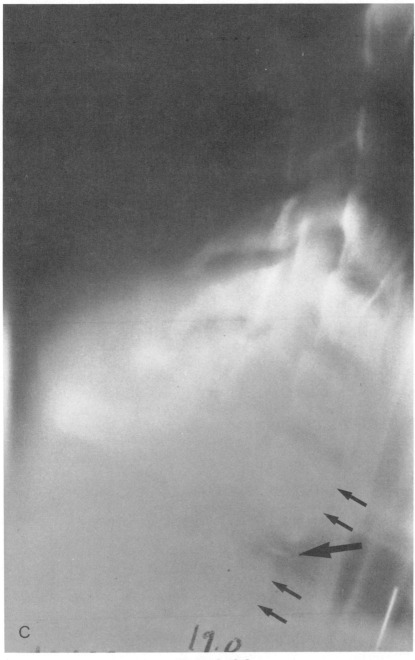

Figure 2.18 C

since it results in decompression of the spinal cord. This is achieved by skull traction at the earliest opportunity.

The indications for spinal decompression are outlined elsewhere in this text with, for the most part, decompression being undertaken anteriorly with reconstitution of the spinal column by means of a bone graft.

Subluxation. This condition is defined as a dislocation of one facet articulation, usually resulting in a locked facet, although a fracture of the facet may occur. The lateral x-ray reveals forward translation of one vertebral body on another by less than 50% (6) (Fig. 2.19). Management of this lesion consists of progressive skull traction of approximately 5 pounds every 15 minutes until the facets unlock. As a rule of thumb, the minimum traction should be approximately 10 pounds with a maximum of 10 pounds for each level of the cervical spine. If at 50 to 60 pounds a reduction is not achieved, a closed manipulation can be undertaken under general anesthesia. The subluxation may spontaneously reduce with the anesthetic, but can be performed with care under image intensifier control by laterally flexing the head away from the lesion while flexing the head forwards and then posteriorly. Failure of reduction will require surgery since an unreduced lesion may lead to late nerve root complications.

Dislocation. This condition exists when both articular facets are dislocated, resulting in displacement of the upper vertebral body by more than 50% of the sagittal diameter (6). Reduction is achieved by skull traction in a similar fashion as a subluxation. Failure to achieve a reduction may require a closed reduction under general anesthesia with image intensifier control, by applying traction and flexing the neck before extending it. If a reduction is not forthcoming, surgery will be necessary.

After the subluxation or dislocation has been reduced, the subsequent treatment varies. It has been suggested that the unilateral locked facet after reduction is a relatively stable injury that need not be fused (28). It is our practice to stabilize the level by means of a halo vest and, at 6 to 8 weeks, evaluate for instability by flexion and extension views under the supervision of a physician. If stable, a collar is prescribed. If unstable, an additional month in the halo vest is advised. We have not operated for instability following this regimen.

Although Holdsworth (36) noted that approximately 35% of patients will develop an interbody fusion following dislocation, we believe that the incidence of spontaneous fusion is lower. If the bodies do not fuse, the probability of late instability with either redislocation or late pain is high (10). We recommend a primary posterior arthrodesis with wiring of a posterior bone graft to stabilize the spine in most dislocations (Fig. 2.6).

Fractures and Fracture Dislocations of the Cervical Spine.

Definitive treatment of unstable injuries includes skull traction to realign the cervical spinal column. If alignment can be well-maintained in a halo

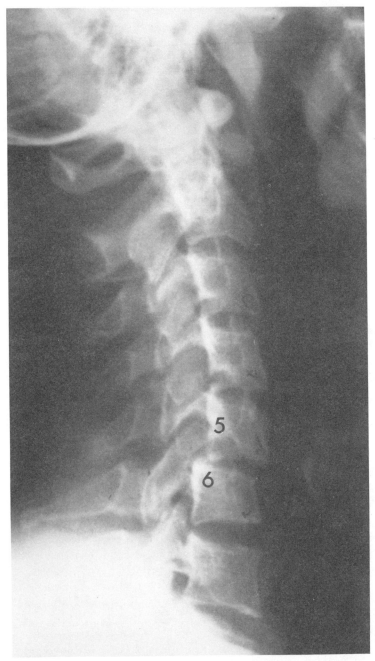

Figure 2.19. Subluxation of C5 on 6. Note the displacement of the vertebral body of C5 is less than 50% of the body width.

vest, we recommend immobilization for 3 to 4 months followed by flexion and extension views to determine the presence of late instability. If a progressive kyphosis develops while in the halo vest as often occurs with adjacent fractures, realignment and posterior stabilization and fusion are recommended (Fig. 2.20).

If anterior interbody fusion has been undertaken for spinal cord decompression, the stability of the spine may be enhanced by anterior internal fixation (Fig. 2.21) but the risk of implant failure is high. We do not recommend internal fixation because of the complications. Supplemental fixation and posterior fusion for anterior decompression and anterior bone block may also be necessary in some very unstable injuries.

Other methods of stabilization of the cervical spine have been recommended, including posterior plates and C-clamps (30, 69). These require considerable experience and expertise in their application but do provide excellent fixation.

To summarize, stable cervical injuries are readily treated by means of an external orthosis for 6 to 12 weeks while unstable injuries require more definitive treatment. We recommend the use of a halo vest for most cervical fractures, including fractures of the odontoid and the C2 pedicle as well as unstable fractures and fracture dislocations of the lower cervical spine as long as alignment can be maintained. If anterior decompression is required for neurosurgical indications, an anterior fusion with or without metal fixation is recommended to stabilize the spine. Occasionally, posterior stabilization and fusion are required to supplement the anterior surgery. Most stabilization procedures can be undertaken posteriorly with wiring of corticocancellous grafts that provide early fixation and subsequent fusion (Fig. 2.22).

Thoracic and Lumbar Fractures and Fracture Dislocations

Unstable injuries of the thoracic and lumbar spine may lead to late deformity and pain (29, 51, 55, 74). Those who advocate the conservative approach do provide definitive treatment for the management of these injuries by means of postural reduction (8, 24, 33, 48, 78). With expert paramedical care, many unstable fractures can be reduced and maintained until fusion occurs. This form of management requires considerable skill in achieving a well-aligned spine and may require up to 3 months of bed rest before ambulation can take place. In spite of this treatment, a significant number of spines will remain ununited or will go on to late instability and pain.

In the past operative management has been unsatisfactory because of inadequate methods of internal fixation (32, 49). Although alignment is obtained, complete bed rest is necessary to maintain the reduction of displaced spinal fractures. When this principle has been ignored and early

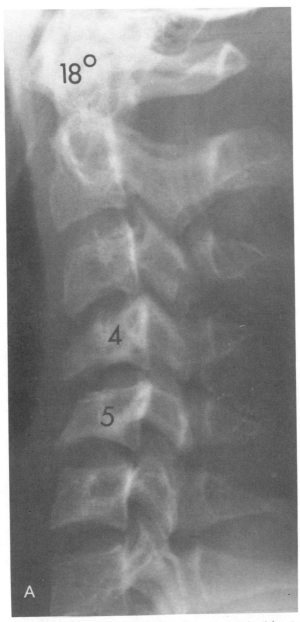

Figure 2.20. Progressive deformity following adjacent vertebral fractures. (*A*) Lateral of the cervical spine demonstrating wedge compression fractures of C4 and C5 with an 18° deformity. (*B*) At 6 weeks the deformity has increased to 20°. (*C*) At 8 weeks there is a 38° angulation. (*D*) Following surgery using rib and interlaminar wiring, the deformity has been reduced to 14°.

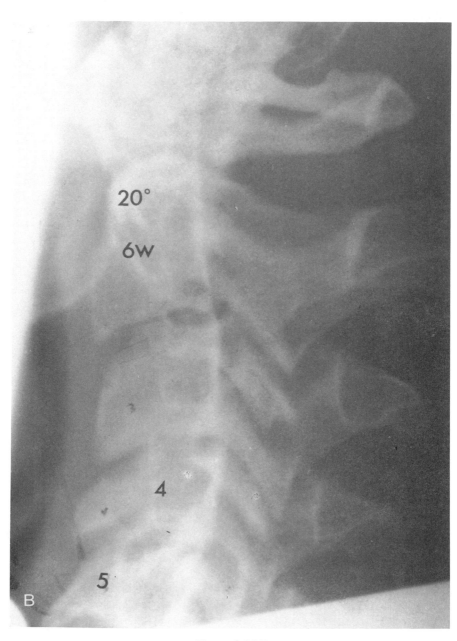

Figure 2.20 B

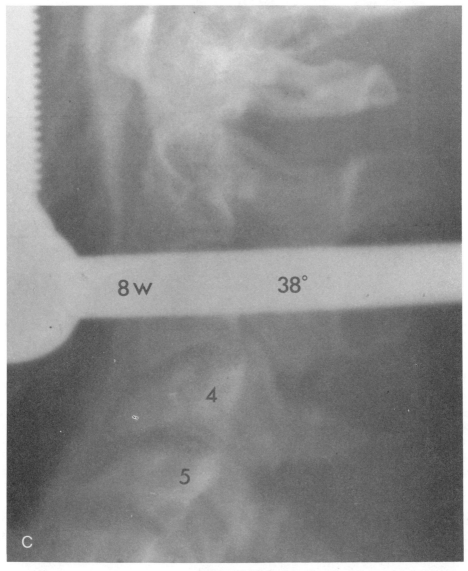

Figure 2.20 C

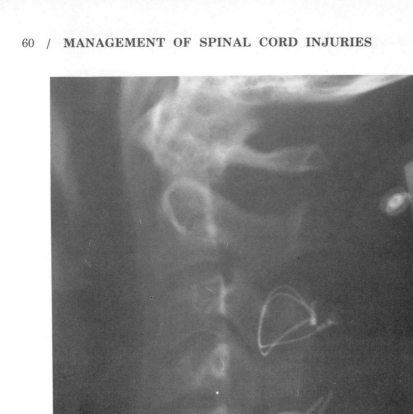

Figure 2.20 D

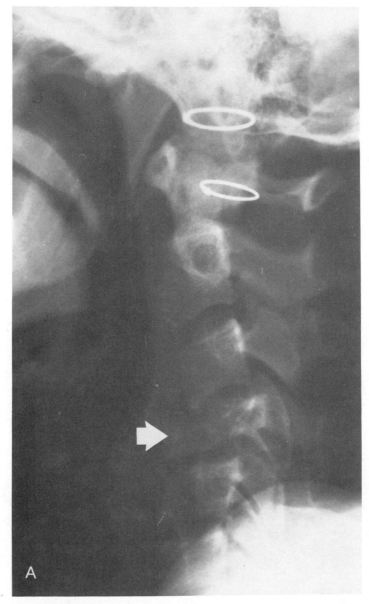

Figure 2.21. Internal fixation for cervical fractures. (*A*) This burst fracture of C4 (arrow) resulted in a partial neurological deficit. Note the widening of the interspinous distance posteriorly between C3 and C4, indicating a very unstable injury. (*B and C*) After anterior decompression and insertion of bone graft from C3 to C5 (arrows), internal fixation has been achieved by two small AO plates and cancellous screws.

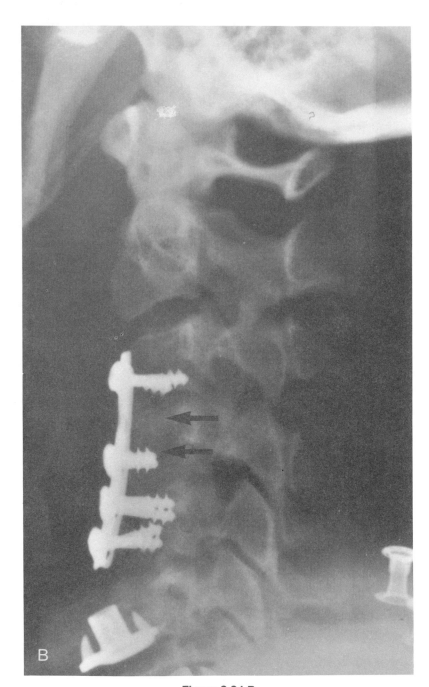

Figure 2.21 B

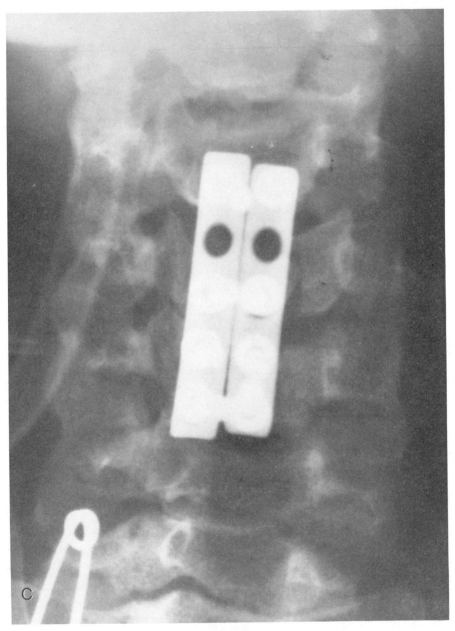

Figure 2.21 C

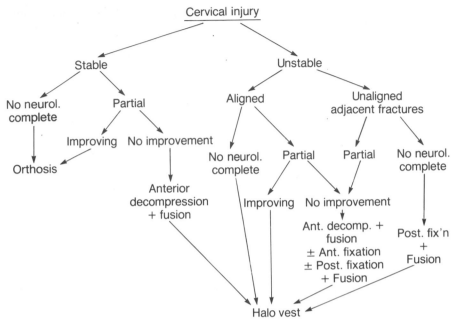

Figure 2.22. Algorithm for the management of cervical injuries.

ambulation instituted, a significant number of unstable injuries have progressed to deformity.

Since the advent of Harrington rods, many of the objections to surgical intervention have been overcome. Spinal alignment and stability as well as early ambulation can be achieved, and earlier discharge to a rehabilitation center is likely (13, 22, 42, 77).

Most unstable injuries are treated operatively at our center. Because of angular deformity and translational malalignment, fractures are stabilized by means of rigid rods inserted two or three levels above and two levels below the fracture for maximum stabilization (40–42, 67). The rods act as internal splints which align the spine and provide three point fixation. Newer fixation devices and segmental fixation, such as Luque rods or wires attached from the laminae to Harrington rods, have been used in the last 3 or 4 years to supplement the fixation (13, 26, 50). Plates such as those described by Roy-Camille (62) have also provided satisfactory fixation for many thoracic and lumbar fractures.

If anterior decompression of the anterior column is necessary, a bone block of corticocancellous bone, usually from the iliac crest, is inserted through a transpleural, retroperitoneal, or combined thoracolumbar approach to realign and provide continuity for the spinal column. Adequate alignment anteriorly, however, is difficult to achieve unless anterior instrumentation is included (46). Because of the persistent angular deformity, we recommend posterior instrumentation to supplement the anterior bone block fusion. This can be done during the same operative procedure or at a later date, 1 to 2 weeks following the primary operation (Fig. 2.23). Anterior decompression can be performed through a posterolateral (costotransverse) approach but the exposure is limited.

In addition to these general comments, specific indications and techniques are worth mentioning.

The Thoracic Spine

Fractures in the upper four to six thoracic vertebrae may not require surgical intervention. Even when the deformity exceeds 30° of angulation or when the loss of height of the vertebral body is greater than 30%, stabilization may not be necessary since the upper thoracic spine does not provide the same weight-bearing function as the lower spine. Furthermore, the ribs tend to stabilize this injury, and late pain is not a common sequela.

For the lower thoracic spine, the principles stated above apply.

Thoracolumbar Injuries

Fractures and fracture dislocations of the thoracolumbar spine are usually treated with open reduction and internal fixation by Harrington distraction or similar rods (16, 22, 29, 40, 43, 77). Besides providing stability, the rods serve to realign the spine, restoring the normal thoracic kyphosis and upper lumbar lordosis. This is achieved by contouring the rods with a slight lordotic curve in the lumbar spine. It is necessary to use square-ended rods with square-holed hooks to prevent the rods from rotating 180° and conforming to the original kyphosis of the injury (Fig. 2.24). Other devices are becoming available that do not require special hooks and rods (39, 40).

Lumbar Fractures

Fractures in the middle and lower lumbar spine are often caused by distraction injuries such as seatbelt injuries (44, 76). This type of lesion (Chance-type fracture) is a distraction injury with fracture or dislocation of the posterior facets, with or without fracture of the vertebral bodies. These injuries are best dealt with by means of Harrington compression rods that reduce the posterior elements. This form of fixation has been found to provide excellent rigidity (41, 67). Furthermore, restoration of the normal lordotic alignment is readily achieved. It is recommended that the fracture be immobilized by means of two hooks above and two hooks below the level of the injury (Fig. 2.25).

Fractures of L5 and the lumbosacral junction are rare and difficult to manage by means of posterior instrumentation (47), although new devices are being developed (40). At this time, these injuries are best treated by means of postural reduction and bed rest since adequate fixation to the sacrum is difficult by operative means.

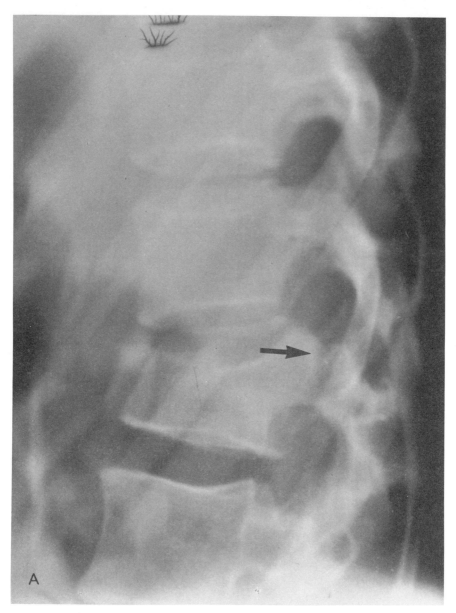

Figure 2.23. Anterior decompression and stabilization. (*A*) Burst fracture of L1 with encroachment of the posterior cortex into the canal (arrow). (*B*) CT scan demonstrating the degree of comminution and displacement of the fracture into the spinal canal. (*C*) CT scan following anterior decompression and insertion of corticocancellous bone graft (arrow). (*D*) Posterior instrumentation and posterior spinal fusion at 1 week following anterior decompression. Note the alignment of the spine has improved. The corticocancellous graft is seen bridging T12 to L1 (arrows).

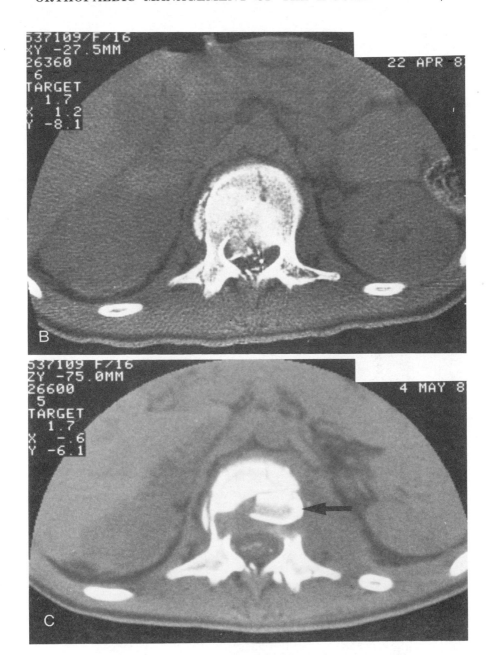

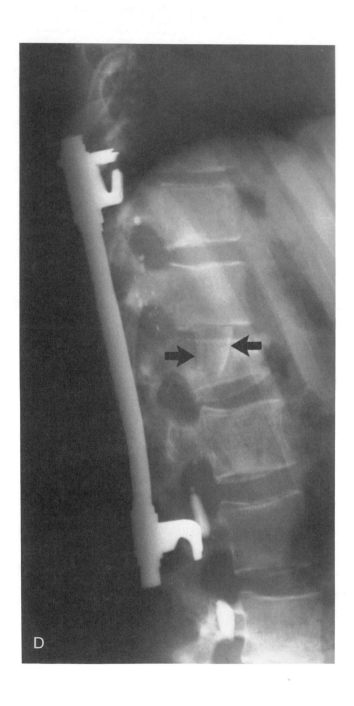

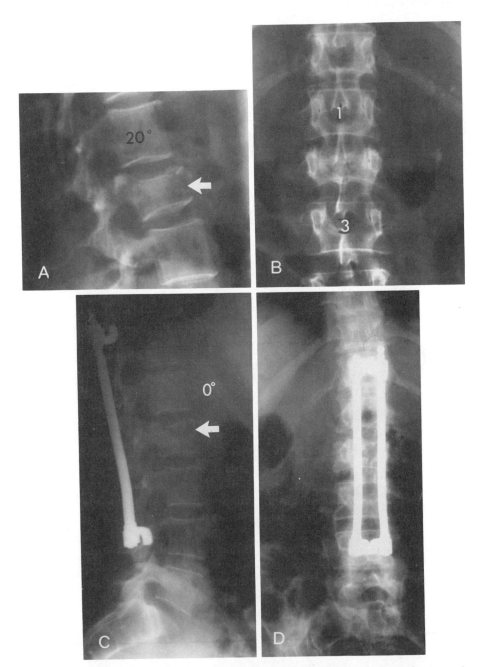

Figure 2.24. Reconstitution of normal vertebral alignment. (*A and B*) Burst fracture of L2 (arrow) with 20° kyphosis between L1 and L2. (*C and D*) Using rods with square ends distally inserted into square holes and contouring the rod into lordosis, the fracture is realigned with 0° angulation. Note the reconstitution of the vertebral height of L2 (arrow).

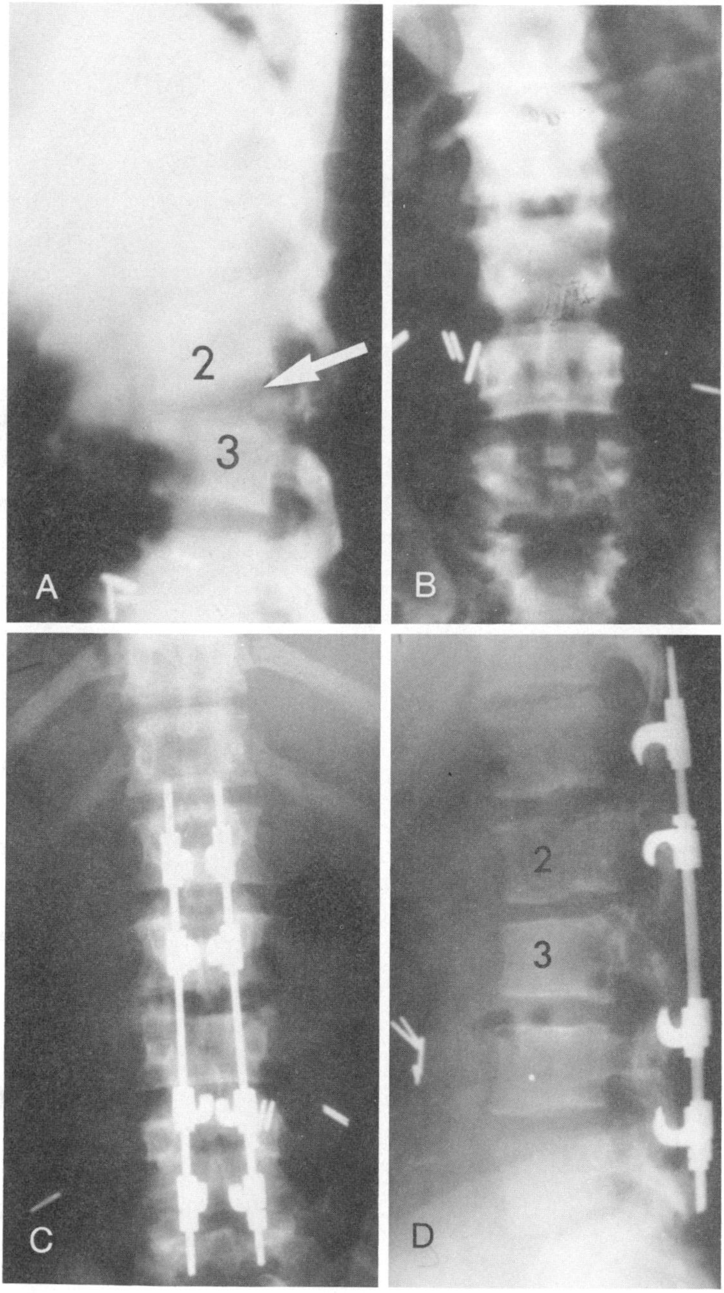

Figure 2.25. Chance fracture. (*A and B*) This distraction injury results in separation of the vertebrae from posterior to anterior at the level of L2–3 (arrow). (*C and D*) Harrington compression rods inserted two levels above and two levels below the injury reducing the L2–3 disruption.

We recommend bone grafting the fracture site, leaving the rest of the instrumented spine unfused. The spinous processes are sufficient for this short fusion since they are readily available. This obviates the need for a second incision with the attendant morbidity associated with bone graft donor sites. Some centers (4, 73) do not supplement the injuries with bone graft if there is significant bony injury. In order to preserve lumbar function, removal of the rods extending below L2 is recommended at 1 year following surgery.

The use of external immobilization, such as a Jewett brace, is recommended for those patients treated by Harrington rods. However, this may not be necessary (73), particularly if the newer modified devices are utilized. Using a Locking-hook rodding device (38, 40), we have not found it necessary to use orthoses for the past 2½ years, except in unusual circumstances. Patients are allowed to sit and ambulate within 3 or 4 days after surgery.

In summary, posterior instrumentation and spinal fusion are recommended for unstable or significantly deformed fractures of the thoracic, thoracolumbar and lumbar spines. The Harrington distraction or similar rods are recommended. Upper thoracic injuries that are relatively unstable may not require surgery. Distraction injuries, such as in the lumbar spine, are treated with compression instrumentation. Lumbosacral fractures and fracture dislocations may require postural reduction, but conservative treatment is recommended (Fig. 2.26).

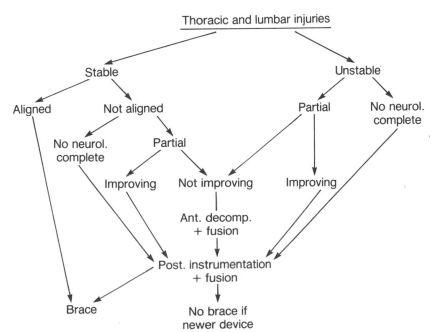

Figure 2.26. Algorithm for the management of thoracic and lumbar fractures.

Deficiencies of Posterior Instrumentation

Numerous instruments have been used in the past for stabilizing the spine posteriorly. Most of these have fallen into disrepute because of their failure to provide rigid fixation (22, 49). Harrington rods, over the past two decades, have been used with good initial results. A review of patients treated at our center (29) has shown that there are deficiencies in the rods that result in some loss of correction and later complications. Harrington rods are not sufficient to control all unstable fractures because they are placed on the tension side of the injury. This results in undue stress to the instrumentation with possible loss of fixation. Furthermore, the difficult insertion has led to technical errors that have resulted in loss of reduction in some cases.

Because of significant loss of height in some injuries, including burst

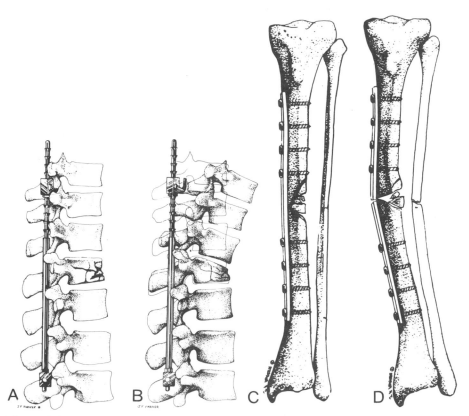

Figure 2.27. Deficiency of posterior instrumentation. (*A and B*) Diagrammatic representation of vertebral fracture reduced by means of Harrington rods. Note the loss of correction due to collapse of the fractured vertebrae. (*C and D*) Failure of the instrumentation can be compared to plating a tibia with a cortical defect on the far side. Eventually, failure will occur as the far defect collapses.

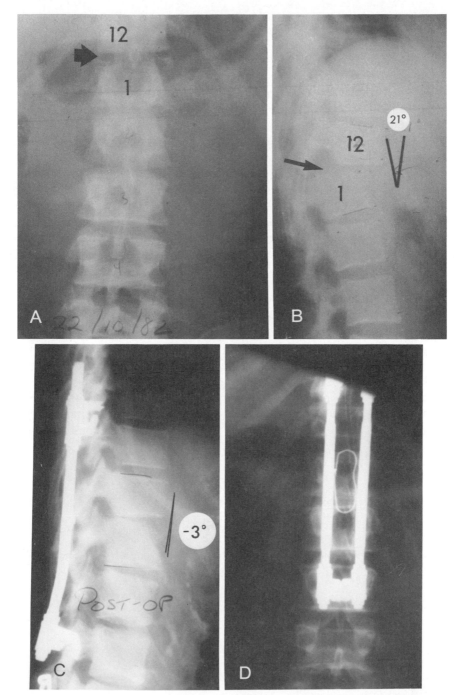

Figure 2.28. A new posterior fixation device. (*A and B*) AP and lateral radiographs of fracture dislocation of T12-L1 (arrows). Note a 21° kyphosis. (*C and D*) The rods have reduced the fracture dislocation to −3° (that is, lordosis) and have restored the vertebral height.

fractures, the restoration of alignment may not allow adequate support in the anterior column (29). If one compares the rods inserted in the spine to a plate applied to a long bone fracture in which there is marked comminution on the far cortex, weight bearing may result in angular deformity and failure of the device (Fig. 2.27). This particular problem requires attention and must be addressed in future studies of instrumentation in spinal fracture treatment. It may be necessary to supplement the posterior instrumentation with an anterior bony block in specific cases.

New instrumentation has been designed to obviate these problems, including the Roy-Camille plates (62) and Luque rods (50), both of which provide segmental fixation. Other devices are being developed, one of which is in current use at our center as part of a multicenter trial (40). Almost 100 patients have been treated with encouraging results using this device (Fig. 2.28).

Conclusions

The approach to management of spinal injuries is based on the degree of instability in the spinal column. Stable injuries can be treated nonoperatively. Although controversy exists as to the appropriate treatment for unstable injuries, our approach has been to operatively stabilize these fractures. In the cervical spine, the halo vest is the treatment of choice for most injuries with posterior stabilization and bone grafting in specific instances. In the thoracic and lumbar spine, posterior instrumentation is recommended not only as primary treatment but also to supplement anterior decompression surgery.

REFERENCES

1. Anderson, L. D. Fractures of the odontoid process of the axis. In: *The Cervical Spine*. J.B. Lippincott Co., Philadelphia, 1983, pp. 206–223.
2. Anderson, L. D., and D'Alonzo, R. T. Fractures of the odontoid process of the axis. *J. Bone Joint Surg., 56A:*1663–1674, 1974.
3. Apuzzo, M. L. J., et al. Acute fractures of the odontoid process. *J.Neurosurg., 48:*85–91, 1978.
4. Armstrong, G. Personal communication.
5. Aymes, E. W., and Anderson, F. M. Fracture of the odontoid process. *Arch. Surg., 72:*377–393, 1956.
6. Beatson, T. R. Fractures and dislocations of the cervical spine. *J. Bone Joint Surg., 45B:*21–34, 1963.
7. Bedbrook, G. M. and Edibam, R. C. The study of spinal deformity in traumatic spinal paralysis. *Paraplegia, 10:*321–335, 1973.
8. Bedbrook, G. M. Treatment of thoracolumbar dislocation and fractures with paraplegia. *Clin. Orthop., 112:*27–43, 1975.
9. Bohlman, H. H. Acute fractures and dislocations of the cervical spine: an analysis of 300 hospitalized patients and a review of the literature. *J. Bone Joint Surg., 61A:*1119–1142, 1979.
10. Bohlman, H. H., and Boada, E. Fractures and dislocations of the lower cervical spine. In: *The Cervical Spine*. J.B. Lippincott Co., Philadelphia, 1983, pp. 232–267.

11. Bradford, D. S., and Thompson, R. C. Fractures and dislocations of the spine. Indications for surgical intervention. Minn. Med., October 7, pp. 711–720, 1976.
12. Burke, D. C., and Murray, D. D. The management of thoracic and thoraco-lumbar injuries of the spine with neurological involvement. J. Bone Joint Surg., 58B:72–78, 1976.
13. Convery, F. R., Ninteer, N. A., Smith, R. W., and Emerson, S. M. Fracture-dislocations of the dorsolumbar spine. Acute operative stabilization by Harrington instrumentation. Spine, 3:160–166, 1978.
14. Davies, W. E., Morris, J. H., and Hill, V. An analysis of conservative (non-surgical) management of thoraco-lumbar fractures and fracture-dislocations with neurological damage. J. Bone Joint Surg., 62A:1324–1328, 1980.
15. Denis, F. Updated classification of thoracolumbar fractures. Orthop. Trans. 6:8–9, 1982.
16. Dickson, J. H., Harrington, T. R., and Erwin, W. D. Results of reduction and stabilization of the severely fractured thoracic and lumbar spine. J. Bone Joint Surg., 60A:799–805, 1978.
17. Donovan, M. M. Efficacy of rigid fixation of fractures of the odontoid process and retrospective analysis of 54 cases. Orthop. Trans. 3:309, 1979.
18. Effendi, B., Roy, D., Cornish, B., Dussault, R. G., and Laurin, C. A. Fractures of the ring of the axis. J. Bone Joint Surg., 63B:319–327, 1981.
19. Ekong, C. U., Schwartz, M. L., Tator, C. H., Rowed, D. W., and Edmunds, V. E. Odontoid fracture: management with early mobilization using the halo device. Neurosurgery, 9:631–637, 1981.
20. Erickson, D. L., Leider, L. L., and Brown, W. E. One stage decompression—stabilization for thoracolumbar fractures. Spine, 2:53–56, 1977.
21. Evans, D. K. Dislocations of the cervicothoracic junction. J. Bone Joint Surg., 65B:124–127, 1983.
22. Flesch, J. R., Leider, L. L., Erickson, D. L., Chou, S. N., and Bradford, D. S. Harrington instrumentation and spinal fusion for unstable fractures and fracture dislocations of the thoracic and lumbar spine. J. Bone Joint Surg., 49A:143–153, 1977.
23. Francis, W. R., Fielding, J. W., Hawking, R. J., Pepin, J., and Hensinger, R. Traumatic spondylolisthesis of the axis. J. Bone Joint Surg., 63B:313–318, 1981.
24. Frankel, H. L., Hancock, D. O., Hyslop, G., Melzak, J., Michaels, S., Ungar, G. H., Vernon, J. D. S., and Walsh, V. J. The value of postural reduction in the initial management of closed injuries of the spine with paraplegia and tetraplegia. Part I. Paraplegia, 7:179–192, 1969.
25. Fried, L. C. Atlanto-axial fracture-dislocations. J. Bone Joint Surg., 55B:490–496, 1973.
26. Gaines, R. W., Munson, G., Breedlove, R., Satterlee, C., and Betten, R. Harrington distraction rods supplemented with sublaminar wires for thoraco-lumbar fracture-dislocations. Experimental and clinical investigation. Proceedings of the 17th Annual Meeting of the Scoliosis Research Society. San Francisco, 1982, pp. 80–81.
27. Garfin, S. R., and Rothman, R. H. Traumatic spondylolisthesis of the axis (hangman's fracture). In: The Cervical Spine. J.B. Lippincott Co., Philadelphia, 1983, pp. 223–232.
28. Gertzbein, S. D. Assessment of cervical spinal instability. In Tator, C. H. (ed.): Early Management of Acute Spinal Cord Injury. Raven Press, New York, 1982, pp. 41–52.
29. Gertzbein, S. D., MacMichael, D., and Tile, M. Harrington instrumentation as a method of fixation in fractures of the spine. J. Bone Joint Surg., 64B:526–529, 1982.
30. Griswold, D. M., et al. Atlantoaxial fusion for instability. J. Bone Joint Surg., 60A:285–292, 1978.
31. Gumley, G., Taylor, D. F. K., and Ryan, M. D. Distraction fractures of the lumbar spine. J. Bone Joint Surg., 64B:520–525, 1982.
32. Guttmann, Sir L. Spinal deformities in traumatic paraplegics and tetraplegics following surgical procedures. Paraplegia, 7:38–49, 1969.
33. Guttmann, Sir L. Spinal injuries, initial treatment of fractures and dislocations in traumatic paraplegia and tetraplegia. In: Folia Traumatologica. Geigy, 1972, pp. 1–16.

34. Guttman, L. Surgical aspects of the treatment of traumatic paraplegia. *J. Bone Joint Surg.*, *31B*:399–403, 1949.
35. Handelberg, F., Bellemans, M. A., Opdecam, P., and Casteleyn, P. T. The use of computerized tomographs in the diagnosis of thoracolumbar injury. *J. Bone Joint Surg.*, *63B*:336–341, 1981.
36. Holdsworth, Sir F. Fractures, dislocations and fracture-dislocations of the spine. *J. Bone Joint Surg.*, *52A*:1534–1551, 1970.
37. Huestis, W. S. Posterior instrumentation for cervical fractures. In Tator, C. H. (ed.): *The Management of Acute Spinal Cord Injury.* Raven Press, New York, 1982, pp. 301–304.
38. Jacobs, R. R., Asher, M. A., and Snider, R. K. Thoracolumbar spinal injures, a comparative study of recurrent and operative treatment in 100 patients. *Spine, 5:*46;3–477, 1980.
39. Jacobs, R. R. Personal communication.
40. Jacobs, R. R., Dayners, L. E., Gertzbein, S. D., Nordwall, A., and Mathys, R. A locking hook-spinal rod: current status of development. *Transactions of the 17th Annual Meeting of the Scoliosis Research Society.* Chicago, 1972, p. 78.
41. Jacobs, R. R., and Ghista, D. N. A biomechanical basis for treatment of injuries of the dorsolumbar spine. In Ghista, D. N. (ed.): *Osteoarthromechanics.* Hemisphere Publishing Corp., McGraw-Hill Book Co, New York, 1983, pp. 435–471.
42. Jacobs, R. R., Nordwall, A., and Nachemson, A. Reduction, stability and strength provided by internal fixation for thoracolumbar spinal injuries. *Clin. Orthop., 171:*300–308, 1982.
43. Katznelson, A. M. Stabilization of the spine in traumatic paraplegia. *Paraplegia, 7:*33–37, 1969.
44. Kaufer, H., and Hayes, A. T. Lumbar fracture dislocations. *J. Bone Joint Surg., 48A:*712–730, 1966.
45. Koch, R. A., and Nickel, V. L. Halo vest: in the evaluation of motion and forces across the neck. *Spine, 3:*103–107, 1978.
46. Kostiuk, J. P. Anterior spinal cord decompression for lesions of the thoracic and lumbar spine. Techniques, new methods of internal fixation, results. *Spine,* In Press, 1983.
47. Kostiuk, J. P., and Hall, B. Complications of spinal fusion to the sacrum in adult scoliosis patients. *Proceedings of the 9th Annual International Society for Study of Lumbar Spine.* 1983, p. 31.
48. Leidholt, J. D., Young, J. J., Hahn, H. R., Jackson, R. E., Gamble, W. E., and Miles, J. S. Evaluations of late spinal deformities and fracture-dislocations of the dorsal and lumbar spine in paraplegics. *Paraplegia, 7:*16–27, 1969.
49. Lewis, J., and McKibbin, B. The treatment of unstable fracture dislocations of the thoracolumbar spine accompanied by paraplegia. *J. Bone Joint Surg., 57B:*603–612, 1974.
50. Luque, E. R., Cassis, N., and Ramirez-Wiella, G. Segmental spinal instrumentation in the treatment of fractures of the thoracolumbar spine. *Spine, 7:*312–317, 1982.
51. Malcolm, B. Spinal deformities secondary to spinal injuries. *Orthop. Clin. North Am., 4:*943–952, 1979.
52. McAfee, P. C., Yuan, H. A., Frederickson, B. E., and Lubicky, J. P. The value of computed tomography in thoracolumbar fractures. An analysis of 100 consecutive cases and a new classification. *J. Bone Joint Surg., 65A:*461–473, 1983.
53. McGraw, R. W., and Rusch, R. M. Atlantoaxial arthrodesis. *J. Bone Joint Surg., 55B:*482–489, 1973.
54. McSweenay, T. Deformities of the spine following injuries to the cord. In: *Handbook of Neurology,* Vol. 26. 1976, pp. 159–174.
55. Nicoll, E. A. Fractures of the dorso-lumbar spine. *J. Bone Joint Surg., 31B:*376–394, 1949.
56. Paradis, G. R., and Janes, J. M. Post-traumatic atlantoaxial instability: the fate of the odontoid process fracture in 46 cases. *J. Trauma, 13:*359–366, 1973.
57. Pierce, D. S., and Barr, J. S., Jr. Fractures and dislocations at the base of the skull and upper cervical spine. In: *The Cervical Spine.* J.B. Lippincott Co., Philadelphia, 1983, pp. 196–206.

58. Post, M. J. D., Green, B. A., Quencer, R. M., Stokes, M. A., Callahan, R. A., and Isemont, F. J. The value of computed tomography in spinal trauma. *Spine, 7*:417–431, 1982.

59. Riska, E. B. Anterolateral decompression as treatment of paraplegia following vertebral fractures in the thoraco-lumbar spine. *Reconstr. Surg. Traumatol., 15*:17–35, 1976.

60. Rivlin, A. S., and Tator, C. H. Effect of duration of acute spinal cord compression in a new cord injury model in the rat. *Surg. Neurol., 10*:38–43, 1978.

61. Rowed, D. W., McLean, J. A. G., and Tator, C. H. Somatosensory-evoked potentials in aute spinal cord injury: prognostic value. *Surg. Neurol., 9*:203–210, 1978.

62. Roy-Camille, R., Saillant, G., Berteaux, D., and Marie-Anne, S. Early mangement of spinal injuries. In: *Recent Advances in Orthopaedics*. Churchill Livingstone, 1979, pp. 57–87.

63. Schatzker, J., Rorabeck, C. H., and Waddell, J. P. Fractures of the dens (odontoid process): an analysis of 37 cases. *J. Bone Joint Surg., 53B*:392–405, 1971.

64. Schellhas, A. P., Latchaw, R. E., Wendling, C. R., and Gold, L. A. J. Vertebrobasilar injuries following cervical manipulation. *J.A.M.A., 244*:1450–1453, 1980.

65. Southwick, W. O. Management of fractures of the dens (odontoid process). *J. Bone Joint Surg., 62A*:482–486, 1980.

66. Stanger, J. K. Fracture dislocations of the thoraco-lumbar spine with special reference to reduction by open and closed operations. *J. Bone Joint Surg., 29*:107–118, 1949.

67. Stauffer, E. S., and Neil, J. L. Biomechanical analysis of structural stability of internal fixation in fractures of the thoracolumbar spine. *Clin. Orthop., 112*:159–164, 1975.

68. Sullivan, J. A., and Bryant, C. H. Management of thoracic and lumbar fractures with harrington rods supplemented with segmented wires. *Proceedings of the 17th Annual Meeting of the Scoliosis Research Society*. Denver, 1982, p. 81.

69. Sweigil, J. F. Halo thoracic brace in the management of odontoid fractures. *Orthop. Trans., 3*:126, 1979.

70. Tator, C. H., and Rowed, D. W. Current concepts in the immediate management of acute spinal cord injuries. *Can. Med. Assoc. J., 121*:1453–1464, 1979.

71. Tupper, J. W., Gunn, D. R., and Mullan, M. P. Double level compression fractures—more unstable than you think. *J. Bone Joint Surg., 56A*:1763, 1974.

72. Waddell, J. P., and Reardon, G. P. Atlanto axial arthrodesis to treat odontoid fractures. *Can. J. Surg., 26*:255–257, 1983.

73. Waddell, J. P. Personal Communication.

74. Watson-Jones, Sir R. Injuries of the Spine. In Wilson, J. N. (ed.): *Fractures and Joint Injuries*, ed. 5. Churchill Livingstone, Edinburgh, 1976, pp. 798–849.

75. White, A. A., Southwick, W. O., and Panjabi, M. M. Clinical instability in the lower cervical spine: a review of past and current concepts. *Spine, 1*:15–27, 1976.

76. White, A. A., and Panjabi, M. M. Practical biomechanics of spine trauma. In: *Clinical Biomechanics of the Spine*. J.B. Lippincott Co., Philadelphia, 1978, p. 115–190.

77. Yosipovitch, Z., Robin, G. C., and Makin, M. Open reduction of unstable thoracolumbar spinal injuries and fixation with harrington rods. *J. Bone Joint Surg., 59A*:1003–1015, 1977.

78. Young, J. S., and Dexter, W. R. Neurological recovery distal to the zone of injury in 172 cases of closed traumatic spinal cord injury. *Paraplegia, 16*:39–49, 1978.

3

The Respiratory System of the Spinal Cord Patient

M. D. L. MORGAN
J. R. SILVER
S. J. WILLIAMS

Respiratory failure and infection are major causes of death and morbidity in spinal injury and especially tetraplegia. A healthy respiratory system depends upon the integrated activity of many nerves and muscles to generate the power to breathe. A knowledge of the mechanisms that govern this activity are of particular importance in spinal injury where neuromuscular paralysis of the respiratory muscles is the primary disorder.

THE RESPIRATORY SYSTEM–NORMAL PHYSIOLOGY

The function of the respiratory system is to remove carbon dioxide from the blood and replenish it with oxygen to be delivered to the tissues. In humans, the two components of this system are a gas exchanger and a pump. The lung, which is the gas-exchanging organ, provides fresh gas for exchange at the blood/air interface. The pump that generates the power to breathe and move the lungs consists of the chest wall and the respiratory muscles. It is easy to understand why physiologists have focused on the lung, especially the behavior of gas flow in the assessment of respiratory function. This is easily measurable, and many common respiratory diseases show characteristic abnormalities in lung function and gas exchange. It is now becoming clear that the function of the lung is inseparable from that of the pump, and many common predominantly intrapulmonary diseases are complicated by chest wall or respiratory muscle abnormalities. Now that our understanding and ability to measure respiratory muscle function have improved, we are able to appreciate their contribution to health or disorder.

The chest wall is the organ that incorporates the rib cage, the diaphragm, and the abdomen. The respiratory muscles comprise three main groups: the diaphragm itself, the intercostal/accessory muscles, and the abdominal muscles. These muscles act upon the chest wall either as prime movers or to strengthen the rib cage and facilitate the action of others. During inspiration they act on the chest wall in an integrated fashion to change its configuration and hence enlarge the thoracic cavity, generating negative intrapleural pressure and inflating the lungs. Enlargement of the thoracic cavity may occur by expansion of the rib cage or by depression of the diaphragm, resulting in displacement of the abdominal cavity. In normal man both mechanisms occur (Fig. 3.1).

The respiratory muscles have been the subject of some excellent recent reviews, and the field is now receiving adequate attention (12, 15–17, 49, 66). The respiratory muscles differ from the other skeletal muscles in some important respects: (a) they must overcome principally resistive and elastic loads rather than inertial loads; (b) they are under both involuntary and voluntary control; and (c) they must contract regularly without prolonged rest for the whole of our lives.

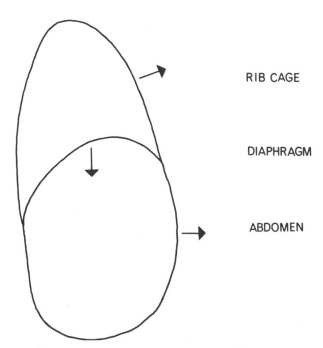

RIB CAGE

DIAPHRAGM

ABDOMEN

Figure 3.1. A schematic representation of the physiological chest wall contains the thoracic and abdominal cavities separated by the diaphragm. The thoracic cavity can enlarge by either expansion of the rib cage or descent of the diaphragm, which will, in turn, distend the abdomen.

In spite of these differences, the function of these muscles still has to be assessed in the conventional way by examining the three variables of force, length, and velocity of shortening. Direct measurements are possible on muscle preparations in vitro and some axial skeletal muscles in life, but because the respiratory muscles have complex origins and insertions, the direct forces produced by muscles in the respiratory system are not usually measured. However, the pressure that they produce *can* be measured: the force divided by the surface area over which the force acts. Changes in fiber length are inferred from changes in volume, and velocity from rate of change of volume or flow. So the basic methods for obtaining information on respiratory muscle function are indirect but include pressure measurements within the thoracic and abdominal cavities and measurements of thoracoabdominal motion or volume change. Sometimes useful information can also be obtained from the EMG of the respiratory muscles. This can be of a simple nature, observing the time of onset and duration of muscle activity, or with quantification of the signals by integration, some measure of the muscles' mechanical output can be obtained (48).

The Diaphragm

The diaphragm is a helmet-shaped sheet of muscle and tendon that separates the thoracic and abdominal cavities. It is the most important inspiratory muscle in the body and is responsible almost entirely for quiet breathing while the other muscles act solely to stabilize the rib cage. The muscle fibers of the diaphragm arise from the lower ribs, run upwards and parallel to the rib cage, and then turn inwards to insert into a central tendon, forming a dome over the abdominal contents. Other muscle fibers originate from the posterior abdominal wall and also insert into the central tendon. This anatomical distinction between two groups of muscle fibers within the diaphragm, the costal and crural portions, may turn out to have functional consequences, though for the present it is convenient to treat the diaphragm as a single functioning organ (21, 22). When the diaphragm contracts, the muscle fibers in apposition to the rib cage shorten, lift the rib cage, and flatten the dome. Inspiration occurs when intrapleural pressure becomes negative following enlargement of the thoracic cavity either by descent of the diaphragm or expansion of the rib cage. When the diaphragm contracts, its radius of curvature flattens as it distends the abdomen and enlarges the thoracic cage. At the same time it also exerts an equal and opposite force, lifting the rib cage (Fig. 3.2).

The shape of the ribs and their articulations are such that cephalad movements of the rib cage enlarge the thoracic cavity in the anteroposterior diameter by the so-called pump-handle action and the transverse diameter by its bucket-handle action. Similarly, caudal movement of the rib cage will make the thoracic cavity smaller and is therefore, expiratory. The efficiency of this dual action of the diaphragm on the abdomen and the rib cage depends heavily on the starting configuration of the dome and the relative compliances of the rib cage and abdomen. All muscles have an optimum starting length and the diaphragm is no exception. Up to a point, the more a muscle is stretched, the stronger it will contract. The pressure developed by the diaphragm when it contracts depends, by Laplace's Law, on the radius of curvature. The higher the dome of the diaphragm when it contracts and the smaller the radius of curvature, the greater will be the transdiaphragmatic pressure (Fig. 3.3). This may be an oversimplification though, because in most normal conditions the diaphragm does not flatten noticeably during its contraction but simply descends. When the diaphragm starts

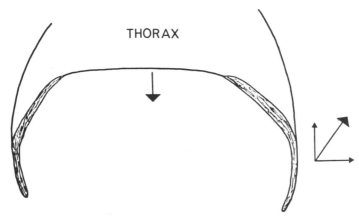

Figure 3.2. The muscle fibers of the diaphragm radiate from the central tendon and lie in apposition to the lower rib cage. When the muscle contracts, the dome of the diaphragm descends and enlarges the thoracic cavity. The abdominal contents offer resistance to diaphragmatic descent and act as a fulcrum. This allows the muscle in apposition to the rib cage to lift and expand the rib cage.

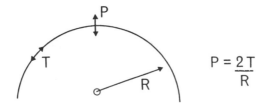

$$P = \frac{2T}{R}$$

Figure 3.3. Laplaces Law states that the pressure difference (P) the diaphragm can generate is proportional to the tension (T) and inversely proportional to the radius of curvature (R). Therefore, the higher the starting position of the diaphragm the more pressure it will be able to generate. This is an oversimplification though, since the diaphragm is not strictly hemispherical.

in this position, most of the muscle fibers are in apposition to the rib cage, and the cephalad, or rib cage lifting, vector will be at its greatest. In 1867 Duchenne realized that the function of the diaphragm could be severely disturbed if the abdominal contents were removed. It is now clearly understood that the effective action of the diaphragm as an inspiratory muscle depends upon the abdominal contents acting as fulcrum (24). Also the relative motion of the rib cage and abdomen will depend upon their compliances.

In summary, the diaphragm is a powerful muscle whose inspiratory action depends upon its configuration and the presence of abdominal resistance to produce expansion of the rib cage. If flattening of the diaphragm should occur, as may happen in pulmonary hyperinflation in emphysema or with loss of abdominal resistance, the diaphragm may lose its inspiratory ability. Indeed, under certain circumstances, it may impede inspiration and have an expiratory action.

The Intercostal/Accessory Muscles

The intercostal muscles have two major functions: (a) they act upon the rib cage to expand or contract it, and (b) they provide tone and stability to the intercostal spaces to allow the thorax to withstand changes in intrapleural pressure. There are two layers of intercostal muscle. The main bulk of the external layer lies posteriorly, and its fibers run diagonally forwards and caudally from one rib to the rib below. The internal intercostals are thicker anteriorly and their fibers slope posteriorly and caudally. The fibers of the thickened anterior portion of the internal layer of the upper ribs run parallel to the sternum and are known as the parasternal intercostals. There have been many theories on the function of intercostal muscles. Until recently, it was felt that the external intercostals and the parasternals were inspiratory in action, and the action of the remainder of the internal intercostals was expiratory. This was primarily based upon the EMG observations of Taylor and a theory of rib movement by Hamberger (41, 78). New light has been shone on the subject by Campbell (12) and more recently by De Troyer. His experiments have shown that both groups of intercostal muscles have inspiratory activity at low lung volumes and expiratory activity at high lung volumes (20). Also he demonstrated that the rib cage compliance varies with inflation, and it is easier to expand the rib cage at low lung volumes and contract it at high lung volumes. Effectively this means that both groups of intercostals are inspiratory in action when the lungs are empty and expiratory when they are full. The different directions of the fiber groups ensure that the different muscles develop optimum efficiency over slightly different phases. The EMG activity in the internal intercostals during expiration is explained as antagonistic activity that strengthens the rib cage rather than assisting expiration.

The accessory muscles comprise the scalenes and the sternocleidomastoids and sundry other groups of primarily postural muscles that can participate in respiratory activity. The scalenes and the sternocleidomastoids both have significant inspiratory activity, especially at high levels of ventilation or in respiratory failure. They are both inserted into the upper rib cage, which they lift and expand when they contract. It is certain that the sternocleidomastoid is a true accessory muscle that contributes to inspiration only during exercise or stress. The function of the scalenes is not so clear. It is possible, as De Troyer suggests, that far from being accessory muscles, the scalenes are necessary even in quiet breathing to stabilize the rib cage when other muscles act upon it.

The Abdominal Muscles

The abdominal respiratory muscles are the recti, the external and internal obliques, and the transversus abdominis. They are predominantly muscles of expiration, and when they contract, they pull the sternum caudally and collapse the rib cage while forcing the diaphragm and abdominal contents up into the thorax to empty it from below. Quiet expiration is largely passive, but at higher levels of ventilation, abdominal muscle assistance becomes necessary. These muscles also provide the explosive expiration necessary for coughing. The abdominal muscles may also facilitate inspiration by contracting to lengthen the diaphragm and decrease its radius of curvature. This may occur at high levels of ventilation in normal patients or in patients with emphysema and flattened diaphragms.

Respiratory Muscle Interaction

To understand the interaction between groups of respiratory muscles, it is helpful to consider the pressures within the thoracic and abdominal cavities. For air to enter the chest during spontaneous ventilation, the pleural pressure (Ppl) must be negative. A negative intrapleural pressure can be achieved by expansion of the rib cage, either accompanied by descent of the diaphragm or with the diaphragm being sucked passively into the thoracic cavity. If the diaphragm contracts, abdominal pressure increases, and the abdominal wall moves out; if the diaphragm is passive, the abdomen is sucked in. The pressure gradient across the diaphragm (Pab-Ppl) is known as the transdiaphragmatic pressure (Pdi). It is an index of mechanical effectiveness of the diaphragm. If negative intrapleural pressure were produced by the rib cage alone, the Pdi would be zero. If the diaphragm contracts and the rib cage is stiff enough to withstand negative pressure, the fall in Ppl is greater with rises in Pdi and Pab that make breathing more efficient (Fig. 3.4).

For the chest wall to inflate the lungs in the most efficient way it should inflate the rib cage along its relaxation curve in order to reverse the motion of passive deflation. In a classic paper, Goldman and Mead argued that the diaphragm alone, through the use of abdominal pressure, was sufficient to

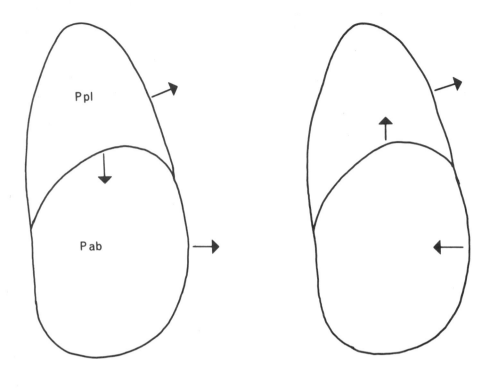

$$Pdi = Ppl - Pab$$

Figure 3.4. The pressure gradient across the diaphragm (Pdi) is a measure of the effectiveness of the diaphragm. It normally descends on inspiration and the Pdi is increased. (*A*) If the diaphragm is weak, the intercostal and accessory muscles can still expand the rib cage but the diaphragm will move passively upwards and the Pdi will be zero (*B*).

expand the rib cage along its relaxation curve in the upright position during quiet breathing (35). This hypothesis has been challenged by Macklem, De Troyer and others on the grounds that electrical activity in the intercostal and accessory muscles is always present and that this activity is necessary to prevent distortion of the rib cage and facilitate the action of the diaphragm. As we shall see when we come to the discussion of spinal injury, it is likely that even in quiet breathing, the integrated activity of many muscles is required for efficient motion of the chest wall.

The Control of Breathing

The control of the respiratory muscles is an exceptionally complex subject that has intrigued physiologists for over a century. In man, the regulation of ventilation must maintain automatic homeostasis over widely different conditions of rest and exercise in sickness and health. In addition, the patterns of breathing are heavily influenced by activities that are not primarily respiratory in nature, such as control of posture, speech, and emotional response. The literature on the subject is very large, but there have been several comprehensive reviews by Newsom-Davies, Berger, and Derenne (1, 7–9, 12, 17). We will discuss aspects of normal control that become relevant after spinal injury.

Central control. The source of organization for respiratory control lies in the medulla where there are several respiratory centers whose neurons are grouped into those with inspiratory activity, expiratory activity, and activity spanning both phases. Efferent pathways leave the centers and travel down the spinal cord to the anterior horn cells, which supply the appropriate respiratory muscles. There is evidence that automatic and voluntary pathways travel in different parts of the spinal cord (65). The cyclical nature of the discharge of the respiratory center forms the basis of respiratory rhythm. This is open to influence from the cortex during voluntary breathing and speech, and also from afferent fibers from the lung and chest wall. The other most important inputs to the respiratory center come from central and peripheral chemoreceptors that are sensitive to hypoxia and hypercapnia.

Spinal integration. The belief that output from the respiratory center was transmitted unchanged to the respiratory muscles was held until relatively recently. It is now clear that spinal mechanisms perform an important function, integrating segmental input from respiratory muscle proprioceptors with the descending drives concerned with respiration and posture. Reflex activity concerned in the control of breathing may stem from chest wall organs, within the lungs themselves, or even from outside the respiratory system.

Chest Wall Reflexes

The relative importance of reflexes originating from the chest wall is still under debate. Muscle spindles and tendon organs are unevenly distributed throughout the respiratory muscles, and it is likely that different muscles have different reflex contributions. The intercostal muscles are rich in muscle spindles while the diaphragm is not. This has been interpreted as indicating that the diaphragm performs the routine act of inspiration, but the intercostals can sense added loads and respond to increased respiratory demands. Stretch reflexes have been demonstrated for the intercostal muscles but not for the diaphragm. So it is likely that the intercostal spindles participate in: (a) the stabilization of the rib cage in case of increased airway resistance; (b) perception of respiratory movement; and (c) postural and antigravitational tone. Reflexes have also been described that originate from intercostal muscle spindles but influence other respiratory muscles indirectly through the respiratory center or alter the respiratory rhythm.

The diaphragm is poor in muscle spindles but rich in golgi tendon organs whose afferent pathways travel up the phrenic nerve. Green has suggested that these receptors are responsible for regulating diaphragmatic tension to adapt to different postures (36). Tonic activity is certainly present within the respiratory muscles, and change in muscle tone is capable of altering lung mechanics. It has been demonstrated in infants and probably in adults that functional residual capacity (FRC) is reduced during REM sleep or anesthesia when tone is suppressed. It is attractive to think that muscle tone is a major determinant of FRC, but this is unlikely to be true, except perhaps in infants with very weak rib cages.

Reflexes Originating from the Lungs

Afferent information from the lungs and airways is transmitted through the vagus nerve. Although the role of the vagus is not as clearly defined in humans as in other species, it appears that reflexes arising in the lungs can influence the timing of inspiration or expiration. Inflation of the lungs can cause apnea or a decrease in respiratory frequency that is abolished by vagotomy, but the classic Hering Breuer reflex is not as strong in man as in animals. Deflation of the lungs below FRC stimulates vagal inhibition of the expiratory muscles, but this of course is likely to be an important mechanism only in extreme circumstances or perhaps in patients with small lung volumes.

Neuromuscular Mechanisms Underlying Cough and Mucociliary Clearance

In health clearance of foreign or unwanted material from the respiratory tract is usually managed quite satisfactorily by pulmonary macrophages and mucociliary clearance. When these systems fail or are overloaded, cough is a fast and powerful clearance mechanism. The cough reflex is a complicated neural arc that is provoked by chemical or mechanical irritation of receptors in the larynx and the first two divisions of the bronchial tree where the major deposition of inhaled particles occurs. After provocation, pulses of positive pressure are applied to the external surfaces of the lungs and bronchial tree that generate high airway flows, clearing the unwanted material.

Cough begins after a rapid inspiration of a volume of gas to about 90% of the total lung capacity. The glottis is closed for about 0.2 seconds while the pressure within the pleural cavity is raised to 50 to 100 mm Hg by respiratory muscle action. The glottis is suddenly opened and expiratory flow at the mouth increases rapidly. Pleural pressure continues to rise after the glottis has opened as a result of continued muscular action. After about 1 liter or less has been expelled, the flow is stopped abruptly by glottic closure or respiratory muscle inhibition. The whole sequence is then repeated several times at lower lung volumes (44, 47).

The effectiveness of cough obviously depends upon the ability of the respiratory muscles to inspire to an adequate starting volume and then to generate the expiratory pressure pulse. The glottis assists in raising the pleural pressure but is not absolutely necessary to achieve expulsive flow. The glottis does, however, contribute to the effectiveness of cough in a different way. It is believed to vibrate the escaping column of gas and dislodge particles that can be carried out on the air flow.

The airways themselves are important in coughing. They are not simply rigid tubes that transmit the pressure pulse, and their caliber gets smaller during the maneuver. Some of this may be due to reflex bronchoconstriction and simple reduction of airway size with lung volume. The most important consideration is dynamic airway compression as discussed by Macklem. Briefly, the Macklem and Mead hypothesis of the equal pressure point states that closure of airways under dynamic conditions occurs when the endobronchial pressure (Palv + Pel) is exceeded by the transmural pressure. This point moves further out to the periphery of the lung as the lung empties. This theory is crucial to the understanding of the cough sequence. Coughs occur in cascades from high to low lung volume because the point of dynamic collapse and the limit of clearance will move further down the bronchial tree as the starting high volume gets smaller (53).

Respiratory Failure and Respiratory Muscle Fatigue

The respiratory system as a whole may fail because of defects in the gas-exchanging system or in the pump. Pump failure can arise in three ways:
1. Lack of central neurological drive such as drug intoxication;
2. Mechanical disorders of the chest wall, e.g. flail chest or scoliosis; or
3. Failure of the muscles to generate the required force, i.e. fatigue.

Obviously there is considerable interaction between the causes of respiratory failure. For example, hypoxia through lung disease will adversely affect central drive or the respiratory muscles. However, it will be valuable for us to examine the relationship between respiratory muscle fatigue and ventilatory failure.

Under normal circumstances, the respiratory muscles work at optimum efficiency to drive the respiratory system. In these conditions, energy demands will comfortably be exceeded by supply. If the system is inefficient, the energy demands of respiratory muscles will increase, and if they outstrip supply, fatigue will ensue until the body can reduce the load or make adaptive responses. The energy demands of the respiratory muscles increase considerably when the respiratory rate or tidal volume increases above the optimum efficiency (59). The work of breathing will also be increased if the lungs are stiff and hard to inflate, or the rib cage compliance is decreased. As we discussed earlier, changes in the configuration of the chest wall such as occurs in hyperinflation also limit the power of the respiratory muscles and reduce efficiency.

The energy requirements of respiratory muscles can be measured as the oxygen cost of breathing (VO_2 resp.) and depend upon blood flow, and oxygen and substrate content. Although there are only 4 to 5 kg of muscle tissue concerned with respiration, the oxygen requirements can be large and, in difficult circumstances, may exceed supply resulting in exhaustion (63). Blood flow to muscles under extreme conditions of stress may be as much as 8 to 10 L/min, and it is not surprising that low output cardiac failure is a portent of respiratory muscle fatigue (4). It is also possible that, like the heart, some respiratory muscles limit their own perfusion during contraction, especially if they are distorted and contracting isometrically. Along with decreased blood flow, reduced oxygen delivery will adversely affect performance, as will lack of substrate in extreme malnutrition or the presence of competing metabolic demands such as fever and sepsis.

Adaptive Responses to Fatigue

If fatigue occurs, the body must act to correct it before ventilatory failure ensues. The type of fatigue that generally occurs in the respiratory muscles is of peripheral type, i.e. failure of muscle contractility. Central fatigue or failure at the neuromuscular junction (as in myasthenia) is not a common problem. At the onset of peripheral fatigue, the muscle becomes refractory to low frequencies of neural stimulation, although it will still respond if the neural drive is increased. This is called low frequency fatigue, and the body can respond by increasing neural stimulation to maintain contraction for a short period only. This type of fatigue is not detectable on the EMG because the excitation of the muscle is normal, but the contractile response is reduced at low frequencies of stimulation.

As the oxygen cost of breathing increases in fatigue, the consumption of the muscles themselves will deprive other tissues of available oxygen. It is likely that the body makes an effort under extreme circumstances to preserve blood flow to the respiratory muscles, as it does to the heart and brain at the expense of other organs.

Lastly the mechanics of breathing can be altered to allow some muscles brief respite and the chance to recover. As we change hands with increasing frequency when we carry a heavy suitcase, there is evidence that the body rotates respiratory muscles under stress. An example of this includes the recruitment and derecruitment of the diaphragm, which manifests itself as inspiratory abdominal indrawing (respiratory paradox) that may become cyclical (respiratory alternans). Another example occurs when long distance runners change stride length to combat fatigue, causing the respiratory rate to alternate between fast and slow rhythms (dirhythmic breathing).

The Detection of Inspiratory Muscle Fatigue

Detection of fatigue depends upon the direct demonstration of diminished respiratory force or a derivative of it.

Clinical Examination. The fatigued patient will have rapid, shallow breathing, perhaps with signs of hypercapnia. Abnormal abdominal movements may be present, and the key to understanding these is palpation of the abdomen. Abdominal muscle contraction in inspiration may have a positive inspiratory action, but passive indrawing indicates diaphragm malfunction. The abdomen may be indrawn in inspiration due to active contraction or passive suction.

Simple Lung Function Measurements. The serial measurement of vital capacity is an excellent guide to inspiratory fatigue and failure. The measurement should be made frequently to predict failure. Static measurement of maximum inspiratory and expiratory mouth pressures (Pi max, Pe max) are an index of respiratory muscle strength. Reduction implies weakness. It is important to remember though, that fatigue can occur before weakness is evident.

Demonstration of Impaired Contractility. Some respiratory muscles are accessible to indirect measurement of the force of contraction following artificial stimulation. Such force/frequency curves have been constructed for the sternomastoid and the diaphragm with low frequency fatigue demonstrated in them (57).

Electromyography. Analysis of the power spectrum to determine the high/low ratio of the frequency components of the inspiratory muscle EMG has been used to detect fatigue (37). The low frequency components increase while high frequency components diminish. A change in the high/low ratios indicates developing fatigue before failure occurs. However, to be useful this change must be observed as it evolves and a single measurement is not useful. This is an abnormality of muscle excitation and is not the same as the demonstration of low frequency fatigue.

Therapeutic Considerations

If fatigue is recognized and the body is failing to correct it, therapeutic intervention is indicated. Primary correction of the underlying cause such as bronchoconstriction, hypercapnia, or heart failure is usually sufficient, but if that fails, ventilatory support and rest is indicated. There is some evidence that the performance of the respiratory muscles can be improved by drugs in the same way that inotropic drugs act on the heart to improve contractility (3). Such a drug is aminophylline, but the evidence for a useful effect in therapeutic doses is still lacking. Finally, if fatigue is not critical and episodic, it is possible that schemes to train the respiratory muscles may be of benefit, but as we see later, improvement after training may be due to many factors other than improved contractility.

THE RESPIRATORY SYSTEM IN SPINAL INJURY— PATHOPHYSIOLOGY

When the spinal cord is damaged, the respiratory muscles below the level of the injury become paralyzed and are devoid of supraspinal control. This interferes with the power and integration of the remaining muscles, reducing their ability to drive the chest wall efficiently. Generally the degree of respiratory disability depends upon the level of injury: the higher the level, the greater the effect. Functionally, the respiratory consequences of spinal injury can be predicted from the level of injury. Patients with cervical spine injury and quadriplegia have the most serious problems while those with lower thoracic and lumbar transections have very little impairment of lung function (Fig. 3.5) unless there are associated chest injuries.

Whether diaphragm function is preserved will depend upon the level of injury to the spinal cord. Transection of the cord at a high level, above C4, leaves the patient with only some of the accessory muscles, mainly the sternocleidomastoid and trapezius, available for use. Survival after such an injury has been documented, but these patients seldom survive long without mechanical ventilatory assistance. On their own, these remaining muscles can inflate the rib cage with a tidal volume of up to 800 ml but do so inefficiently (14). In addition, all afferent nerves from the rib cage and

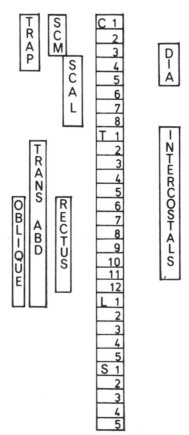

Figure 3.5. The segmental innervation of the major respiratory muscles.

diaphragm are destroyed, and vagally mediated reflexes can only respond to large changes in lung volume. As a consequence, the sensation of respiratory rhythm is disturbed, and these patients are subject to apnea (28). Since the accessory muscles are primarily postural muscles, there is evidence that they do not maintain cyclical activity during sleep. This may be the reason why many of these high cervical patients die during sleep in spite of adequate ventilation during the day. Cervical transection below C4 will preserve partial or complete diaphragm function as well as preserve the scalenes. These patients are at risk from respiratory complications arising from poor function during the early stages of their injuries, but once they recover, they can be independent of mechanical assistance. As we know that the diaphragm contributes 65% of the vital capacity in the normal person, it ought to be sufficient to cope with the meagre ventilatory requirements of the resting tetraplegic (15).

Patients with high thoracic lesions have some intercostal muscle preservation but paralysis of the abdominal muscles. Inspiratory capacity rapidly approaches normal as the level of the lesion descends below the first few segments. Paralysis of the abdominal muscles alone will have a small effect on inspiration but a larger effect on expulsive expiration. Damage to the cord and cauda equina following lumbar spine injury produces little effect on lung function.

LUNG VOLUMES AND SPIROMETRY

Since the importance of the respiratory system in determining survival has been recognized, there have been several surveys of lung function in these patients (10, 11, 27, 31, 32, 42, 51, 77). Not surprisingly, many of them have concentrated on lung function in the quadriplegic patient. For many reasons, the acutely injured patient is delicate and difficult to study. Nearly all the investigators have examined stable patients many months or years after their injuries. Only a few studies have been made in the acute phase of injury even though respiratory insufficiency is likely to be at its greatest then (46, 52). We will look at these results in terms of lung volumes, gas exchange, and lung mechanics.

For gas exchange to occur, ventilation of the alveolus must be efficient. During a breath, gas is drawn down the bronchial tree until it contacts the gas-exchanging surface. In a breath of 700 ml, about 130 ml will not reach the functioning alveolus but remain in the trachea and main bronchi. This is called dead space and is fixed. The tidal volume (Vt) can never fall below a critical level where encroachment of the dead space (Vd) reduces alveolar ventilation (Va). The alveolar ventilation equation is: $VT = Va + Vd$.

The vital capacity (VC) is the largest amount of gas that we can expire after taking a full breath in. It is normally about nine times the tidal volume. We use the vital capacity as a measure of ventilatory reserve, and as this reserve gets smaller, the tidal volume must remain fixed. As the ratio of VT to VC increases, it implies that the ventilatory reserve is being used up.

The natural volume at which we stop breathing out and begin to breathe in is determined by the balance between the force of the elastic recoil tending to collapse the lungs and the outward recoil of the chest wall. This is known as the functional residual capacity (FRC). A normal person can squeeze out a little more air (the expiratory reserve volume) with the expiratory muscles but can never empty the lungs completely as there is always some gas left (the residual volume, RV). The vital capacity is the difference between the full lung at total lung capacity and the emptiest possible lung at residual volume. It is a good test of muscular weakness because it tests both inspiratory and expiratory power (Fig. 3.6).

The results of the measurements of several investigators of lung volumes and spirometry following spinal injury are shown in Table 3.1. We have also summarized the data for patients with cervical and high thoracic lesions (Table 3.2).

For patients with cervical injury below C4, the vital capacity falls on average to 58% of normal with considerable individual variation (Fugl-Meyer reports 28% to 64%). The total lung capacity is reduced to 74% of normal, and the residual volume rises. There is some loss of inspiratory capacity, but the vital capacity is reduced largely at the expense of the expiratory reserve volume. This is not surprising since all expiratory muscles are paralyzed and the FRC should be the same as the residual volume. Most investigators did however demonstrate that there is some expiratory capacity beyond FRC, but as Bergovsky (10) discovered, this is due to the movement of the shoulder girdle and change in position rather than true expiratory muscle activity. It is abolished if the patient is supine. The reduction in these lung volumes can easily be explained by the loss of action of some inspiratory and expiratory muscles. It is of interest though that the

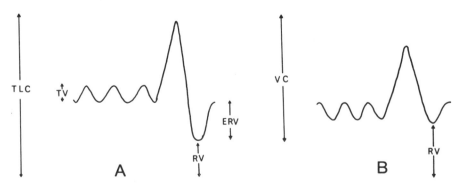

Figure 3.6. (*A and B*) Spirometric records during the tidal breathing and a vital capacity in a normal (*A*) and a tetraplegic (*B*) subject. The vital capacity is reduced in the tetraplegic because of the reduction in inspiratory capacity and also because all the major expiratory muscles are paralyzed and the residual volume is raised to the same level as the functional residual capacity.

Table 3.1.
Lung Volumes and Spirometry

	Level	n	Position	VC	FEV₁/VC	RV	TLC	FRC	ERV	PEFR	PIFR
Cameron 1955	C5–8	11	supine	65%	—	—	—	—	—	—	—
						RV/TLC n 25%					
Hemingway 1958	C4–8	29	sitting	65%	—	41%	—		50%	—	—
	T1–12	14	sitting	83%	—	36%			100%	—	—
	L1–5	21	sitting	100%	—	33%			100%	—	—
Bergovsky 1964	C5	10	sitting	65%	84%	—	—		132 ml sit.	40% sup.	—
Stone & Ketts 1963	C4–7	9	sitting	53%	—	123%	73.6%	98%	32.6%	—	—
	T3–10	6	sitting	75%	—	96%	81.5%	85%	80.33%	—	—
McKinley 1969	Cervical	8	supine	65%	84%	—	—	—	—	—	—
	Below T6	4	sitting	100%	—	—	—	—	—	—	—
Fugl-Meyer 1971	C4–7	26	sitting	42%	85%	168%	69%	90%	23%	65%	75%
	T1–6	4	sitting	62%	81%	136%	79%	87%	50%	—	—
	T6–12	6	sitting	78%	84%	79%	77%	72%	73%	—	—
	L1–5	4	sitting	95%	78%	117%	99%	97%	83%	—	—
Forner 1980	C5–8	42	sitting	51%	82%	132%	74%	78%	33%	47%	—
McMichan 1980	C4–8	22	supine	54%	82%	141%	78%	92%	38%	50%	62%

Table 3.2.
Summarized Lung Volumes and Spirometry on Chronic Patients (% Normal)

	VC	FEV$_1$/VC	RV	FRC	TLC	ERV	PEFR	PIFR
Cervical injury C4–8	57.5%	83.4%	141%	89.5%	73.7%	(sitting) 35.3%	54%	68.5%
Thoracic injury T1–6	73.3%	81.0%	116%	85%	80.25%	65%	—	—

FRC should fall in all the studies. If the FRC were simply determined by the balance of the mechanical forces of elastic and rib cage recoil, it should not change if the intercostals are paralyzed. This can be seen as evidence of resting muscle tone in the intercostals. The peak inspiratory and expiratory flow rates, which are effort dependent, are reduced; expiration is more affected than inspiration. There is no evidence of airway obstruction, and the FEV1/VC ratio is normal or high.

In high thoracic lesions the pattern of abnormality is similar, but the reduction in values is less. The vital capacity averages 73% of normal, though this is also variable especially at the highest level. As the level of injury descends, the values of all lung volumes approaches normal, and lumbar spine injuries cannot be expected to significantly reduce any values.

Effect of Body Position on Lung Volumes

In normal man, the vital capacity and other lung volumes are reduced by about 5% when supine. In 1955 Cameron tipped tetraplegic patients to discover if they could stand postural drainage physiotherapy. He was most surprised to discover that the vital capacity actually improved by 6% when the patient was tipped 15° head down and fell 7% when tipped head up. This work was repeated in detail by Fugl-Meyer, who found that the vital capacity fell by 45% when patients were tipped almost vertical. The residual volumes and the FRC also increased proportionately, but there was no change in the total lung capacity. This, of course, has important consequences for the patients when they first sit up. The mechanisms will be discussed later.

Vital Capacity Following Acute Injury

In quadriplegia, even when the diaphragm is intact, the vital capacity soon after injury may be much reduced, falling to as little as 300 ml. Acutely injured patients are delicate to study and may even find it difficult to perform the tests, but there have been two recent studies of spirometry in these patients that have demonstrated this early defect, following it to recovery. McMichan followed 22 patients (C4–8) and found that the vital capacity averaged 30% immediately after injury and rose to 54% at 4.5 months. Ledsome and Sharp followed flow/volume curves and showed similar results (Table 3.3). Soon after injury, the vital capacity is reduced to the point where it is almost equivalent to tidal volume; the patient must make a maximal effort with each breath. This improves quickly between the third and fifth weeks to achieve stable, safe values. Peak inspiratory mouth pressures and maximum flow rates also improve, but expiratory mouth pressures do not increase beyond those expected from the improvement in lung volume.

Table 3.3.
Improvement of Vital Capacity Following Injury

	Initial	3/52	5/52	9/52	3/12	4/12	5/12
McMichan 1980							
Mean VC LS	1.5%	—	—	2.3L%	—	2.7L%	—
Pimax cm H_2O	46%	—	—	73%	—	77%	—
Pemax cm H_2O	44%	—	—	55%	—	53%	—
Ledsome & Sharp 1981							
Mean VC L	1.5%	1.5%	2.2%	—	2.4%	—	2.8%
PEFR L/S	2.7%	3.2%	3.4%	—	3.6%	—	3.7%

ABNORMALITIES OF THORACOABDOMINAL MOTION

In spite of the belief that the diaphragm can drive the respiratory system along its relaxation curve, it has been known for a long time that the thoracoabdominal movements of the quadriplegic are abnormal. This implies that although the diaphragm has normal activity, it cannot inflate the lungs in the most efficient way. The work of breathing has been shown to be increased. These abnormal movements of the rib cage have been described by many authors in the chronic patient (55, 56, 71). In the sitting position, the anteroposterior (AP) and lateral diameters of the lower rib cage may expand normally while the upper AP rib cage diameters are reduced in amplitude or even move slightly inward on inspiration. In the supine posture, this paradoxical motion of the rib cage is increased. Meanwhile, abdominal excursion is exaggerated in the supine posture and reduced when upright.

Any mechanism that prevents the rib cage from expanding or moves it paradoxically will make inspiration inefficient. The rib cage may fail to expand for many reasons. It may have lost mobility through stiffness or ankylosis of the rib cage joints or because of spastic intercostal muscle tone. But if the rib cage moves paradoxically, it must do so through the action of the diaphragm. This can occur by two mechanisms. First, if the rib cage wall is weak and distensible, it will be unable to withstand the negative intrapleural pressure generated by the action of the diaphragm. Second, the part of the rib cage that is in apposition to the diaphragm is normally expanded directly, and it will only be subject to paradoxical motion if the configuration of the diaphragm flattens and constricts the lower ribs (Fig. 3.7).

A convenient way to display these abnormal movements is by the rib cage/abdomen motion plot devised by Konno and Mead (45). The abnormal movements can then be compared to the idealized relaxation characteristics. In Figure 3.8, we see these plots applied to magnetometer measurements made by Danon and Sharp in a C1 quadriplegic whose breathing was driven by a phrenic pacemaker or temporarily by his sternocleidomastoid and trapezii alone. The movements are compared to a relaxation curve obtained during mechanical ventilation. When the patient is sitting and using his neck muscles, the rib cage expands in the correct direction but the passive motion of the diaphragm is reflected by the inward abdominal motion. When the neck muscles are silent and the diaphragm is active, the abdominal motion is appropriate with some expansion of the rib cage, though it is not entirely normal since it has to spring back to the relaxation curve to deflate in expiration. When the patient is supine, the system behaves in the same way when driven by the neck muscles. But when the diaphragm is paced, there is obvious rib cage paradox.

A similar analysis has been applied to patients with lower cervical (C5–

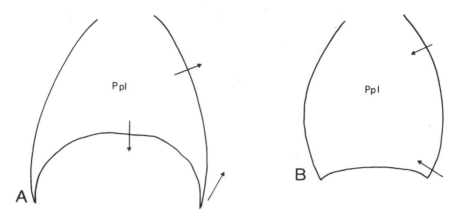

Figure 3.7. (*A and B*) Expansion of the thorax usually occurs through the combined action of the respiratory muscles. The intercostals and accessory muscles expand the upper rib cage and the diaphragm descends and also expands the lower rib cage (*A*). Abnormal, inward motion of the thorax in inspiration (*B*) can occur in the upper rib cage because it is too weak to withstand the negative pressure and in the lower rib cage when the diaphragm is flat and constricts it.

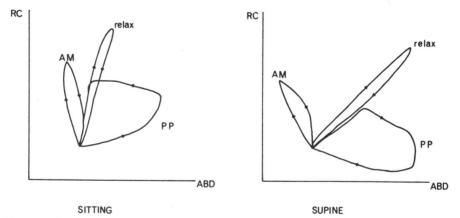

SITTING   SUPINE

Figure 3.8. A plot of rib cage motion against abdominal motion in a C1 tetraplegic while using accessory muscles alone or a phrenic pacemaker. When the accessory muscles are active (AM), they expand the rib cage by cephalad motion alone and the abdomen is sucked in passively. During phrenic pacing (PP) in the supine posture, the rib cage movements are paradoxical while the abdomen expands. Both movements will enlarge the thorax but neither is efficient enough to move the thorax along its relaxation curve (relax). Redrawn from Danon, J., Druz, W. S., Goldberg, N. B. and Sharp, J. T. Function of the isolated paced diaphragm and the cervical accessory muscles in C1 quadriplegics. *Am. Rev. Respir. Dis. 119:*909, 1979.

6) lesions by Mortola and Sant Ambrogio (55). They examined lateral and AP rib cage motion in supine and upright positions (Fig. 3.9). All movement takes place to the right of the relaxation curve, indicating that the system is driven by the diaphragm. Again in the sitting position, the AP rib cage motions are almost normal but the transverse expansion is reduced. In the

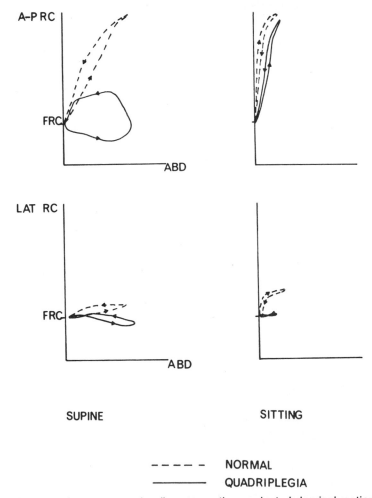

Figure 3.9. Plots of anteroposterior rib cage motion against abdominal motion (upper) and lateral rib cage against abdomen (lower). The upper rib cage moves paradoxically in the supine position but almost normally in the sitting position. The lateral rib cage dimensions begin by moving appropriately but change midway through the breath and begin to move inwards. Abdominal motion is much less marked in the sitting position. Redrawn from Mortola, J. P., and Sant'Ambrogio, G. Motion of the rib cage and the abdomen in tetraplegic subjects. *Clin. Sci. Mol. Med.*, 54:25–32, 1978.

supine position, the AP rib cage movements are always paradoxical in inspiration while the lateral diameter starts appropriately but changes direction midway through inspiration. It seems inconsistent that, as we have seen earlier, ventilation is more difficult in the sitting position when the thoracoabdominal motions are more appropriate. The reasons for this will be dealt with in a separate section.

Mortola and Sànt Ambrogio also made a second observation about the motion of the chest wall (Fig. 3.10). They noticed that not only did the rib cage distort during inspiration but it sprang back to its relaxation position at the beginning of expiration. This results in a delay of expiration while volume is redistributed between the abdomen and the rib cage. Only when the rib cage is settled in its relaxation position will air flow begin. In summary, the consequences of these observations are that, in the sitting position, the accessory muscles can expand the rib cage by their pump

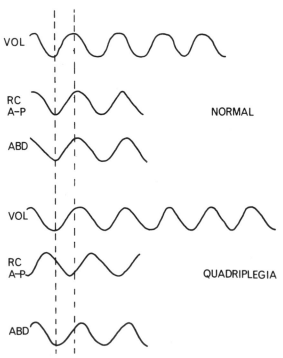

Figure 3.10. In the normal person the changes in thoracoabdominal dimensions are synchronous with air flow and volume change. In the tetraplegic subject, the rib cage is distorted during inspiration and has to spring back to its relaxation position before airflow occurs in expiration. This redistribution of volume is manifested in asynchrony of rib cage and abdominal motion. Redrawn from Mortola, J. P., and Sant'Ambrogio, G. Motion of the rib cage and the abdomen in tetraplegic subjects. *Clin. Sci. Mol. Med.*, 54:25–32, 1978.

handle action and the diaphragm can also expand it by the bucket handle action. However, in the supine position, unnecessary energy is expended in distorting the rib cage during inspiration. When the stored energy is released in early expiration, it can interfere with air flow.

Measurements of thoracoabdominal motion have proved invaluable in understanding how the chest wall functions in these patients, but many authors have found difficulty in making these measurements because of the delicate state of many tetraplegic patients, especially in the acute stage. In addition, most measurements of rib cage and abdominal dimensions are single point measurements and may not always reflect the overall pattern. We have recently developed a noninvasive optical method of analyzing chest wall motion that is particularly suitable for studying tetraplegic subjects at any stage without discomfort (54). So far we have confirmed the findings of previous authors. Figure 3.11 shows a recently injured tetraplegic (8) in whom the characteristic abdominal pattern of respiration is seen together with a clear demonstration of inspiratory rib cage paradox and distortion.

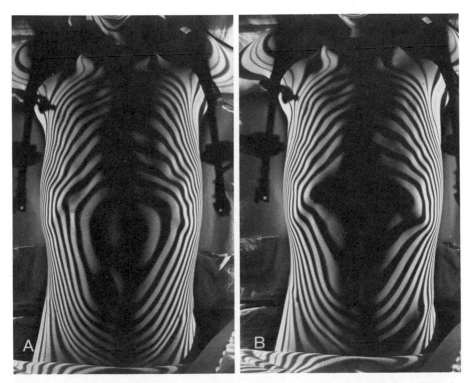

Figure 3.11. Optical contour maps of the supine torso of a tetraplegic subject in inspiration (A) and expiration (B). The contour lines are produced by the body distorting a projected pattern and defining its shape and motion. On inspiration the number of contour lines increases as the abdomen distends while the rib cage actually collapses under negative pressure.

THORACOABDOMINAL PRESSURES AND COMPLIANCE

The measurement of pressure within the thorax and abdomen of the quadriplegic has helped us understand more about the function of the respiratory muscles and the mechanical properties of the lungs and chest wall. Minimal pleural pressures are generally reduced to about 27% to 75%, as are mouth pressures. The maximum pleural pressures obtained during forced expiration are very much reduced, amounting to the elastic recoil of the lung only. Transdiaphragmatic pressure has been measured by De Troyer and found to be within the normal range in the sitting position (19).

The product of respiratory muscle action in the quadriplegic will depend on how easily the relative parts of the system can be inflated and on changes in the compliances of the three components of the respiratory system. The lung, the rib cage, and the abdomen have importance consequences. The pulmonary compliance has been measured in quadriplegics, and some authors have found it reduced. A fall in pulmonary compliance occurs in respiratory muscle weakness from other causes also and probably results from microatelectasis and fibrosis (18, 33). This is made worse in quadriplegia by the rib cage distortion that destabilizes some lung units. The variation in detection by different authors may reflect a number of differences in the choice of subjects, such as freedom from infection or effective physiotherapy.

The mobility of the rib cage is very important in determining how it will move, and there is evidence that the joints of the rib cage in many quadriplegics stiffen through disuse or possibly heterotopic ossification after injury (31, 82). The degree of muscle tone that returns to the intercostal muscles will also alter rib cage compliance, causing some variation between patients. Direct measures of rib cage compliance have recently been made in quadriplegics (26a).

The abdomen itself is not a passive structure, and abdominal muscle tone in the quadriplegic will determine its compliance, which may vary considerably. In most patients, the abdominal compliance is increased because the wall is floppy. In some patients, it is reduced through spastic tone. It must be remembered that the diaphragm must work against some abdominal resistance in order to work efficiently, though too much resistance may be detrimental, as in generalized spasm or gross obesity.

TONE, REFLEX ACTIVITY, AND SPASTICITY

There is evidence for a level of resting tone within the respiratory muscles (80). This tone provides stabilization of the rib cage during inspiration and can also be adjusted to compensate for postural changes. There is also evidence that tone in the diaphragm alters to optimize length-tension relationships in different postures (81). After transection of the spinal cord, removal of tone will increase rib cage and abdominal compliance in the same way anesthesia does, although the regulation of the diaphragm is maintained through the phrenic nerve (5). There seems to be some variability in the activity of denervated muscle as it recovers. After spinal shock has subsided, tone returns to the respiratory muscles as elsewhere, and they may become spastic. The degree of spasticity is unpredictable though it will, of course, make a difference to the compliances.

It is possible to feel the tone in the intercostal spaces or even observe its absence when the intercostal spaces are indrawn in inspiration (39). Electromyography clearly demonstrates the spectrum of activity that occurs in quadriplegic muscles. Often there is no activity at all, and sometimes there is constant tonic spasm. An interesting finding was made by Silver and Guttmann, who observed phasic discharges in the intercostal spaces in several quadriplegics and proposed that there was a stretch reflex present in denervated intercostal muscle that assists inspiration. Phasic activity in the upper intercostal muscles has also been demonstrated by De Troyer, who noted that it was associated with greatly improved respiratory performance (19). There is still debate as to whether this phasic activity is truly reflex or simply represents some residual or recovered voluntary activity. Whatever its cause, its presence confers considerable advantage.

Uncontrolled reflex spastic activity can occur in all limb muscles that have intact reflex arcs after injury, and it would be surprising if it did not occur within the respiratory muscles as well. It is likely that spastic tone may vary according to distant stimulation or bowel or bladder dysfunction. Patients who have incomplete lesions with preservation of sensation often describe spasm of the rib cage muscles that they perceive as a tightening around the chest. But this does not interfere with ventilatory function; on the contrary, stiffening may improve it. In those patients with partial damage to the diaphragm, it is possible that some spastic units are subject to reflex spasms spreading in the same way (72, 73). In summary, the degree of spastic tone that returns to the respiratory muscles will in general improve the stability of the rib cage and decrease the compliance of the abdomen. However, sudden variations in tone occurring in spasms may introduce incoordinate activity into the chest wall.

THE MECHANICS OF POSTURE CHANGE

We can now consider why there should be a reduction in ventilation when the tetraplegic patient sits up. In the normal person, several reflex events serve to preserve or improve ventilation when standing upright. In the supine position, the compliance of the abdomen is greater than the rib cage in spite of the weight of the abdominal contents that push the diaphragm up into the thorax and produce a more favorable configuration. Thus, when the diaphragm descends, it displaces the abdominal contents but does not expand the rib cage very much. When we stand up, the effect of gravity is replaced by increased abdominal muscle tone, and the contraction of the diaphragm produces greater rib cage expansion, assisted by the recruitment of intercostal and neck muscles. At the same time, the tendency for blood to leave the chest through pooling in leg veins is reversed by sympathetic correction.

In the supine quadriplegic, the diaphragm is aided by the weight of the abdominal contents that improve its configuration and performance. However, during the course of its descent, the relatively compliant abdomen allows the diaphragm to flatten, which compresses the lower rib cage and explains the late inspiratory paradox in this position. The upper rib cage paradox simply follows intrathoracic pressure. In the upright or sitting position, the abdominal contents are unsupported and postural tone correction in the abdominal muscles does not occur because the belly sags and the starting position of the diaphragm is flatter. However, the abdomen has reached its elastic limit and is less compliant. Therefore the rib cage lifting vector will be greater and the motion more appropriate. Also, the starting configuration is flatter and the product of diaphragm contraction will be less.

So, the ability of the diaphragm to generate inspiratory force is greater in the supine position primarily through its optimum configuration, but much of its energy in this position will be used to distort the rib cage. The overall performance can be much improved if the initial abdominal sag is prevented and its compliance decreased by use of a binder or corset. Patients with abdominal muscle spasm are likely to have an advantage in this respect.

ACUTE/CHRONIC MECHANICAL CHANGES

We are also now able to understand why the ventilatory capacity is so poor in the acute stages of injury in spite of a functioning diaphragm and why it should improve without the recovery of any further voluntary muscle function. After injury, muscle tone is flaccid and the rib cage joints are still mobile. These patients are, of course, always nursed supine, and the distortion of the rib cage will be greatest in this position. It is our experience that the distortion of the rib cage is greatest soon after injury and becomes less as the intercostal tone recovers and the joints stiffen (54a). The diaphragm then expends a proportion of its energy in distorting the rib cage and not producing air flow until the rib cage stabilizes. During this time the diaphragm is under stress, and its own performance may improve through a training mechanism. One other influence is that partial recovery may occur while the level of the lesion descends as edema of the cord recedes. This is particularly relevant to the diaphragm when the lesion may be asymmetrical and temporary hemidiaphragm paralysis may occur. Under normal circumstances, half a diaphragm works almost as well as the whole, but this requires the preservation of other muscles as well (25).

COUGH

The ability to cough is seriously impaired in the quadriplegic but less so in lower levels of injury. The generation of expiratory force in the quadriplegic is entirely derived from the elastic recoil of the lung produced by the previous inspiration (67). This reduces maximal expiratory flow rates to 65% of normal but the flow rates at lower lung volumes are better preserved (MEF 25% = 80% N). Maximal pleural pressures during cough are considerably reduced and in some cases may never become positive (19, 27, 32). The pleural pressure rise produces dynamic compression of the airways downstream of the equal pressure point and increases the linear velocity of gas flow and the removal of foreign material. Therefore in the quadriplegic, although bulk gas flow is near normal, the paralyzed expiratory muscles fail to produce dynamic compression and increase the linear velocity of the gas. Gas flow itself is also delayed by the outward inspiratory recoil of the rib cage in expiration with this biphasic action affecting flow profiles and interfering with expulsive effort (Fig. 3.12).

Lastly, because the cascades of cough cannot include the maximum lung volumes, the equal pressure point will never reach the largest airways, as in a curarized subject (2). Therefore the reduced coughing ability of the

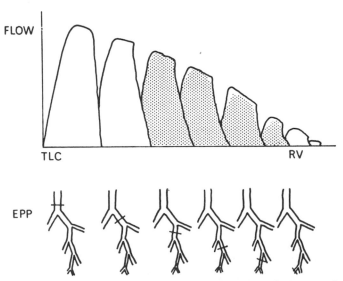

Figure 3.12. The flow volume curves during cough. Maximum flow rates diminish with starting lung volume. Tetraplegics (speckled area) are not able to achieve the highest or the lowest lung volumes. The equal pressure point (EPP) moves peripherally with fall in lung volume. The tetraplegic cannot therefore achieve high linear gas flows in proximal airways.

quadriplegic will probably only allow him to clear the smaller airways, with secretions lodging in the main airways and trachea.

GAS EXCHANGE

Of the many factors that influence gas exchange, alveolar ventilation, membrane diffusion, and blood flow/ventilation matching are important. Many studies of blood gases in the stable quadriplegic have shown them to be normal. Only one study has demonstrated hypoxia in chronic patients, and this was attributed to alveolar hypoventilation in view of the raised arterial $PaCO_2$ (10). Measurement of diffusing capacity by carbon monoxide transfer in the same study was normal.

By contrast, hypoxemia is a well recognized complication of acute injury in high spinal injury. Ledsome and Sharp found that the average PaO_2 in patients with C5–6 lesions was 73 mm Hg (N = 90 mm Hg), and 4 of 11 patients had levels below 60 mm Hg in the first week (46). In two patients with injury at a higher level (C4), artificial ventilation was required for hypoxemia in spite of an adequate vital capacity. Another study of blood gases in acute injury confirmed that hypoxia was present in 44% of the injured, falling below 60 mm Hg in 8% (75).

The mechanism for this hypoxia is not inadequate alveolar ventilation since the $PaCO_2$ is normal. There is, however, a large alveolar-arterial gradient implying that ventilation perfusion mismatch is responsible. The most likely causes for this are areas of microatelectasis resulting from incomplete expansion. A further mechanism may be similar to the V/Q mismatch seen after head injury, which is believed to be due to sensitivity to circulating catecholamines, producing patchy, noncardiogenic pulmonary edema (61, 64). This acute hypoxia is relatively short-lived and will improve rapidly as ventilation improves and the lung compensates.

SENSATION OF BREATHING

We have seen how the fine control of breathing depends upon sensory information from the lungs, the diaphragm, and the intercostal muscles. Although the intercostal muscles are rich in muscle spindles, they do not play a major role in the perception of breathing. Spinal cord transection or anesthesia below the level of T1 do not impair breath-holding or sensation of load (26). In addition, the neural response to added respiratory load is normal in the quadriplegic so that immediate adaptation can still take place (5, 28). With higher levels of injury, presumably when there is partial damage to the diaphragm or phrenic nerve, there is reduced ability to perceive elastic loads, though this is variable. Interestingly, McKinley found that those who could not perceive elastic loads were also those who did not sigh (51). Sighing is important to prevent microatelectasis, and indeed, those patients who did sigh were less susceptible to respiratory infection.

With high cervical injury the breath-holding time is prolonged and terminated only by hypoxia (58) whereas it is terminated by chest wall reflexes in the healthy person. Sensation of elastic loads is much reduced, but resistive loads may still be felt. Such perception is mediated through large airway receptors and the vagus. It is also possible for them to perceive large changes in lung inflation, especially at extremes of lung volume. The reduction of the drive to breathe may make patients susceptible to sudden death in spite of adequate accessory muscle ventilation (28).

SUSCEPTIBILITY TO FATIGUE

As far as we are aware, there have not been any studies yet that have demonstrated respiratory muscle fatigue as a contributing factor to ventilatory failure following spinal injury. It is, however, highly likely that this should occur.

Following the acute injury, we have seen how the work of breathing is increased and the ventilatory reserve is reduced at the same time the body has fewer muscles to recruit. The metabolic demands of the diaphragm are likely to be high while oxygen and nutrient delivery is reduced, and further hypoxic damage to the cord may reduce diaphragm function. Failure to clear secretions will result in respiratory infection, which will increase the respiratory load and at the same time increase the metabolic demands. Fatigue of this nature may precipitate catastrophic respiratory failure without warning. Since the body is unable to rotate respiratory muscles, some of the physical signs will be absent. Under these circumstances, early mechanical ventilation is indicated, which allows rest until stabilization and may reduce cord damage by withdrawing the competing demands of the respiratory muscles.

In the stable patient, the situation is much improved and there is some ventilatory reserve. The work of breathing is still increased, but the metabolic demands of the respiratory muscles are normal (70). However, during intermittent illness and infection, fatigue and failure may still be a risk.

PRACTICAL MANAGEMENT OF RESPIRATORY PROBLEMS RESULTING FROM ACUTE MUSCULAR PARALYSIS

Initial Assessment—Physical Examination

The respiratory system should be examined as soon as possible after injury and a full history of previous chest disease obtained. The physical examination should take account of any associated chest injury and document any abnormalities of thoracoabdominal motion such as asymmetrical abdominal expansion, which may signify partial phrenic damage. It may be difficult to examine the chest thoroughly on one visit because the patient's back may be inaccessible and the examination should be completed after the patient has been turned. The level of the neurological lesions should be noted, and any change should help anticipate respiratory problems.

Chest Radiograph

All patients should have a chest radiograph on admission. The physician should remember that the appearance of some features, such as pleural effusion, are altered in the supine position, and a lateral decubitus film is helpful.

Diaphragm Screening

The extent of remaining voluntary activity of the diaphragm can be determined and quantified by fluoroscopy. In the normal person, appropriate movement of the diaphragm in the upright posture does not by itself confirm normal function (1). In the tetraplegic, however, there is unlikely to be any confusion but the excursion of the diaphragm can be measured and any asymmetry noted. Further examinations should be performed if the phrenic segments are at risk. Video records are useful.

Lung Function

Serial measurements of the vital capacity are a good guide to respiratory muscle weakness, and this measurement should be made on admission and several times a day thereafter. A single reading is not by itself very useful except where it is very low, requiring ventilatory support (46). Also, the actual value may be less accurate because of difficulty in performing the test due to the patient's lack of coordination. However, bedside measurements should be made with a suitable instrument, such as the Wright's respirometer, repeated frequently to observe the trend. This measurement ought to be repeated in every position that the patient is likely to be in in case there are postural variations (68), which are especially likely if there is unilateral phrenic damage.

Arterial Blood Gases

These should be taken on admission and regularly through the early stages of treatment. Hypoxia may occur through hypoventilation, V/Q imbalance, or pulmonary edema. If ventilation is satisfactory, the $PaCO_2$ is normal or low and hypoxia is most likely to be due to ventilation/perfusion mismatch resulting from microatelectasis or pulmonary edema. In these cases, the pO_2 may be low without a great reduction in vital capacity (46). A raised $PaCO_2$ indicates that hypoxia is due to hypoventilation and appropriate measures will be necessary. It is most important to keep patients well oxygenated because hypoxia will predispose to respiratory muscle fatigue and may also extend the neurologic lesion. The PaO_2 ideally should be kept above 65 mm Hg (8.7 Kpa), and the inspired FiO_2 can be titrated against blood gases. Ear oximetry, if it is available, may be used to measure the oxygen saturation, and transcutaneous measurement of the trend of $PaCO_2$ can be useful. However, transcutaneous measurement should be used with caution because the heated electrodes can produce burns on anesthetic skin.

Positive Pressure Ventilation

Some patients with high cervical injury require artificial ventilation as a temporary measure at some stage. In one series all patients whose last normal segment was C4 needed ventilation. The indications for intervention are ventilatory failure, hypoxemia that cannot be corrected, and impending fatigue precipitated by the increasing metabolic demands of sepsis, etc. These patients are usually easy to ventilate and require only standard equipment and normal ventilator settings. Care must be taken when the patients are put on a ventilator because they lack normal sympathetic vascular tone and large alterations in blood pressure occur (29). One difficulty lies in securing the airway because manipulation of the neck during intubation may exacerbate the cord injury. In such cases intubation can be achieved with a fiberoptic bronchoscope or intubating laryngoscope.

Access to the airway allows direct suction and clearance of the major bronchi and helps prevent infection and atelectasis. Care must be taken with instrumentation in the airway since stimulation of unopposed vagal activity may precipitate extreme bradycardia and cardiac arrest. This can be prevented with atropine and correction of associated hypoxia. If an endotracheal tube or a tracheostomy is in place, the inspired gases should be humidified. This is often forgotten if the patient is breathing spontaneously, especially during transfers between hospitals. Failure to humidify may result in atelectasis.

Clearance of Secretions and Prevention of Respiratory Infection by Physiotherapy

Sputum retention occurs in patients with both high cervical and thoracic lesions because they are unable to cough effectively. They are also at risk from minor atelectasis because they cannot sigh and open up basal airways. Active physiotherapy plays an important role in the management of spinal patients. McMichan advised that acute tetraplegic patients should be repositioned every 2 hours, including turning them prone. Also helpful are four hourly deep breathing exercises, incentive spirometry, and chest physiotherapy with assisted coughing (52). Finally, if lobar collapse occurs, the lobe can be reexpanded with fiberoptic bronchoscopy, suction, and lavage. With this sort of policy, McMichan claims a reduction in the number of patients requiring ventilation and a significant fall in mortality.

LUNG PROBLEMS RELATED TO INJURY BUT NOT RESULTING FROM MUSCULAR PARALYSIS

Neurogenic Pulmonary Edema Following the Acute Injury

Some degree of pulmonary edema may be found in up to 50% of spinal cord injuries (61) immediately after injury. Mechanical trauma to the spinal cord rapidly initiates a short-lived but explosive autonomic discharge accompanied by bradycardia, hypertension, and the development of many bizarre arrhythmias (79). This results in a marked increase in peripheral vascular resistance, causing a shift of blood into the relatively more compliant pulmonary circulation. As a result of the extreme increases in pulmonary vascular pressure, the pulmonary capillary integrity may be lost with resultant protein leakage into the lungs. Because the restoration of capillary integrity is not immediate, the pulmonary edema persists after the pressure has returned to normal. The systemic and pulmonary hypertension may be of short duration, explaining the normal pressures recorded many hours after the development of pulmonary edema. Attempts to raise the blood pressure by crystalloid infusion may only produce hemodilution and a further fall in plasma oncotic pressure (76). Monitoring the central venous pressure (CVP) is of little use because spinal cord injured patients often show a disproportionate rise in the pulmonary wedge pressure before such a rise occurs in the CVP. In the presence of leaking capillaries, high left atrial pressures will produce edema at an early stage (50). The heart itself may also be damaged by associated blunt trauma or catecholamine-induced degeneration and may contribute to the problem. As a rule, this type of pulmonary edema is short-lived and reversible, and supplementary oxygen or IPPV should tide the patient over if necessary. Large doses of diuretic are unlikely to help and will only impair the circulating volume. Occasionally, the pulmonary edema will be intractable, with ensuing adult respiratory distress syndrome.

Associated Trauma

Many patients with traumatic cord injuries will have associated chest problems. Silver found that 48% had other injuries or aspiration pneumonia (69). The common injuries included rib fractures and flail segments, pneumothorax, hemothorax, and pulmonary contusion. Rib cage injuries are particularly likely in association with thoracic spine injuries, and immediate intercostal drainage will be necessary for pneumothorax or hemothorax and IPPV for flail segments. Hall et al recorded rupture of the diaphragm in 11% of patients presenting with thoracic spine and rib cage trauma (40).

Distant injuries may also have an effect. Associated head injury is common, and loss of consciousness may lead to aspiration and loss of respiratory drive while neurogenic pulmonary edema is more common. Fracture of the large bones may initiate fat emboli as well as make the patient difficult to care for. The fat causes microvascular blockage of the pulmonary capillaries and respiratory failure with hypoxemia. A clue to this cause may come from systemic overspill of fat to produce petechiae and cerebral dysfunction. Intraabdominal problems such as paralytic ileus or gastrointestinal hemorrhage are also common and may interfere with breathing.

Deep Vein Thrombosis and Pulmonary Embolism

Patients with acute spinal cord injuries are prone to develop deep vein thrombosis and pulmonary embolus. The reported incidence of venous thrombosis varies according to the diagnostic technique used. Clinical examination can detect 14%, impedance plethysmography 60%, and I131 labelled fibrinogen uptake has reported a 100% incidence. The diagnosis of pulmonary embolism is 14% with clinical examination and plain radiograph, 35% with isotope scans, and 36% at autopsy (62). The meticulous and regular measurement of calf and thigh circumferences is a simple method for detecting a deep vein thrombosis and can be followed up by a venogram. The diagnosis of pulmonary embolus is more difficult in spinal injury patients. The usual symptoms may be absent, and it may also occur in the absence of clinical evidence of a DVT in up to 50% of patients. It is usually associated with a paucity of physical symptoms, usually dyspnea accompanied by hypocapnic hypoxemia and some abnormalities of the chest radiograph, ECG, or isotope scan. The tendency to intravascular coagulation is increased by trauma, immobility, and distant sepsis. The presence of endotoxins in the blood are known to be associated with intravascular coagulation, and the high incidence of urinary infection in spinal patients may be a factor.

It has been shown that prophylactic anticoagulation therapy begun within a few days of admission prevents pulmonary emboli and does not hinder the patient's management (74). Other measures include passive mobilization, massage of the lower limbs, and elastic stockings. Since dislodgement of thrombi with consequent pulmonary embolism has been described during passive exercise, it is reasonable to withhold exercises during the first 72 hours and limit their use until anticoagulation has been stabilized. The required period of anticoagulation varies between individuals, and most patients are susceptible for about 12 weeks with some at risk for much longer. Factors to be taken into account when discontinuing treatment include the time from injury, the degree of spasticity in the lower limbs, ambulation, the presence of infection, previous episodes of thromboembolism, and any evidence of recent intravascular coagulation.

Associated Lung Disease

The patient with spinal injury may, of course, have a preexisting lung disease such as asthma or COPD which influences their management. These chest diseases are usually managed in the standard way, but particular care must be taken with certain drugs. For example, severe hypotension has been reported following subcutaneous administration of terbutaline in patients with evidence of autonomic dysfunction (60).

Long Term Ventilation and Phrenic Pacing

Some patients with high spinal injury may prove impossible to wean from mechanical ventilation, and some will require continued ventilation at night. In some of these patients, diaphragmatic pacing may be considered. A paralyzed diaphragm may be electrically stimulated if the lower motor neurons in the phrenic nerves are intact and the cell bodies in the C3–4–5 segments of the spinal cord are viable. Diaphragm pacing is possible if partial or complete respiratory paralysis requiring artificial ventilation has been present and stable for at least one month, the phrenic nerves are viable, the diaphragm responds well to electrical stimulation, and cerebral function is normal. Continuous pacing of one or both hemidiaphragms results in diaphragm fatigue, which if prolonged may irreversibly damage the muscle. In adults then, full-time ventilatory support can be achieved by pacing the two hemidiaphragms alternately for 12 hour periods of rest and stimulation. In those in the under-10 age group or in patients with subnormal diaphragm function, unilateral pacing may not be sufficient and bilateral simultaneous stimulation will be necessary, alternating with periods of mechanical ventilation. The stimulating electrodes used to be placed in the neck, but a thoracic approach to the phrenic nerve is now favored. In a series of 20 patients Glenn has provided full- or part-time support of respiration for up to 10 years. In some patients it was possible to achieve ultimate independence even though diaphragm function was subnormal at the outset through periodic conditioning of the muscle (34).

If diaphragmatic pacing is not possible in these patients then long term ventilation is best achieved by IPPV. Negative pressure ventilation, for example with a cuirass is not usually suitable because chest wall anesthesia predisposes the skin to pressure sores. For this reason, the cuirass has been unpopular in the United Kingdom, but there is no other reason why it cannot be used successfully in expert hands. Each ventilator-dependent patient requires three ventilator systems: a bedside unit, a portable battery operated ventilator, which may be attached to his wheelchair, and an Ambu bag for emergencies (23).

Respiratory Muscle Training

Training may improve the strength or endurance of the respiratory muscles in normal subjects and also in patients with tetraplegia. An improvement in performance should be of benefit in the prevention of respiratory failure resulting from excessive demands upon the respiratory system or the compromising of the respiratory system itself. Studies of training in tetraplegia have used techniques aimed at either increasing lung volume or increasing the strength and endurance of muscle fibers in the diaphragm. Improvement in lung volume will increase the ventilatory capacity, and make cough and sputum clearance more efficient, while endurance training may provide a potential increase in ventilatory reserve under conditions of stress. Methods of muscle training that have been used include incentive spirometry (13), loaded breathing against inspiratory and expiratory resistances, isocapnic hyperventilation, and lung volume expansion by insufflation or glossopharyngeal breathing. Fugl-Meyer (30) and later Hultgren (43) demonstrated a lasting improvement in lung volumes and mouth pressures (a measure of respiratory muscle strength) after a combination training program of loaded breathing and mechanical insufflation for 15 minutes per day over 30 days. Gross and associates used loaded inspiration for 16 weeks and showed a significant and progressive increase in strength and endurance of the diaphragm as judged by increasing mouth pressures and avoidance of EMG changes of a diaphragm fatigue following hyperventilation (38). On the present evidence, it seems that training schemes produce improvement in either strength and volume or endurance, and that strength and volume training is the easiest to perform with the most useful and long lasting benefit.

CONCLUSION

We have seen how patients with spinal injury may have considerable respiratory problems that will influence their survival and quality of life. In recent years a positive approach to the management of these problems has greatly decreased the mortality in tetraplegia (68). We anticipate that continued efforts to understand the nature of respiratory paralysis and new methods of improving residual function will improve their outlook and their comfort.

REFERENCES

1. Alexander, C. Diaphragm movements in the diagnosis of diaphragm paralysis. *Clin. Radiol.*, *17:*79, 1966.
2. Arora, N. S., and Gal, T. J. Cough dynamics during progressive expiratory muscle weakness in healthy curarised subjects. *J. Appl. Physiol.*, *51:*494–498, 1981.
3. Aubier, M., De Troyer, A., Sampson, M., Macklem, P. T., and Roussos, C. Aminophylline improves diaphragmatic contractility. *N. Engl. J. Med.*, *305:*249–252, 1981.
4. Aubier, M., Trippenbach, T., and Roussos, C. Respiratory muscle fatigue during cardiogenic shock. *J. Appl. Physiol.*, *51:*499–508, 1981.
5. Axen, K. Ventilatory responses to mechanical loads in cervical cord-injured humans. *J. Appl. Physiol.*, *52:*748–756, 1982.
6. Banzett, R. B., Inbar, G. F., Brown, R., Goldman, M., Rossier, A., and Mead, J. Diaphragm electrical activity during negative lower torso pressure in quadriplegic men. *J. Appl. Physiol.*, *51:*654–659, 1981.
7. Berger, A. J., Mitchell, R. A., and Severinghaus, J. W. Regulation of respiration (part I). *N. Engl. J. Med.*, *297:*92–96, 1977.
8. Berger, A. J., Mitchell, R. A., and Severinghaus, J. W. Regulation of respiration (part II). *N. Engl. J. Med.*, *297:*138–143, 1977.
9. Berger, A. J., Mitchell, R. A., and Severinghaus, J. W. Regulation of respiration (part III). *N. Engl. J. Med.*, *297:*194–201, 1977.
10. Bergofsky, E. M. Mechanism for respiratory insufficiency after cervical cord injury. *Ann. Intern. Med.*, *61(3):*435–447, 1964.
11. Cameron, G. S., Scott, J. W., Jousse, A. T., and Botterell, E. M. Diaphragmatic respiration

in a quadriplegic patient and effect of position on his vital capacity. *Ann. Surg., 141:*451–456, 1955.

12. Campbell, E. J. M., Agostini, E., and Newsom-Davies, J. *The Respiratory Muscles. Mechanics and Neural Control,* Second ed., Lloyd Luke, London, 1970.
13. Cheshire, J. E., and Flack, W. J. The use of operant conditioning techniques in the respiratory rehabilitation of the tetraplegic. *Paraplegia, 16:*162–174, 1979.
14. Danon, J., Druz, W. S., Goldberg, N. B., and Sharp, J. T. Function of the isolated paced diaphragm and the cervical accessory muscles in C1 quadriplegics. *Am. Rev. Respir. Dis., 119:*909, 1979.
15. Derenne, J.-P. M., Macklem, P. T., and Roussos, C. H. The respiratory muscles: Mechanics, control and pathophysiology. Part I. *Am. Rev Respir. Dis., 118:*119–133, 1978.
16. Derenne, J.-P. M., Macklem, P. T., and Roussos, C. H. The respiratory muscles: Mechanics, control and pathophysiology. Part II. *Am. Rev. Respir. Dis., 118:*373–390, 1978.
17. Derenne, J.-P. M., Macklem, P. T., and Roussos, C. M. The respiratory muscles: Mechanics control and pathophysiology. Part III. *Am. Rev. Respir. Dis., 118:*581–601, 1978.
18. De Troyer, A., Borenstein, S., and Cordier, R. Analysis of lung volume restriction in patients with respiratory muscle weakness. *Thorax, 35:*603–610, 1980.
19. De Troyer, A., and Heilporn, A. Respiratory mechanics in quadriplegia. The respiratory function of the intercostal muscles. *Am. Rev. Respir. Dis., 121:* 591, 1980.
20. De Troyer, A., Kelly, S., and Zin, W. A. Mechanical action of the intercostal muscles on the ribs. *Science, 220:*87–88, 1983.
21. De Troyer, A., Sampson, M., Sigrist, S., and Macklem, P. T. Action of costal and crural parts of the diaphragm on the rib cage in dogs. *J. Appl. Physiol., 53:*30–39, 1982.
22. De Troyer, A., Sampson, M., Sigrist, S., and Macklem, P. T. The diaphragm: two muscles. *Science, 213:*237–238, 1981.
23. Dingmans, L. M., and Hawn, J. M. Mobility and equipment for the ventilator dependent tetraplegic. *Paraplegia, 16:*175–183, 1978.
24. Duchenne, G. B. A. Physiologie dés movements démontrée a l'aide de l'éxperimentation électrique et de l'obsérvation clinique, et applicable a l'étude des paralysies et dés déformations. Translation in Kaplan, E. B., *Physiology of Motion,* J. B. Lippincott, Co., Philadelphia, 1949, pp 443–503.
25. Easton, P. A., Fleetham, J. A., De La Rocha, A., and Anthonisen, N. R. Respiratory function after paralysis of the right hemidiaphragm. *Am. Rev. Respir. Dis., 127:*125–128, 1983.
26. Eisele, J., Trenchard, D., Burki, N., and Guz, A. The effect of chest wall block on respiratory sensation and control in man. *Clin. Sci., 35:*23–33, 1968.
26a. Estenne, M., Heilporn, A., Delhez, L., Yernault, S. C., and De Troyer, A. Chest wall stiffness in patients with chronic respiratory muscle weaknesss. *Am. Rev. Respir. Dis., 128:*1002–1007, 1983.
27. Forner, J. V. Lung volumes and mechanics of breathing in tetraplegics. *Paraplegia, 18:*258–266, 1980.
28. Frankel, H. L., Guz, A., and Noble, M. Respiratory sensation in patients with cervical cord transection. *Paraplegia, 9*(3):132–136, 1971.
29. Frankel, H. L., Matthias, C. J., and Spalding, J. M. K. Mechanisms of reflex cardiac arrest in tetraplegic patients. *Lancet, 2:*1183–1185, 1975.
30. Fugl-Meyer, A. R. A model for the treatment of impaired ventilatory function in tetraplegic patients. *Scand. J. Rehabil. Med., 3:*168–177, 1982.
31. Fugl-Meyer, A. R. Effects of respiratory muscle paralysis in tetraplegic and paraplegic patients. *Scand. J. Resp. Dis., 3:*141, 1971.
32. Fugl-Meyer, A. R., and Grimby, G. Ventilatory function in tetraplegic patients. *Scand. J. Rehabil. Med., 3:*151–160, 1971.
33. Gibson, G. J., Pride, N. B., Newsom-Davies, J., and Loh, L. C. Pulmonary mechanics in patients with respiratory muscle weakness. *Am. Rev. Respir. Dis., 115:*389–395, 1977.
34. Glenn, W. W. L., Hogan, J. F., and Phelps, M. L. Ventilatory support of the quadriplegic

patient with respiratory paralysis by diaphragm pacing. *Surg. Clin. North Am., 60:*1055, 1980.

35. Goldman, M. D., and Mead, J. Mechanical interaction between the diaphragm and rib cage. *J. Appl. Physiol., 35:*197–204, 1973.
36. Green, M., Mead, J., and Sears, T. A. Effects of loading on respiratory muscle control in man. In: *Loaded breathing.* Edited by Pengelly, L. D., Rebuck, A. S., and Campbell, E. J. M., Longman, Inc., 1974, pp. 73.
37. Gross, D., Grassino, A., Ross, W. R. D., and Macklem, P. T. Electromyogram pattern of diaphragmatic fatigue. *J. Appl. Physiol., 46:*1–7, 1979.
38. Gross, D., Ladd, M. W., Riley, E. J., Macklem, P. T., and Grassino, A. The effect of training on strength and endurance of the diaphragm in quadriplegia. *Am. J. Med., 68:*27–35, 1980.
39. Guttmann, L., and Silver, J. R. Electromyographic studies on reflex activity of the intercostal and abdominal muscles in cervical cord lesions. *Paraplegia, 3:*1–22, 1965.
40. Hall, J. C., Douglas, M. C., and Burke, D. C. Rupture of the diaphragm associated with spinal cord injury. *Aust. N.Z. J. Surg., 51:*594–597, 1981.
41. Hamberger, G. E. De respirationis mechanismo. Jena. 1727.
42. Hemingway, A., Bors, E., and Hubby, R. P. An investigation of the pulmonary function of paraplegics. *J. Clin. Invest., 37:*773–782, 1958.
43. Huldtgren, A. C., Fugl-Meyer, A. R., Jonasson, F., and Bake, B. Ventilatory dysfunction and respiratory rehabilitation in post traumatic quadriplegia. *Eur. J. Respir. Dis., 61:*347–356, 1980.
44. Irwin, R. S., Rosen, M. J., and Braman, S. Cough, a comprehensive review. *Arch. Intern. Med. 137:*1186–1191, 1977.
45. Konno, K., and Mead, J. Measurement of the separate volume changes of rib cage and abdomen during breathing. *J. Appl. Physiol., 22:*407–422, 1967.
46. Ledsome, J. R., and Sharp, J. M. Pulmonary function in acute cervical cord injury. *Am. Rev. Respir. Dis., 124:*41, 1981.
47. Lieth, D. E. Cough. In: *Respiratory defence mechanisms:* Part II. Edited by Brain, J. D., Proctor, D. F., and Reid, L. M. Dekker, New York/Basel, pp 545–592, 1977.
48. Lourenco, R. Y., and Mueller, E. P. Quantification of electrical activity in the human diaphragm. *J. Appl. Physiol., 22:*598–600, 1967.
49. Luce, J. M. Respiratory muscle function in health and disease. *Chest 81:*82–90, 1982.
50. Mayer, G. A., Berman, I. R., Dotty, D. B., Moseley, R. V., and Gutierrez, B. S. Haemodynamic responses to acute quadriplegia with or without chest trauma. *J. Neurosurg., 34:*168–177, 1971.
51. McKinley, A. C., Auchincloss, J. M., Gilbert, R., and Nicholas, J. J. Pulmonary function, ventilatory control and respiratory complications in quadraplegic subjects. *Am. Rev. Respir. Dis., 100:*526–532, 1969.
52. McMichan, J. C., Michel, L., and Westbrook, P. Pulmonary disfunction following traumatic quadriplegia. *J.A.M.A., 243:*528–531, 1980.
53. Mead, J., Turner, J. M., Macklem, P. T., and Little, J. B. Significance of the relationship between lung recoil and maximum expiratory flow. *J. Appl. Physiol., 22:*95–108, 1967.
54. Morgan, M. D. L., Gourlay, A. R., and Denison, D. M. An optical method of studying the shape and movement of the chest wall in recumbent patients. *Thorax* (in press).
54a. Morgan, M. D. L., Gourlay, A. R., Silver, J. R., Williams, S. J., and Denison, D. M. The contribution of the rib cage to breathing in tetraplegia. *Thorax, 40:*613–617, 1985.
55. Mortola, J. P., and Sant'Ambrogio, G. Motion of the rib cage and the abdomen in tetraplegic subjects. *Clin. Sci. Mol. Med., 54:*25–32, 1978.
56. Moulton, A., and Silver, J. R. Chest movements in patients with traumatic injuries of the cervical cord. *Clin. Sci., 39:*407–422, 1970.
57. Moxham, J., Morris, A. J. R., Spiro, S. G., Edwards, R. H. T., and Green, M. Contractile properties and fatigue of the diaphragm in man. *Thorax, 36:*164–168, 1981.
58. Newsom-Davies, J. High cervical cord transection. *Am. Rev. Respir. Dis., 119(2)* pt 2: 69,

1979.
59. Otis, A. B., Fenn, W. O., and Rahn, M. Mechanics of breathing in man. *J. Appl. Physiol.* 2:592–607, 1950.
60. Pingleton, S. K., Schwartz, O., Szymanski, D., and Ebstein, M. Hypotension associated with terbutaline therapy in acute quadriplegia. *Am. Rev. Respir. Dis., 126:*723–725, 1982.
61. Poe, R. H., Reisman, J. L., and Rodenhouse, T. G. Pulmonary oedema in cervical spinal cord injury. *J. Trauma, 18:*71–73, 1978.
62. Purkash, A., Prakash, V., and Purkash, I. Experience in managing thrombo embolism in patients with spinal cord injury—Part I; Incidence, diagnosis and role of some risk factors. *Paraplegia, 16:*322, 1978.
63. Roussos, C., and Macklem, P. T. The respiratory muscles. *N. Engl. J. Med., 307:*786–797, 1982.
64. Schumacker, P. T., Rhodes, G. R., Mewell, J. C., et al. Ventilation-perfusion imbalance after head trauma. *Am. Rev. Respir. Dis., 119:*33–43, 1979.
65. Sears, T. A. The respiratory motor neurones. Integration at spinal segmental level. In *Breathlessness.* Edited by Howell, J. B., and Campbell, E. J. M., Blackwell, Oxford. pp 33, 1966.
66. Sharp, J. T. Respiratory muscles. A review of old and newer concepts. *Lung, 157:*185–199, 1980.
67. Siebens, A. A., Kirby, N. A., and Poulos, D. A. Cough following transection of the spinal cord at C6. *Arch. Phys. Med., 45:*1, 1964.
68. Silver, J. R. The immediate management of spinal injury. *Br. J. Hosp. Med., 29:*412–425, 1983.
69. Silver, J. R. Chest injuries and complications in the early stages of spinal cord injury. *Paraplegia, 5:*226–228, 1968.
70. Silver, J. R. Oxygen cost of breathing in tetraplegic patients. *Paraplegia, 1:*204, 1963.
71. Silver, J. R., and Abdel-Halim, R. E. Chest movements and electromyography of the intercostal muscles in tetraplegic patients. *Paraplegia, 9:*72, 1971.
72. Silver, J. R., and Lehr, R. P. Dyspnoea during generalised spasms in tetraplegic patients. *J. Neurol. Neurosurg. Psychiatry, 44:*842–845, 1981.
73. Silver, J. R., and Lehr, R. P. Electromyographic investigation of the diaphragm and intercostal muscles in tetraplegics. *J. Neurosurg., 44:*837–841, 1981.
74. Silver, J. R., and Moulton, A. Prophylactic anticoagulant therapy aganst pneumonary emboli in acute paraplegia. *Br. Med. J., 2:*338–340, 1970.
75. Simha, R. P., Ducker, T. B., and Perot, P. L. Arterial oxygenation. Findings and its significance in central nervous system trauma patients. *J. A. M. A., 224:*1258–1260, 1973.
76. Staub, N. C. State of the art-Pathogenesis of pulmonary oedema. *Am. Rev. Respir. Dis., 109:*358–372, 1974.
77. Stone, D. J., and Keltz, H. The effect of respiratory muscle dysfunction on pulmonary function. Studies in patients with spinal cord injuries. *Am. Rev. Respir. Dis., 88:*621–629, 1963.
78. Taylor, A. The contribution of the intercostal muscles to the effort of respiration in man. *J. Physiol., 151:*390–402, 1960.
79. Theodore, J., and Robin, E. D. Speculations on neurogenic pulmonary oedema. *Am. Rev. Respir. Dis., 113:*405–511, 1976.
80. Tusiewicz, K., Bryan, A. C., and Froese, A. B. Contributions of changing rib cage diaphragm interactions to the ventilatory depression of halothane anaesthesia. *Anesthesiology, 47:*327–337, 1977.
81. Vellody, V. P. S., Nassery, M., Balasaraswathi, K., Goldberg, N. B., and Sharp, J. T. Compliances of human rib cage and diaphragm—abdomen pathways in relaxed versus paralysed states. *Am. Rev. Respir. Dis., 118:*479–491, 1978.
82. Wharton, G. W., and Morgan, T. M. Ankylosis in the paralysed patients. *J. Bone Joint Surg.* pp. 105–112, 1952.

4

The Management of the Neurogenic Bladder

S. HERSCHORN AND R. G. GERRIDZEN

Man's ability to exercise complete volitional control over voiding is taken for granted until an insult to the nervous system, such as a spinal cord injury, alters detrusor control.

ANATOMY AND PHYSIOLOGY

The bladder normally acts as both a storage vessel, by accommodating increasing volumes of urine, and as an organ of expulsion, which, by coordinated muscle contraction and sphincter relaxation, will completely and efficiently empty its contents at a socially acceptable time.

The bladder muscle or *detrusor*, a meshwork of interlacing smooth muscle bundles, is innervated by the parasympathetic nervous system, originating at sacral cord segments S2, S3, and S4.

The urethral sphincter mechanisms can be divided into proximal and distal components. The proximal urethral sphincter in the male is found in the region of the vesical neck and prostatic urethra, as smooth muscle fibers course through the vesical neck and terminate as far distally as the verumontanum. These fibers are continuous with smooth muscle of the detrusor, with some traversing the prostate gland itself. Smooth muscle distal to the verumontanum is surrounded by the external sphincter. The latter is composed of striated muscle and surrounds the membranous urethra. It is under voluntary control by way of the pudendal nerve from cord segments S2, S3, and S4.

In the female, the proximal sphincteric mechanism is formed by smooth muscle bundles that course from the bladder and are continuous with the urethra. Elastic fibers are interspersed within the smooth muscle, more abundant at the vesical neck. There is also thought to be a vascular cushion effect. The external sphincter in the female extends into the anterior wall of both the proximal and distal third of the urethra but is deficient posteriorly in these areas (12). The external sphincter in the female is relatively weak when compared to its counterpart in the male.

Understanding the development of reflux requires a brief but important discussion of the anatomy of the ureterovesical junction. The musculature of the ureter is laid down in a helical fashion until it enters the bladder wall (intravesical ureter). Here the musculature of the ureter continues in a longitudinal fashion and forms the lateral border of the superficial trigone and the interureteric ridge. The adventitia of the ureter has two layers in its intravesical course: the inner one originating from the ureter itself and the outer layer from the bladder. The space between, known as "Waldeyer's space," allows for some ureteral mobility.

Factors important in the prevention of reflux in normal individuals include the position and morphology of the ureteric orifice, an adequate length of intravesical and submucosal ureter, adequate detrusor muscle buttressing posteriorly, and normal bladder and sphincteric function.

NEUROPHYSIOLOGY

The detrusor muscle itself is supplied by parasympathetic outflow from sacral cord segments S2, S3, and S4. There is asymmetry of its innervation and usually functional nerve root dominance. There are sympathetic receptors in the bladder whose distribution is important. Alpha receptors are found predominantly in the trigone, vesical neck, and proximal urethra. Beta receptors, on the other hand, are predominant in the detrusor body. The distal urethral smooth muscle is primarily under alpha-adrenergic control while the periurethral striated muscle is supplied by fibers from the pudendal nerve, originating from sacral cord segments S2, S3, and S4. The act of normal micturition is initiated by cortical control. The brain receives afferent signals from the bladder and urethra through the posterior columns, spinothalamic and spinocerebellar tracts and descending motor pathways travelling in the corticospinal and reticulospinal tracts.

URODYNAMIC INVESTIGATIONS

The need for functional assessment in the urological management of the spinal cord injured patient is evident. The intravenous pyelogram, cystogram, and cystoscopic examination are static, structural tests, while the lower urinary tract is a dynamic system. Dynamic and quantitative evaluation of urological function is therefore essential for diagnosis and follow-up. Urodynamics is the branch of urology that quantifies bladder and urethral function in either or both the storage and voiding phases. Table 4.1 shows the tests used, while Figures 4.1 and 4.2 illustrate the information necessary to plan appropriate urologic treatment.

CLASSIFICATION OF NEUROLOGIC VOIDING DYSFUNCTION

As the physiology of micturition becomes better understood and diagnostic methods become more critical, so must our classifications alter while the traditional classifications are still referred to for historic reasons (Table

Table 4.1.
Urodynamic Tests

Storage Phase	Voiding Phase
Cystometrogram	Free-flow rate
Urethral pressure profilometry	Pressure/flow
Electromyography	Electromyography
Catheter cystrogram	Intraurethral pressures
	Voiding cystourethrography

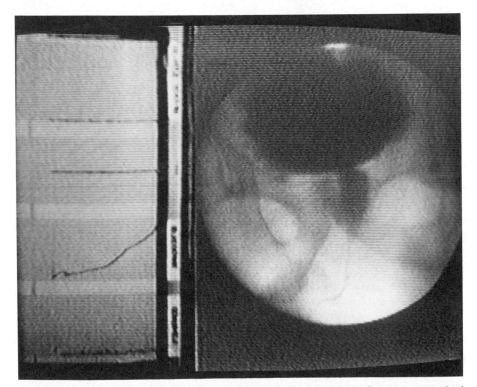

Figure 4.1. A 61-year-old male with complete C6–7 quadriplegia 2 years postspinal cord injury, complaining of recurrent lower urinary tract infections. The urodynamic recording shows a heavily trabeculated bladder with a capacity of 250 cc. During the voiding phase, the pressure is 92 cm H_2O and the external sphincter is in spasm (detrusor-sphincter dyssynergia). The patient underwent a successful external sphincterotomy.

4.2) (4, 27). More recently, a new, functional urodynamic classification has been proposed that correlates bladder and urethral function together (Table 4.3) (26). Wein (60) has proposed an alternate simple but relevant classification, which is clinically useful in the treatment of neurogenic bladder resulting from spinal cord injury (Table 4.3). The system distinguishes

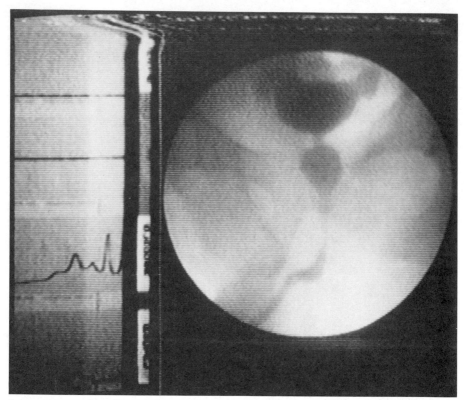

Figure 4.2. A 53-year-old male with complete C5–6 quadriplegia 1 year post-spinal cord injury, complaining of symptoms of autonomic dysreflexia during voiding. The urodynamic recording shows a small capacity bladder with diverticula. The voiding phase is seen and the pressure is intermittently elevated to 70 cm H_2O, with tightness at both the bladder neck and external sphincter. Treatment consisted of a bladder neck incision and external sphincterotomy to achieve a low pressure voiding system.

Table 4.2.
Traditional Classification of Neurogenic Bladder

Lapides	Bors
Uninhibited neurogenic bladder	Incomplete upper motor neuron lesion
Reflex neurogenic bladder	Complete upper motor neuron lesion
Autonomous neurogenic bladder	Complete lower motor neuron lesion
Sensory neurogenic bladder (paralytic)	Lower motor neuron lesion (sensory mainly)
Motor paralytic bladder	Lower motor neuron lesion (motor mainly)

between bladders that fail to store and those that fail to empty. Basing this classification on urodynamic findings as well as clinical manifestations makes it easier to understand the subsequent acute and chronic urological management of the spinal cord injured patient. Our further modification of

Table 4.3.
Recent Classifications of Neurogenic Bladder

Functional Classification – Wein

Failure to store:
  Because of the bladder
  Because of the outlet
Failure to empty:
  Because of the bladder
  Because of the outlet

Urodynamic Classification – Krane and Siroky

Detrusor hyperreflexia (or normoreflexia)
  Coordinated sphincters
  Striated sphincter dyssynergia
  Smooth muscle sphincter dyssynergia
  . Nonrelaxing smooth muscle sphincter
Detrusor areflexia
  Coordinated sphincters
  Nonrelaxing striated sphincter
  Denervated striated sphincter
  Nonrelaxing smooth muscle sphincter

Modified Urodynamic Classification	
Bladder	Sphincter (Proximal and/or distal)
High pressure (>60 cm H$_2$O) }	{ Obstructive
Low pressure (<60 cm H$_2$O) }	{ Non-obstructive

this classification system (Table 4.3) is based on urodynamics, specifying the pressure of the system in relation to the presence or absence of outflow obstruction.

THE MANAGEMENT OF THE ACUTE PHASE

Following acute suprasacral spinal cord injury, there is often a period of spinal bladder shock with loss of bladder tone, detrusor areflexia, and a closed vesical neck (52). Since its advent in 1947 by Guttman and Frankel, intermittent catheterization has been the mainstay of early bladder management in most centers. Lapides (1972) modified the procedure by performing clean rather than sterile intermittent catheterization. Clean intermittent catheterization should be safe if the procedure is done in an atraumatic fashion, if the bladder is not allowed to become overdistended, and if host resistance is able to deal with any bacteria introduced by the procedure (28, 29). Lapides believes therefore that increased susceptibility to bacterial invasion is secondary to decreased blood flow in the bladder wall and urethelium, usually caused by bladder overdistension. Although the bladder is hypotonic and areflexic, this is not so with the external sphincter. Nanninga and Meyer studied 44 patients with spinal cord injury within 72 hours of their accidents. All those with suprasacral lesions had a positive bulbocavernosus reflex, and 30 of 32 had increased sphincter activity during bladder filling, despite an areflexic detrusor (41). Rossier and associates also concluded that the external sphincter does not decrease activity in spinal shock but its activity may increase with recovery (52, 53). This has been confirmed by Downie and Awad (9). Koyanagi and co-workers have demonstrated a 39% dissociation in the electromyogram of the anal and urethral sphincters. One should not therefore rely completely on anal electromyography (25). Because of increased external sphincter activity and a closed vesical neck in the acute phase, the Crede maneuver is of no benefit in the early management of suprasacral cord injuries (52) and may in fact be dangerous.

Fam and associates studied 120 patients with spinal cord injuries for whom sterile intermittent catheterization was performed early (10). Seven percent of patients with incomplete lesions and 24% of those with complete lesions had infected urine at the time of discharge. However, only 43% had sterile urine after 8 weeks of drainage with a suprapubic cystostomy catheter. Cook reports no major complications in 41 patients treated with percutaneous suprapubic cystostomy with 43% retaining sterile urine after 7 weeks (8).

The authors believe that for accurate urine output measurement or prevention of detrusor overdistension following surgical procedures, indwelling catheter drainage may be advisable during the initial period following injury. Intermittent catheterization should however be instituted as early as possible as the treatment of choice in acute spinal cord injury.

CHRONIC MANAGEMENT

Improving longevity and quality of life as well as preserving renal function are important goals of modern urologic management of neurogenic bladder in spinal cord injuries. The advent of clinical urodynamic studies, especially in combination with video cystourethrography, provides the facility to quantitatively study lower urinary tract function, thus offering the best management.

O'Flynn states that urination will become more normal as the spinal cord injury is less complete (43). In Hackler's study of World War II and Korean War Veterans there was a 49% mortality at 25 years follow-up, with 43% of all deaths being kidney related. Forty percent had pathological evidence of renal amyloidosis, and 23% had pyelographic evidence of chronic pyelonephritis, the worst upper tract lesions being seen in those patients with cervical and high thoracic cord injuries managed with indwelling urethral catheters (16). Jacobs studied 59 veterans: 25 patients had indwelling urethral catheters for longer than 10 years, 25 had catheters less than 10 years, and 9 did not have catheters (22). The results were not unexpected. The creatinine clearance was significantly reduced in those with indwelling catheters for more than 10 years, 76% having abnormal upper tracts. Fifty-two percent of patients with a catheter less than 10 years had abnormal upper tracts, the most common abnormalities being renal scarring and calculi. Of the 50 patients with catheters, 15 (30%) had renal calculi and 29% had major urethral complications related to the catheter. There was a 100% infection rate in the urine of those with chronic urethral catheters (42).

Clearly, chronic urethral indwelling catheters as forms of permanent management are less than ideal except under certain circumstances. These include: (a) retention or incontinence in seriously ill and debilitated patients for whom intermittent catheterization is not feasible; (b) when surgical intervention to relieve obstruction is medically contraindicated, as in certain patients with upper urinary tract deterioration or vesicoureteral reflux; and (c) total incontinence in females for whom surgical or conservative procedures are not feasible (23).

The ideal goal in long-term management is the development of a balanced bladder that the patient can most easily manage. The criteria for a balanced bladder are: (a) the patient voids no more frequently than every 2 hours; and (b) residual urine is less than 100 ml (13). The main stipulation is that this balanced bladder must be part of a low pressure rather than a high pressure system. A strong detrusor can overcome an obstructive sphincter and give a false sense that there is a balance in the system. Such a patient may develop problems in the future, emphasizing the need for urodynamic assessment.

According to Graham, 57% to 70% of patients can achieve a balanced bladder with no specific urologic intervention (22). Perlow and Diokno have commented on the prediction of function of the urinary tract and noted that spinal shock may last from 1 week to 3 months. They conclude generally that patients with lesions above T7 develop reflex neurogenic bladders, those with lesions below T11 have lower motor neuron bladders, and lesions in the T8, T9, and T10 range are in a clinically unpredictable grey area (48). Our results in 136 spinal cord injured patients showed that high pressure voiding predominated in patients with lesions above T7 while 35% of patients with lesions below T7 also had high pressure voiding.

The ideal management avoids any specific intervention apart from intermittent catheterization while a balanced bladder develops, but 30% of patients will require pharmacologic manipulation or surgery.

Intermittent Catheterization

Clean intermittent catheterization has become a well-accepted part of management and may be combined with pharmacotherapy as discussed later. Frequency of catheterization is the most important factor in its success (40, 44). Orikasa and associates followed 26 patients on intermittent catheterization with no instances of upper tract deterioration (44). In the Lapides group of 218 patients, there was only one episode of acute pyelonephritis, and urine was sterile in 48% of the patients (28). Perkash had a 98% catheter-free rate in his group, with 68% free of infection (45). Moloney and co-workers studied 16 patients on intermittent catheterization and found no difference between saline and chlorhexidine as prep solutions to prevent recurrence of infection. They also noted that infection is heralded by urethral or paraurethral colonization (37). Nanninga and associates followed 85 patients, 33% of whom had reflux and/or hydronephrosis or ureterectasis. Most were treated by simply increasing the frequency of intermittent catheterization (40).

Pharmacotherapy

Pharmacologic agents used in the urinary tract can be divided into three main groups: drugs that act on the bladder, the internal sphincter, or the external sphincter (Table 4.4).

Bladder-stimulating agents are generally cholinergic or parasympathomimetic drugs of which the prototype is bethanechol chloride. Bladder-relaxing drugs such as propantheline or oxybutynin generally have anticholinergic properties. Oxybutynin chloride was shown to provide a 97% improvement in bladder capacity and a 77% improvement in delayed onset of first sensation to void (6). The drug had to be stopped in one-third of patients because of adverse effects (6). The drug possesses a direct smooth muscle relaxant effect as well as anticholinergic properties and is especially useful in incontinent female patients with reflex bladders who are on intermittent catheterization. The use of cholinergic or bladder-stimulating agents in suprasacral cord injuries is generally detrimental and discouraged. Light and Scott studied bethanechol chloride and found no change in appearance of the detrusor contraction after a 5 mg subcutaneous injection. Urinary flow rate was significantly reduced with increased outflow resistance (32). Yalla has confirmed an increase in intrasphincteric pressure and enhanced arrhythmic activity in the external sphincter following bethanechol administration (62).

The second major group of agents are those affecting the internal sphincter mechanism. These again can be subclassified as either enhancing or

Table 4.4.
Action of Pharmacologic Agents

	Contraction	Relaxation
Bladder:	bethanechol, carbachol	atropine, propantheline, oxybutynin, dicyclomine, flavoxate, imipramine, salbutamol
Internal Sphincter:	imipramine, ephedrine, phenylephrine, phenyl-propanolamine	phenoxybenzamine, prazosin
External Sphincter:	bethanechol, carbachol	baclofen, diazepam, dantrolene

reducing sphincter activity. Agents that enhance internal sphincter mechanism activity are generally alpha-adrenergic agonists, such as ephedrine sulphate, phenylpropanolamine and pseudoephedrine. These agents have little role in the management of the spinal cord injured bladder. The prototype of internal sphincter-relaxing drugs is phenoxybenzamine, an alpha-blocking agent that binds irreversibly to alpha receptor sites and prevents norepinephrine binding (55). At a dose of at least 30 mg per day, it has been shown to decrease residuals in 90% of sacral injuries (lower motor neuron bladders) (54). Its use in suprasacral injuries is limited and probably unnecessary. Most of the sphincter problems in suprasacral lesions are related to external sphincter spasticity and detrusor contraction pressure inadequate to open the vesical neck (52).

At present, external sphincter-relaxing agents generally play little role in the physician's armamentarium. Baclofen acts specifically on the spinal cord with a depressant action on the spinal cord interneurons, pyramidal tract neurons, and Purkinje cells. It may also inhibit mono- and polysynaptic reflexes by presynaptic hyperpolarization. Major side effects are often prohibitive and may include somnolence in quadriplegics and upper limb weakness in paraplegics (31). Dantrolene sodium acts on the sarcoplasmic reticulum of muscle fibers by interrupting excitation contraction coupling. In Hackler's study, approximately 50% of patients failed to show improvement and 12 of 15 complained of generalized weakness. Hepatotoxicity may be a problem as a high drug level is necessary to have an effect on micturition (18). The major aim in developing a balanced bladder is to keep the voiding pressure under 60 cm of water to help prevent reflux, hydronephrosis, bladder wall thickening, trabeculation, and autonomic dysreflexia. In general, a few basic statements can be made concerning pharmacotherapy:

1. Anticholinergic (bladder-relaxing) agents are useful in suprasacral cord lesions to decrease detrusor pressure and increase capacity and continence interval in those on intermittent catheterization.
2. Cholinergic (bladder-stimulating) agents are contraindicated in the presence of detrusor sphincter dyssynergia.
3. External sphincter pharmacomanipulation is of limited practical usefulness at the present time.

THE CONCEPT OF DETRUSOR SPHINCTER DYSSYNERGIA

As previously stated, external sphincter activity does not decrease with spinal shock and in fact may be enhanced with bladder recovery. Generally, the higher the cord lesion, the higher the incidence of detrusor-sphincter dyssynergia (DSD). Detrusor-sphincter dyssynergia is defined as a condition that exists when simultaneous contraction of the detrusor muscle and external sphincter oppose each other. Pontine-mesencephalic reticular formation activity is necessary for coordinated voiding to take place, and therefore, DSD is only seen in suprasacral cord injuries (3). Blaivas has classified DSD into three types (3). Type I, accounting for 30% of DSD, consists of an increase in sphincter activity at the peak of detrusor contraction with sudden sphincter relaxation as detrusor pressure drops. Type II is typified by clonic contractions of the sphincter during detrusor contraction with interrupted voiding occurring in about 15% of patients. Type III, contraction of the sphincter persisting through the entire detrusor contraction with obstructed flow or essentially no voiding, is seen in 55% of patients and puts these patients in the highest risk group (3). There is purported to be no correlation between the type of DSD and the level of suprasacral injury (3). DSD is the most common cause of unbalanced bladder (52). At this juncture, a discussion of autonomic dysreflexia is necessary.

Autonomic dysreflexia occurs with suprasacral cord injuries above the T7 level (55). Afferents in the vesical neck and posterior urethra act as stimuli, triggering the onset of dysreflexia (47). The major signs and symptoms are sweating, sudden pressor response, and headache. Phenoxybenzamine has been shown to decrease the pressor response and headache, but does not alter the sweating (55). Perkash has demonstrated a mean systolic and diastolic blood pressure rise of 77 and 44 mm of mercury respectively during urodynamic studies on quadriplegics with DSD and lesions above the T5 level (47). A significant improvement is seen with external sphincterotomy, which will be discussed later.

The authors feel that a very precise way of diagnosing DSD is by urodynamics combined with simultaneous video cystourethrography (Figure 4.1) (21). Bladder neck obstruction alone or with DSD can also be demonstrated by this technique (Figure 4.2).

External Sphincterotomy

We have described the various types of DSD and identified it as the most common cause of an unbalanced bladder in spinal cord injuries. With DSD present, voiding is initiated by involuntary detrusor reflex rather than urethral relaxation (3). Radiologic findings during video urodynamics include a tightness in the region of the external sphincter during detrusor contraction, a dilated posterior urethra, seminal vesicle reflux, or filling of the prostatic ducts (30).

There are two main interventions for DSD and its attendant problems. Intermittent catheterization in combination with anticholinergic agents will decrease detrusor pressure and increase bladder capacity. Where there is high residual urine, upper tract deterioration, vesicoureteral reflux, detrusor sphincter dyssenergia on urodynamic testing, and autonomic dysreflexia, surgical sphincterotomy is indicated.

The two major types of sphincterotomy presently employed are the bilateral and anteromedian sphincterotomy. These may be combined with a transurethral incision of the vesical neck or prostatectomy if indicated for obstruction at that particular level. The bladder neck incision is preferred over resection to avoid postoperative contracture. Perkash reported 90% success with first operation and noted improvement in all of nine patients with neurogenically induced reflux (46). Morrow and Bogaard noted reduction of hydronephrosis on IVP in seven of eight patients following sphincterotomy and bladder neck incision (38). Madersbacher has stated that the anteromedian sphincterotomy is the best anatomic operation since both the circular striated fibers and the longitudinal fibers of the external sphincter are strongest in the anterior region. Of 17 patients studied, only 2 required reoperation (34). Yalla's series of 31 patients undergoing anteromedian sphincterotomy demonstrated that blood transfusions were not required and there was no loss of erection postoperatively (61). Morrow and Scott report complete loss of erection in 3.9% of 131 patients undergoing bilateral sphincterotomy (39). Herschorn and associates have shown that postoperative impotence is not as dependent upon the type of initial sphincterotomy as on the number of the sphincterotomies required (20). Sphincterotomy has been suggested as the procedure of choice in reflux secondary to neurogenic bladder in spinal cord injury (10, 13, 46). Golji, reporting on 53 patients with chronic suprasacral spinal cord injury, had over 70% success in removing indwelling urethral catheters following sphincterotomy (11).

In summary, sphincterotomy has become a standard and very successful procedure in the urologic management of DSD associated with suprasacral cord injuries. As a result, many patients are living catheter-free without urinary diversion.

Urinary Diversion

Although urinary diversion was once a more accepted mode of management, it is now a last resort procedure. It is still indicated however in progressive irreversible hydronephrosis and intractable incontinence in the female who has failed to respond to other means of management (17). It is certainly easier to manage an ileal conduit stoma than bilateral nephrostomies. Moeller followed 31 patients with spinal cord injuries who underwent ileal conduit urinary diversion (36). The average follow-up period was 5 years and only one-half of patients had a fair to good result. In the 31 patients, there were 8 major complications and deaths, 5 of these in the cervical cord injured group.

In general, ileal loop diversion still has a limited place in management but only after all other efforts have failed. Colonic conduits have become more popular in the authors' clinical setting as they can be constructed with an antireflux ureteral anastomosis.

Artificial Sphincter

The artificial inflatable urinary sphincter is another alternative in the management of neurogenic incontinence. Specific indications and contraindications do exist. Light and Scott (33) reported on 49 patients with spinal cord injury and neurogenic bladder who underwent implantation. While the overall success rate was 70%, patients with areflexic bladders did better than patients with hyperreflexic or low-compliance bladders. Males with outflow obstruction required transurethral procedures, and females with obstruction underwent bladder flap urethroplasties in preparation for the sphincter. To achieve the 70% success rate, multiple operations were necessary in the majority of patients due to mechanical and infective complications. If, however, bladder emptying is deficient, intermittent catheterization can be utilized safely (2).

Nerve-Blocking Techniques

Nerve blocks and sectionings have been used to increase the bladder capacity by abolishing or reducing hyperreflexia. They have also been utilized to decrease the urethral resistance due to external sphincter spasm. Rockswold and Bradley (50) used sacral nerve blocks in 50 patients, guided by air cystometry and sphincter electromyography. In 26 patients the detrusor reflux was abolished with a unilateral S3 or S4 lidocaine block. This technique can be followed by either permanent phenol block or sacral nerve sectioning provided no significant adverse effects result. It is a time-consuming and difficult procedure to undertake and must be accompanied by simultaneous urodynamic testing.

Pudendal nerve blocks or neurectomy have been attempted in the past to achieve voiding. Bilateral blocks, however, are necessary to effectively inactivate the external urethral sphincter (50). The procedure is also technically difficult and the risk of impotence is significant. Lack of perianal and perivaginal sensation in the area of the block as well as bowel incontinence can result (49).

Electrical Stimulation Techniques

Electrical stimulation techniques have been reported by many investigators to simulate normal bladder function. Both phases of lower urinary tract function have been studied to either prevent uninhibited contractions or to cause bladder evacuation. Various kinds of electrical implants have been tried for emptying the bladder. These have involved electrodes on the bladder wall (19, 56), on the sacral nerves (5, 15), or on the conus medullaris (14). The initial enthusiasm for direct bladder stimulation subsided for several reasons. Direct bladder stimulation required strong currents that occasionally caused pelvic floor, abdominal wall, or lower limb spasms, and pain in patients with incomplete lesions. Device failure was due to electrode breakage and migration with bladder movement. Conus medullaris stimulation (14) has resulted in voiding in a number of patients but does require a high stimulus amplitude. Associated autonomic responses of piloerection, adductor spasm, increased skin temperature, occasional penile erection, and diffuse pelvic pain were some of the side effects of conus medullaris stimulation. These two latter modalities could not reliably cause the external sphincter to relax during the voiding phase.

Tanagho and Schmidt (58) described a canine model for selective sacral root stimulation. External sphincter relaxation and effective voiding were achieved by applying the electrode to the ventral root, sectioning the dorsal root to eliminate the spread of stimuli to the spinal cord, and selectively sectioning somatic fibers of that particular sacral root before it joins the other sacral roots to form the pudendal nerve. Brindley and co-workers (5) reported on 11 spinal injured patients in whom electrodes were placed around S2-4 anterior roots and voiding was achieved. By delivering strong bursts of stimulation, the external sphincter is activated intermittently; with short intervals of stimulation, the detrusor, which is simultaneously activated, will contract continuously. Ten patients now void by this method and the eleventh had a previous sphincterotomy. Sacral nerve root stimulation holds promise for the future if detrusor-sphincter dyssynergia can be overcome.

Externally applied stimulation devices have been used for many years in the treatment of incontinence. Anal or vaginal plugs with external stimulators can promote continence by either inhibiting the detrusor reflex or causing sphincter contraction (57). This modality has met with limited acceptance due to patient intolerance of anal plugs and unsatisfactory performance of various battery-powered devices (35). Cutaneously applied nerve stimulation has been described by McGuire and associates (35). Detrusor contractility was inhibited effectively by stimulating the common peroneal or posterior tibial nerve in one lower limb and grounding the opposite side. Four spinal cord injured patients were kept dry with this method. The authors theorized that the current traverses the spinal cord and that afferent as well as antidromic efferent activity induced in the posterior tibial nerve caused inhibition of detrusor activity. This method will undoubtedly be investigated further.

Electrical stimulation techniques may possibly be very common modalities in the urologic management of the spinal cord injured patient in the future. At this time, however, they are not widely available and the more traditional forms of treatment are still preferred.

Other Measures

Trigger voiding measures are aimed at inducing a detrusor contraction in patients with hyperreflexic bladders. Stimulation of the lumbosacral dermatomes, such as suprapubic tapping, pulling of the pubic hairs, stroking of the glans penis, and anal sphincter stretching (24), may result in bladder contraction and external sphincter relaxation. Valsalva maneuver may also be required.

Voiding by Crede maneuver can be carried out by patients who have hyporeflexic bladders and nonobstructive sphincters. Abdominal straining can be done by patients with lower lesions as long as the technique does not induce reflex contractions of the external sphincter.

FOLLOW-UP

The importance of regular, long-term follow-up cannot be over-emphasized (40, 51). The authors' patients are assessed with video urodynamics, consisting of subtracted bladder pressure measurements and video cysto-urethrography. These studies are performed approximately every 4 months during the first year following injury and every 6 months to 1 year thereafter, when the bladder has stabilized. Comarr has stated that residual urine estimations are still an important tool in monitoring bladder function (7). Rosen and associates have warned of the development of silent hydronephrosis, which in most cases occurred when detrusor pressure was high (greater than 60 cm of water) and adequate follow-up was lacking. Male patients are easier to manage since they are easily fitted with external appliances. Penile implants have been used for patients who have difficulty in maintaining condoms (59). Even a simple procedure, such as circumcision, can make appliance management much easier.

Proper and regular urologic care can lead not only to increased quantity but also quality of life for the spinal cord injured patient. The achievement of a low pressure urinary system can maintain the patient free of morbidity and mortality from the urinary tract (Figure 4.3) (1). Urodynamic studies

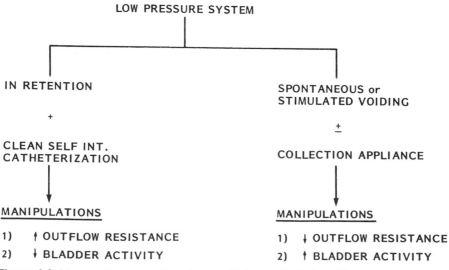

Figure 4.3. Manipulations used in spinal cord injury patients to achieve a low pressure system.

are a guide to management based on the pressures and findings at various times in the postinjury course. All the above mentioned modalities have to be considered in order to achieve a low pressure system; failures often mean permanent indwelling catheterization or urinary diversion.

REFERENCES

1. Barkin, M., Dolfin, D., Herschorn, S., Bharatwal, N., and Comisarow, R. The urologic care of the spinal cord injury patient. *J. Urol.*, *129:*335, 1983.
2. Barrett, D. M., and Furlow, W. L. The management of severe urinary incontinence in patients with myelodysplasia by implantation of the AS 791/792 urinary sphincter device. *J. Urol.*, *128:*484, 1982.
3. Blaivas, J. G., Sinha, H. P ., Zayed, A. A. H., and Labib, K. B. Detrusor-external sphincter dyssynergia: a detailed electromyographic study. *J. Urol.*, *125:*542–545, 1981.
4. Bors, E., and Comarr, A. E. *Neurological Urology*. University Park Press, Baltimore, 1971, pp. 129–135.
5. Brindley, G. S., Polkey, C. E., and Rushton, D. N. Sacral anterior root stimulators for bladder control in paraplegia. *Paraplegia*, *20:*365, 1982.
6. Brooks, M. E., and Braf, Z. F. Oxybutynin chloride (Ditropan)—Clinical uses and limitations. *Paraplegia*, *18:* 64, 1980.
7. Comarr, A. E., and Peha, L. J. Further cinecystourethrography studies among spinal cord injury patients. *Urol. Int.*, *29:*34, 1974.
8. Cook, J. B., and Smith, P. H. Percutaneous suprapubic cystostomy after spinal cord injury. *Br. J. Urol.*, *48:*119, 1976.
9. Downie, J. W., and Awad, S. A. The state of urethral musculature during the detrusor areflexia after spinal cord transection. *Invest. Urol.*, *17:*55, 1979.
10. Fam, B. A., Rossier, A. B., Blunt, K., Gabilondo, F. B., Sarkarati, M., Sethi, J., and Yalla, S. V. Experience in the urologic management of 120 early spinal cord injury patients. *J. Urol.*, *119:*485, 1978.
11. Golji, H. Urethral sphincterotomy for chronic spinal cord injury. *J. Urol.*, *123:*204, 1980.
12. Gosling, J. The structure of the bladder and urethra in relation to function. In: *Urologic Clinics of North America Symposium on Clinical Urodynamics*, *6:*35, 1979.
13. Graham, S. D. Present urological treatment of spinal cord injury patients. *J. Urol.*, *126:*1, 1981.
14. Grimes, J. H., Nashold, B. S., and Anderson, E. E. Clinical application of electronic bladder stimulation in paraplegics. *J. Urol.*, *113:*338, 1975.
15. Habib, H. N. Experience and recent contributions in sacral nerve stimulation for voiding in both human and animal. *Br. J. Urol.*, *39:*73, 1967.
16. Hackler, R. H. A 25-year prospective mortality study in the spinal cord injured patient: Comparison with the long term living paraplegic. *J. Urol.*, *117:*486, 1977.
17. Hackler, R. H. Surgical treatment of neurogenic bladder dysfunction. In: *Clinical Neuro-Urology*. Edited by R. J. Krane, and M. B. Siroky. Little, Brown & Co., Boston, 1979, pp. 197–212.
18. Hackler, R. H., Broeker, B. H., Klein, F. A., and Brady, S. M. A clinical experience with dantrolene sodium for external urinary sphincter hypertonicity in spinal injured patients. *J. Urol.*, *124:*78, 1980.
19. Halverstadt, D. B., and Parry, W. L. Electronic stimulation of the human bladder 9 years later. *J. Urol.*, *113:*341, 1975.
20. Herschorn, S., Barkin, M., Dolfin, D., and Comisarow, R. Videourodynamics and transurethral sphincterotomy in spinal cord injury patients. Presented at the Canadian Urological Association Meeting, Ottawa, June 1982.

21. Herschorn, S., Barkin, M., Dolfin, D., and Comisarow, R. Transurethral sphincterotomy—factors influencing success. In press.
22. Jacobs, S. C., and Kaufman, J. M. Complications of permanent bladder catheter drainage in spinal cord injury patients. *J. Urol.*, *119:*740, 1978.
23. Khanna, O. P. Nonsurgical therapeutic modalities. In: *Clinical Neuro-Urology.* Edited by R. J. Krane and M. B. Siroky. Little, Brown & Co., Boston, 1979, p. 160.
24. Kiviat, M. D., Zimmermann, T. A., and Donovan, W. H. Sphincter stretch: a new technique resulting in continence and voiding in paraplegics. *J. Urol.*, *114:*895, 1975.
25. Koyanagi, T., Arikado, K., Takamatsu, T., and Tsuji, I. Experience with electromyography of the external urethral sphincter in spinal cord injury patients. *J. Urol.*, *127:*272, 1982.
26. Krane, R. J., and Siroky, M. B. Classification of neuro-urologic disorders. In: *Clinical Neuro-Urology.* Little, Brown & Co., Boston, 1979, pp. 143–158.
27. Lapides, J. Neuromuscular vesical and ureteral dysfunction. In: *Urology*, ed. 3, vol. 2. Edited by M. F. Campbell and J. H. Harrison, W. B. Saunders Co., Philadelphia, 1970, pp. 1343–1378.
28. Lapides, J., Diokno, A. C., Gould, F. R., and Lowe, B. S. Further observations on self-catheterization. *J. Urol.*, *116:*169, 1979.
29. Lapides, J., Diokno, A. C., Silber, S. J., and Lowe, B. S. Clean intermittent self-catheterization in the treatment of urinary tract disease. *J. Urol.*, *107:*458, 1972.
30. Leriche, A., Archimbaud, J. P., Bedard, E., Minaire, P., and Bourret, J. Differential diagnosis and limitations of external sphincterotomy. *Paraplegia*, *13:*280, 1976.
31. Leyson, J. F. J., Maring, B. F., and Sporer, A. Baclofen in the treatment of detrusor-sphincter dyssynergia in spinal cord injury patients. *J. Urol.*, *124:*82, 1980.
32. Light, J. K., and Scott, F. B. Bethanechol chloride and the traumatic cord bladder. *J. Urol.*, *128:*85, 1982.
33. Light, J. K., and Scott, F. B. Use of the artificial urinary sphincter in spinal cord injury patients. *J. Urol.*, *130:*1127, 1983.
34. Madersbacher, H. The twelve o'clock sphincterotomy: technique, indications, and results. *Paraplegia*, *13:*261, 1976.
35. McGuire, E. J., Shi-chun, Z., Horwinski, E. R., and Lytton, B. Treatment of motor and sensory detrusor instability by electrical stimulation. *J. Urol.*, *129:*78, 1983.
36. Moeller, B. A. Some observations of 31 spinal cord injury patients on whom the Bricker operation was performed. *Paraplegia*, *15:*230, 1977–78.
37. Moloney, P. J., Doyle, A. A., Robinson, B. L., Fenster, H., and McLoughlin, M. G. Pathogenesis of urinary infection in patients with acute spinal cord injury on intermittent catheterization. *J. Urol.*, *125:*672, 1981.
38. Morrow, J. W., and Bogaard, T. P. Bladder rehabilitation in patients with old spinal cord injuries with bladder neck incision and external sphincterotomy. *J. Urol.*, *117:*164, 1977.
39. Morrow, J. W., and Scott, M. B. Erections and sexual function in post sphincterotomy bladder neck patients. *J. Urol.*, *119:*500, 1978.
40. Nanninga, J. B., and Hamilton, B. Long-term intermittent catheterization in the spinal cord injury patient. *J. Urol.*, *128:*760, 1982.
41. Nanninga, J. B., and Meyer, P. Urethral sphincter activity following acute spinal cord injury. *J. Urol.*, *123:*528, 1980.
42. O'Flynn, J. D. Early management of neuropathic bladder in spinal cord injuries. *Paraplegia*, 12:83, 1974.
43. O'Flynn, J. D. Early and late management of the neuropathic bladder in spinal cord injury patients. *J. Urol.*, *120:*726, 1978.
44. Orikasa, S., Koyanagi, T., Motomura, M., Kudo, T., Togashi, M., and Tsuji, I. Experience with non-sterile intermittent catheterization. *J. Urol.*, *115:*141, 1976.
45. Perkash, I. Intermittent catheterization and bladder rehabilitation in spinal injury patients. *J. Urol.*, *114:*230, 1975.
46. Perkash, I. Detrusor-sphincter dyssynergia and dyssynergic responses: recognition and

rationale for early modified transurethral sphincterotomy in complete spinal cord injury lesions. *J. Urol.*, *120:* 469, 1978.

47. Perkash, I. Pressor response during cystomanometry in spinal injury patients complicated with detrusor-sphincter dyssynergia. *J. Urol.*, *121:*778, 1979.
48. Perlow, D. L., and Diokno, A. C. Predicting lower urinary tract dysfunctions in patients with spinal cord injury. *Urology*, *18:*531, 1981.
49. Raz, S., and Bradley, W. E. Neuromuscular dysfunction of the lower urinary tract. In: *Campbell's Urology*, ed. 4, Vol. 2. W. B. Saunders Co., Philadelphia, 1979, p. 1253.
50. Rockswold, G. L., and Bradley, W. E. The use of sacral nerve blocks in the evaluation of neurogenic bladder disease. *J. Urol*, *118:*415, 1977.
51. Rosen, J. S., Nanninga, J. B., and O'Connor, V. J. Silent hydronephrosis, a hazard revisited. *Paraplegia*, *14:*124, 1976.
52. Rossier, A. B., and Fam, B. A. From intermittent catheterization to catheter freedom via urodynamics: A tribute to Sir Ludwig Guttman. *Paraplegia*, *17:*73, 1979.
53. Rossier, A. B., Ott, R., and Roussan, M. S. Urinary manometry in patients with spinal cord injury: Neurological considerations in the rehabilitation of acute and chronic neurogenic bladder. *Arch. Phys. Med. Rehabil.*, *56:*187, 1975.
54. Scott, M. B., and Morrow, J. W. Phenoxybenzamine in neurogenic bladder dysfunction after spinal cord injury. I. Voiding dysfunction. *J. Urol.*, *119:*480, 1978.
55. Scott, M. B., and Morrow, J. W. Phenoxybenzamine in neurogenic bladder dysfunction after spinal cord injury. II. Autonomic dysreflexia. *J. Urol.*, *119:*483, 1978.
56. Stenberg, C. C., Burnette, H. W., and Bunts, R. C. Electrical stimulation of human neurogenic bladders: experience with four patients. *J. Urol.*, *97:*79, 1967.
57. Suhel, P., and Kralj, B. Treatment of urinary incontinence using functional electrical stimulation. In: *Female Urology*. Edited by S. Raz. W. B. Saunders Co., Philadelphia, 1983, p. 215.
58. Tanagho, E. A., and Schmidt, R. A. Bladder pacemaker: scientific basis and clinical future. *Urology*, *20:*614, 1982.
59. Van Arsdalen, K. N., Klein, F. A., Hackler, R. H., and Brady, S. M. Penile implants in spinal cord injury for maintaining external appliances. *J. Urol.*, *126:*331, 1981.
60. Wein, A. J. Classification of neurogenic voiding dysfunction. *J. Urol.*, *125:*605, 1981.
61. Yalla, S. V., Fam, B. A., Gabilondo, F. B., Jacobs, S., DiBenedetto, M., Rossier, A. B., and Gittes, R. F. Anteromedian external urethral sphincterotomy: technique, rationale, and complications. *J. Urol.*, *117:*489, 1977.
62. Yalla, S. V., Rossier, A. B., Fam, B. A., Gabilondo, F. B., DiBenetto, M., and Gittes, R. F. Functional contribution of autonomic innervation to urethral striated sphincter: studies with parasympathomimetic, parasympatholytic, and alpha-adrenergic blocking agents in spinal cord injury and control male subjects. *J. Urol*, *117:*494, 1977.

5

Gastrointestinal Complications in Spinal Cord Injuries

T. SEATON
R. HOLLINGWORTH

Gastrointestinal problems frequently complicate spinal cord injuries (11, 32). With most spinal cord injuries being caused by trauma, the acute phase assessment of other intraabdominal injuries is often difficult. Similarly, the assessment of acute intraabdominal emergencies, either associated with "stress" of a spinal cord injury or quite unrelated, is complicated by the loss of some traditional clinical signs associated with intraabdominal catastrophe (11, 44, 54). This problem continues in the chronic phase of spinal cord paralysis with intraabdominal emergencies accounting for up to 10% of the overall mortality (7, 22, 44).

During the chronic phase of spinal cord injury, gastrointestinal problems are primarily those of altered motility and control of bowel function related in some way to the disruption of extrinsic nervous pathways to the gut. This creates a major hurdle for the rehabilitation patient desiring functional independence.

The understanding of gastrointestinal physiology has been slow to develop, possibly because of problems in access and methodological difficulties. The physiology of gut motility is best understood in the esophagus and stomach at the upper end and the rectum at the lower end, with the small bowel and most of the large bowel lagging way behind. Similarly, the effects of various foods on motility and the action of fiber and various drugs such as laxatives are still poorly understood and controversial. Gastrointestinal problems after a spinal cord injury change with time, although they do overlap. This discussion will therefore be divided into the traditional "acute" and "chronic" phases of spinal cord injury. A full review of the current understanding of control of gut motility is beyond the scope of this chapter, but it will be outlined briefly as an integral part of the section on the chronic phase of spinal cord injuries.

G.I. PROBLEMS IN THE ACUTE PHASE OF SPINAL CORD INJURY (SCI)

During the initial phase of SCI, disorders of the G.I. tract may occur secondary to the abrupt change in nervous control, the neuroendocrine response to stress, or as a result of coincidental trauma to abdominal structures.

Gastric dilatation and *ileus* are seen more often in cervical and high thoracic lesions and can be life threatening if unrecognized (32, 45, 52). Acute gastric dilatation is usually associated with loss of large amounts of fluid into the stomach and the precipitation of hypovolemic shock. In patients with SCI, acute gastric dilatation may compromise respiratory function further by limiting diaphragmatic movements and may also expose the patient to the danger of aspiration.

Acute gastric dilatation is easily detected clinically and radiologically, and warrants prompt decompression with nasogastric suction and intravenous fluid replacement. Cholinergic agents such as metoclopramide hydrochloride have been reported as being useful, but their role in gastric stasis following spinal cord injury has not been established (43). Intestinal ileus usually recovers more quickly than gastric stasis, but may complicate nutritional support in the acute phase.

Gastroduodenal ulceration and bleeding are important complications in all traumatized patients (17, 38, 50). Often referred to as "stress ulceration," this complication has been reported in from 0.5% to 22% of patients with spinal cord injuries (39). Hemorrhage from the G.I. tract following spinal cord injury has been associated with high mortality in the past, however, this rate appears to be falling in later reported series (11, 39, 41). Early diagnosis, improved critical care management, and possibly the use of H-receptor antagonists may be contributing to the falling mortality rate. Bedside endoscopy has been shown to be a safe and useful procedure in patients with SCI (53). It should have an accuracy rate of 85% or better in diagnosing the site of upper gastrointestinal bleeding.

Shock, catecholamines, and steroids have been implicated in the pathogenesis of acute gastroduodenal ulceration, though conclusive evidence is lacking (14, 23, 38, 50). Similarly, the role of H-blockers in prophylaxis and treatment remains controversial.

Cimetidine is the most popular of the H-antagonists, and although its side effects are few, they are particularly relevant to patients with spinal cord injuries. If there is associated head injury, central nervous system depression with cimetidine may obscure evaluation in the acute phase. This is particularly important if there is coexistent renal or hepatic dysfunction. (This is not usually an issue in young and otherwise fit patients.) The metabolism of various drugs handled by the liver via the phase I pathway of mixed function oxydase microsomal enzymes may be impaired by cimetidine, thus prolonging drug half-life. Specifically, warfarin sodium, diazepam, and anticonvulsants, often used in patients with multiple trauma, should be monitored carefully if used in conjunction with cimetidine. Newer H-antagonists (ranitidine hydrochloride) do not share this phase I inhibition and also appear to have fewer CNS effects (49).

During traumatic spinal cord injury, there may be coincidental gastrointestinal trauma producing ruptured viscus, infarcted bowel, or pancreatitis (10, 11, 32). Later on, patients may present with acute surgical emergencies such as appendicitis, cholecystitis, or perforated or infarcted bowel. Evaluation of these patients is particularly difficult because of the impaired sensory input from the parietal peritoneum. In one study, all cases of appendicitis in patients with SCI were found to have perforated and were associated with abscess by the time they were diagnosed and had surgery (11). Although no prospective studies have been reported, a number of series describing general surgical problems in patients with spinal cord injury point to a higher mortality in this group of patients than would be expected in the general population (7, 11, 44). Clinical clues such as anorexia, tachycardia, shoulder tip pain, and vague abdominal discomfort, although nonspecific, warrant close scrutiny and prompt investigation in this group of patients (44). Some investigations such as abdominal ultrasound may be of limited value in many SCI patients because of increased amounts of intraluminal gas. A high index of suspicion and the early use of investigative procedures cannot be overemphasized (33, 44, 54).

Nutrition

During the 1970's, the degree of malnutrition among hospitalized patients was identified. This occurs in up to 50% of general medical and surgical patients. Efforts were made to define nutritional markers that would lead to early diagnosis and encourage preventive intervention (6, 9). Spinal cord injury patients are at risk for several reasons. Their injuries often result from multiple trauma. In addition to the hypermetabolic state in the acute phase, a long period of hospitalized general medical and surgical management often involves extended periods of decreased nutritional intake. Associated intercurrent illnesses and disturbances in gut motility also work against the establishment of adequate nutritional intake.

Traditional methods of nutritional assessment involve anthropomorphic measurements, estimates of ideal body weight, and biochemical assessments, including serum proteins, creatinine height ratios, etc. These have now been shown to be of limited value in other hospitalized patients, but the problem in spinal cord injury patients is compounded by the muscle atrophy associated with denervation, further undermining the interpretation of some of these measurements (40, 46). There are now more sophisticated techniques available for body composition analysis, including isotope and neutron activation studies, which can assess total body content of individual elements, allowing more objective measurements in these patients.

Nutritional support in the acute phase, when the patient may be quite ill, is further complicated by some of the metabolic alterations associated with trauma. Of particular importance is the respiratory system where excessive carbohydrate calorie loads may result in respiratory failure. This is an issue of quadriplegic paralysis affecting the intercostal muscles where respiratory reserve may be quite limited. The strategy should be to estimate total caloric and protein needs and to meet these rather than to arbitrarily provide large nutritional loads either intravenously or via the G.I. tract.

Clinicians responsible for feeding these patients in the acute phase need to be aware of disturbed gastric motility. If vomiting is a problem, tube feeding may be successfully achieved by utilizing weighted tubes that are advanced into the small bowel before the infusion is started.

During the acute phase of spinal cord shock, paralytic ileus may preclude the use of enteral feeding. Total parenteral nutrition should be started initially with the patient weaned toward full enteral feeding as the clinical progress dictates (27).

G.I. PROBLEMS IN THE CHRONIC PHASE OF SPINAL CORD INJURY

Following recovery from the acute injury, the problems in the chronic phase are dominated by disturbances in motility of the G.I. tract and, to a lesser extent, general consequences of injury such as residual nutritional deficiencies, rarely amyloidosis, and incidental G.I. problems.

Effect of SCI on the Intestinal Motility

Normal motility requires coordinated activity to move luminal contents distally in the gut. This activity is mediated by longitudinal and circular muscle layers, and controlled by intrinsic and extrinsic nervous systems as well as the influence of regulating peptides (29). Disturbances in any of these factors may result in disordered motility, translated into altered transit time and other symptoms.

The *extrinsic* nerve supply of the gut comprises the central nervous system as well as the autonomic outflow. The autonomic nervous system consists of the familiar sympathetic and parasympathetic divisions. The sympathetic nervous system has its outflow from the central nervous system in the thoracolumbar region (T4 to L2). Its ganglia are located in chains in the paravertebral region and close to the aorta. Postganglionic fibers follow the arteries to the gut. Sympathetic outflow to the gut is often disrupted in spinal cord injury, depending on the level of neurological deficit.

The parasympathetic supply is via the vagus for most of the gut, down to the level of the right or transverse colon, and sacral outflow is via the nervi erigentes that supply the rectum and left colon. In spinal cord injury, much of the parasympathetic supply to the G.I. tract is left intact.

The enteric nervous system consists of the submucosal (Meissner's) and muscular (Auerbach's) plexuses. It is a unique nervous supply in that it is able to act independently of extrinsic nervous supply from the central nervous system or the autonomic nervous system. This autonomous function however can be modulated by the extrinsic input as well as regulatory peptides acting locally or centrally. The enteric nervous system is large and complex, with about as many neurons as are in the spinal cord. Its activity in man or in the experimental animal is not significantly altered by sympathectomy or vagotomy (29, 30). Although the relationship between the levels of the neuronal network have been investigated in various animal models, the influence of the higher nervous centers on gut motility in man is not yet fully understood (26, 29, 57).

Various techniques have been used for measuring intestinal motility at different levels of the G.I. tract with varying success. Such technical difficulties as irreproducibility of results, lack of standards for normal function, and other measurement artifacts have been major obstacles in reaching a better understanding of altered gastrointestinal physiology in intact patients as well as those with cord lesions. The three major areas of investigation have been electromyography, manometry, and radiological techniques. Only a few studies have been able to correlate two of these modalities. The upper gastrointestinal tract as well as the distal colon and rectum have been studied most extensively, largely because of their accessibility to intubation. Unfortunately, little is known about the motility of the small bowel and much of the colon.

Upper G.I. Motility

Although motility of the esophagus is probably the best understood area in the gastrointestinal tract, no study has looked at the alterations in esophageal motility in patients with spinal cord injury. There is radiological evidence that these patients have a higher prevalence of gastroesophageal reflux and hiatus hernia than normal (32). Prolonged supine position, depressed diaphragmatic function, and chronic constipation may be contributing factors to gastroesophageal reflux in these patients.

Motility patterns in the stomach and small bowel depend on whether they are examined after a meal or in the fasting state. During feeding, gastric motility is active and appears to serve the function of mixing the ingested material with gastric juice. In the antrum, coordinated contractions propel aliquots of the gastric content into the duodenum at intervals and eventually empty the stomach. This activity is modified by the type of food ingested (protein vs fat etc.) and even the amount of liquid in the meal. It appears to be controlled by the intrinsic nervous system but also is greatly influenced by gastrointestinal hormones.

In the fasting state, beginning in the proximal stomach, contractions occur intermittently and move in an aboral direction down the entire small bowel. This activity is referred to as a migrating myoelectric complex (MMC) or interdigestive motor complex (IDMC). It is also controlled by the intrinsic nervous system and is felt to have a role in moving residual ingested material distally as well as controlling bacterial population within the lumen ("housekeeper role").

Fealey and associates reported in abstract form the effect of spinal cord transection on human upper G.I. motility (26). Five patients with high cord lesions were studied in comparison with three patients with low cord lesions and four healthy volunteers. There were no significant differences among the different groups for the duration or cycle lengths of the interdigestive motor complexes. There also seemed to be no significant alteration in postprandial motility although the patients with high cord lesions had some delay in gastric emptying compared to normal patients with low cord lesions (26). Whether these are clinically significant changes or can be modified by drugs is unknown.

Colonic Motility

Functionally, three types of movement appear to be present in the large bowel:

1. Segmental movement that seems to serve in a mixing function;
2. Retrograde movement that is present particularly in the right colon as well as the rectal sigmoid area. This decreases colonic transit, thereby allowing full storage of feces and allowing appropriate time of defecation; and
3. Mass movement occurring as waves of contractions throughout the length of the colon, allowing for propulsion of large amounts of colonic content.

Studies of colonic motility in patients with spinal cord injury have been mainly anecdotal and subject to a variety of interpretations. One group, however, has repeatedly reported abnormalities in pressure-volume relationships (compliance) in the colon of patients with spinal cord injuries. Glick, Meshkinpour, and their colleagues have shown that for a given distending volume, the colonic pressure is much higher in patients with spinal cord injuries than normal controls (31, 42). It is not known whether this observation is responsible for any clinical problems or whether it can be modified by diet or drugs.

The Anal Sphincters and the Control of Continence

The control and function of the anal sphincters and the rectum have received considerable attention. As early as 1877, the relaxation of the internal anal sphincter in response to distention of the rectum was described (33).

Continence at rest is largely dependent on the action of the anal sphincters. The internal anal sphincter is composed of smooth muscle and is really an expanded portion of the enteric muscle coat of the colon. The external anal sphincter consists of striated muscle with contributions from the muscles of the pelvic floor.

The internal anal sphincter maintains its tone at rest but relaxes to rectal distention (the anorectal reflex) (19, 28, 33, 59). In the normal state, the external anal sphincter also maintains tonic activity. As rectal distention increases and the internal anal sphincter relaxes, the external anal sphincter tone increases further. This now allows for voluntary control of evacuation of the rectum as the external anal sphincter is under CNS control via its striated muscle component. There is a rich supply of sensory nerves to the distal portion of the anal canal that respond to pain, pressure, temperature, and stool consistency. This allows for monitoring of the process of defecation. Defecation is normally achieved by voluntary relaxation of the external anal sphincter and increased intraabdominal pressure by fixing the diaphragm and contracting the abdominal muscles (58). Defecation can, of course, be achieved even if this "straining" is voluntarily suppressed.

Following spinal cord injury, changes occur affecting the control of anorectal function. The anorectal reflex described above is preserved (19, 31, 57, 59). This is controlled by the enteric nervous system and therefore it is independent of the level of the spinal cord injury. The major problem lies in the disruption of the CNS input to the external anal sphincter.

Afferent sensory input to the brain is disrupted. However, unless otherwise damaged, the intact spinal reflex continues to control the external sphincter. In both normals and patients with spinal cord injury, rectal distention above the conus medullaris produces an initial rise in the tone of the external anal sphincter, but this soon relaxes in SCI patients, causing automatic defecation. In the intact patient, voluntary control of the external sphincter allows for suppression of the urge to defecate to a much greater distention of the rectum (28).

The reflex relaxation of the internal sphincter by rectal distention can be utilized to maintain normal bowel habits in patients with spinal cord injury, initiating defecation with suppositories or digital stimulation. Regular timing of meals, adequate fiber intake, and assumption of a vertical posture as soon as possible are helpful in the rehabilitation of normal bowel habits. Unfortunately, the spontaneity and ease of defecation tends to deteriorate with time, resulting in the need for laxatives and enemas. It appears that careful maintenance of normal bowel habits may retard this deterioration (34).

Parasympathetic Disturbances

The parasympathetic supply to the upper G.I. tract is via the vagus. This nerve supplies the small bowel and possibly the right and transverse colon.

The exact extent of vagal supply to the colon is uncertain (18, 21). The rectum and distal colon are supplied by the nervi erigentes that originate from the second, third, and fourth sacral nerves.

Truncal vagotomy has no regularly demonstrable effect on gut motility. Trauma to the lumbar spine and pelvis, however, may result in damage to the parasympathetic supply to the distal colon and rectum, and these injuries as well as surgical resection of the nervi erigentes have been reported to cause abnormal anal reflexes and chronic constipation (18, 20, 21). A few patients have been treated successfully by surgically bypassing the distal colonic segment (20, 21).

CONSTIPATION

Chronic constipation, with or without spurious diarrhea, occurs frequently in patients with spinal cord injury. Treatment and prevention of this complication plays a major part in management of these patients. Procedures range from manual disimpaction through a variety of enema preparations to laxatives. Many of these preparations are ancient, and their mode of action is poorly understood. Some preparations are frankly dangerous and should be abandoned. All this may present particular problems in patients with spinal cord injury.

There has been renewed interest in the physiology of laxative action in recent years, and as the clinical pharmacology becomes unraveled, the old classification will need to be changed. In this discussion we will use the old classification but will refer to some of the current theories on the physiological bases of the specific laxative actions (2, 24).

Enemas

Soapsud Enemas

Enema preparations using various concentrations of soapsuds have no place in modern medicine. They have been widely reported to cause mucosal damage and deliver large amounts of sodium and potassium to the colon, which may result in severe electrolyte imbalance and hypovolemic shock.

Tap water enemas are usually safe but should be given with caution in patients who have renal impairment because of the problem of possible water intoxication.

Saline Enemas

A variety of enemas use saline or hypertonic concentrations of sodium phosphate-biophosphate. When administered carefully, these are usually mild enemas that act by irrigating the colon and breaking up the particles of stool. Sodium absorption may be a problem, especially if there is impaired renal function.

Oil Retention Enemas

Enemas using various volumes of mineral oil have been popular for severe constipation. Once again, this mode of action seems to be entirely mechanical, with the oil having a lubricant action on the particles of stool.

There is a suggestion that mineral oil, especially when taken orally, may coat the stool and therefore inhibit the action of the colon in absorbing fluid and dehydrating the stool. Mineral oil is messy, unpleasant to use, and has been reported to cause lipoid pneumonia when taken orally. It is another product that is obsolete and should be abandoned.

Laxatives

The traditional classification of laxatives is based on what was considered to be their mode of action. The current theories are not established well enough to allow for a change in this now somewhat descriptive classification (55).

Bulk Laxatives

There is controversy about the action of fiber and the consequences of fiber deficient diets. Low fiber diets have been implicated in causing "many of the diseases of civilization" (12), such as gallbladder disease, coronary artery disease, diabetes, and colon cancer. There is significant controversy as to whether some of these problems are due to the Western diet being low in fiber or too high in other components, such as saturated fats. There is no doubt, however, that a high fiber diet is effective in preventing and managing constipation.

Unfortunately, even the definition of what types of fiber are important is somewhat controversial, and the effects of various constituents of dietary fiber differ. Wheat fiber in various preparations of bran contains cellulose as well as lignin and various gums. Other preparations, such as psyllium hydrophilic mucilloid (Metamucil), are mainly cellulose and hemicellulose.

The action of all the fiber preparations seems to be based on their ability to hold water in the stool. This results in an expanded and softened stool, which is associated with reduced intracolonic pressure and decreased gastrointestinal transit time. The African stool (associated with a high fiber diet) has about four times the volume of an English or North American stool, and it passes through the G.I. tract twice as rapidly (8).

Bran as a cereal preparation is the cheapest and most physiological way of preventing or treating simple constipation. Unfortunately, bran cereals tend to be unpalatable, and there are a variety of commercial preparations of bran as cookies or compressed pellets designed to make it easier to take. The target is to increase the dietary fiber to 10 to 20 gm per day.

There are other bulk-forming agents whose mode of action is similar to bran. The most popular is psyllium, presented in a variety of commercial preparations (Metamucil, Prodiem). Other less commonly used preparations include Ispaghula and Sterculia gum extracts.

Stimulants

This group of laxatives was thought to act by irritating or stimulating the gut and increasing motility. It now seems much more likely that the increased motility is due to the stimulation of active fluid secretion into the gut lumen (24). There are three commonly used types: the diphenylmethane laxatives, the anthracene glycosides, and Castor Oil.

Diphenylmethane Laxatives. *Phenolphthalein.* Phenolphthalein is the active ingredient in many of the over-the-counter laxatives. It is tasteless, odorless, and commonly used in various chocolate preparations. The drug is absorbed from the gut and gets involved in the enterohepatic circulation. It is excreted in bile as the glucuronide and has its laxative action in this form. Although listed as a "stimulant laxative," phenolphthalein appears to act in the experimental animal by accumulation of fluid and electrolytes in the intestinal lumen. Phenolphthalein had been used as an indicator in organic chemistry, and its presence in the stool can be detected by adding alkali (sodium hydroxide) to the stool, which results in an immediate color change. This drug is moderately potent with relatively few side effects. However, because of its wide availability, it is commonly abused (52).

Oxyphenisatin. This drug, related to phenolphthalein, has been shown to cause chronic active hepatitis. It is no longer available in North America but may still be available elsewhere. It should not be used (16).

Bisacodyl. This drug is effective both as a suppository and as an oral preparation. Free bisacodyl is absorbed from the small bowel and the colon and is reexcreted in the bile as the glucuronide. The glucuronide is not absorbed in the small bowel and is deconjugated by bacterial action in the colon. Deconjugation and presentation of the drug to the colon was considered essential for its action, but this has now been questioned (56). On the contrary, this is another drug that appears to act by net accumulation of fluid and electrolytes in the small bowel (25).

Anthracene Glycosides (Anthraquinones). The commonly used Anthraquinones include senna, cascara sagrada, and danthron. Senna and cascara sagrada are both more potent than phenolphthalein or danthron. Both these substances are glycosides, and the molecule requires hydrolysis by colonic bacteria for its action. These compounds have been demonstrated to stimulate peristalsis in the colon after direct application to the mucosa, and the effects can be prevented by application of a topical local anesthetic (35).

These drugs also have been shown to produce net sodium and water accumulation in the gut (30). The relative importance of the effects on the colon and those on water and electrolyte secretion is yet to be determined.

Chronic use of senna may cause pigmentation of the colonic mucosa (melanosis coli). This is reversible with withdrawal of the drug, but chronic use may actually cause bowel damage.

Danthron. Unlike senna and cascara sagrada, Danthron is not a glycoside and is somewhat less potent. It is absorbed in the small bowel and detoxified in the liver. It may color the urine pink or orange.

Castor Oil. Castor oil is a very potent laxative that has been extensively investigated in recent years. The active principle is ricinoleic acid, a hydroxy fatty acid. It has potent effects on fluid secretion into the bowel, similar to the action of cholera toxin in stimulating cyclic AMP in the small bowel (41). Castor oil has a very unpleasant taste, is potent with a rapid onset of action, and is associated with violent cramps. It is best avoided in routine clinical practice.

Stool Softeners

Dioctyl Sodium Sulfosuccinate. Dioctyl sodium sulfosuccinate is widely promoted as a laxative because of its detergent effect in softening of the stool. Its action is similar to that of castor oil in producing net water accumulation in the intestine which appears to be accomplished by inhibition of Na-K-ATPase and stimulation of adenyl cyclase (5, 48). The detergent-like action of dioctyl sodium sulfosuccinate causes some disruption of the gastric and intestinal mucosa (1, 13). It would appear to increase the intestinal absorption of other drugs concurrently administered and may increase their toxicity (60).

Osmotic Laxatives

The mechanism of action of osmotic laxatives is thought to be the simple retention of osmotically active small molecules that retain water in the bowel lumen. Compounds such as magnesium sulfate and sodium phosphate-biphosphate are commonly used in this way. This simple explanation for their action has been questioned (20). Magnesium compounds release cholecystokinin, which may account for some of the laxative action (36, 37). All saline laxatives should be used with caution in patients who have impaired renal function.

Lactulose. Lactulose is a synthetic disaccharide that is not split by intestinal enzymes. In the colon, the compound is broken down by bacteria to acetic, lactic, and other organic acids. Acidification of the stool results in reduced ammonia absorption and provides symptomatic improvement in patients with portal-systemic encephalopathy (15).

Water and electrolytes are retained in the small bowel by the osmotic effect of the unabsorbed disaccharide. This osmotic effect is augmented in the colon where the Lactulose is broken down into many smaller components by bacterial action.

Lactulose is an effective and relatively safe laxative (47, 58). The dose is adjusted to produce the desired consistency and frequency of stool. In encephalopathic patients, 20 to 30 gm three times a day can produce two to three soft stools daily. The usual dose in constipation is 2 to 7½ gm once or twice daily.

Practical Considerations

In general, the most important consideration in using laxatives, especially in the long term, is to try to avoid those that will produce discomfort or have harmful side effects. The most physiological way to maintain regular bowel habits is to ensure adequate fiber in the diet. An addition of 10 to 20 gm of fiber per day as bran is a reasonable first step in a program of maintenance of normal bowel habits. Patients who find bran unpalatable can be tried on psyllium mucilloid in one of the preparations such as Metamucil® or Prodiem®. It is important to ensure an adequate fluid intake because these products as well as the osmotic laxatives act by holding fluid within the lumen of the gut.

Lactulose is a reasonable product to add if fiber alone is ineffective. It is not a very potent laxative, but the dose of syrup can be adjusted over a fairly wide range to produce the desired degree of laxation. The stimulant laxatives are best avoided on the long term.

If a suppository is used to stimulate the defecation reflex, a plain glycerin suppository should be tried. If ineffective, bisacodyl should be the second choice.

There is a need for further investigation of the effects of these agents in patients with denervated gut. Whether they respond differently from patients who have an intact nervous system is not known. Also the implications of some of the observations, such as decreased colonic compliance for the use of high fiber diets in patients with spinal cord injury, need to be assessed.

CONCLUSION

In the acute phase of the spinal cord injury, most of the gastrointestinal complications are related to general surgical problems and nutritional support. The surgical principles of management are the same as in intact patients, and there is no real evidence presented in the literature that patients with spinal cord injuries are more prone to these complications than other patients with other injuries. Because of altered sensory input from the parietal peritoneum, there is a greater potential for delaying diagnosis in patients with spinal cord injury. Clinicians therefore have to be very aggressive with early investigation based on subtle symptoms and signs.

The pathophysiology of disturbed intestinal function in neurologically intact patients is still poorly understood. The irritable bowel syndrome is one of the most common clinical problems seen by a gastroenterologist. It is still not settled whether that disorder is caused by disturbed intestinal motility, impaired nervous or hormonal control of the gut, or is purely functional. Management is therefore still largely empirical. It is even more difficult to draw solid conclusions from the literature on the alterations in bowel function after spinal cord injury. Clinical research on the effects of different diets and drugs on intestinal motility in spinal cord injury is clearly very desirable. It would make a contribution not only to the management of spinal cord patients but would also help clinicians to understand some of the problems in gut motility in intact patients.

REFERENCES

1. Bernier, J. J., et al. Cell loss under laxatives in human jejunum. *Gastroenterology, 76:*1099a, 1979.
2. Biender, J. H., and Donowitz, M. A new look at laxative action. *Gastroenterology 69:*1001–1005, 1975.
3. Binder, H. J. Pharmacology of laxatives. *Annu. Rev. Pharmacol. Toxicol., 17:*355–367, 1977.
4. Binder, H. J., Dobbins, J. W., and Whiting, D. S. Evidence against the importance of altered mucosal permeability in ricinolic acid induced fluid secretion. *Gastroenterology, 72:*1029, 1977.
5. Binder, H. J., and Donowitz, M. Effect of dioctyl sodium sulphasuccinate on colonic fluid & electrolyte movement. *Gastroenterology, 69:*941–950, 1975.
6. Blackburn, G. L., Bistran, B. R., Main, B. S., et al. Nutritional and metabolic assessment of the hospitalized patient. *JPEN, 1:*11–22, 1979.
7. Breithaup, D. J., Jousse, A. T., and Wynn-Jones, M. Late causes of death and life expectancy in paraplegia. *Can Med. Assoc. J., 85*(July 5):73–77, 1961.
8. Burkitt, D. P., Walker, A. R. P., and Painter, N. S. Effect of dietary fibre on stools and transit-times and its role in the causation of disease. *Lancet 2:*1408–1411, 1972.
9. Butterworth, C. E., and Blackburn, G. L. Hospital malnutrition & how to assess the nutritional status of a patient. *Nutrition Today 2:*8, 1975.
10. Carey, M. E., Nance, F. C., and Kirgis, H. D. Pancreatitis following spinal cord injury. *J. Neurosurg., 47:*917–922, 1977.
11. Charney, K. J., Juler, G. L., et al. General surgery problems in patients with spinal cord injuries. *Arch. Surg., 110(9):*0, 1975.
12. Cleave, T. L. The Saccharine Disease. Wright & Sons Ltd., Bristol, 1974.
13. Cochran, K. M., Nelson, L., Russell, R. I. et al. Laxative & gastric mucosal damage - the danger of dioctyl sodium sulphosuccinate. *Gut, 18:*422, 1977.
14. Conn, H. O., and Blitzer, B. L. Non association of adrenocorticosteroid therapy and peptic ulcer. *N. Engl. J. Med., 294:*473–479, 1976.
15. Conn, H. O., et al. Comparison of lactulose & neomycin in the treatment of chronic portal-systemic encephalopathy. *Gastroenterology, 72:* 573–583, 0000.
16. Cooksley, W. G. E., Cowen, A. E., and Powell, L. W. The incidence of oxyphenisatim ingestion in chronic active hepatitis: a prospective controlled study of 29 patients. *Aust. N. Z. J. Med., 3:*124, 1973.
17. Czaja, M. A., McAlhany, J. E., and Pruitt, B. A. Acute gastroduodenal disease after thermal injury; an endoscopic evaluation of incidence & natural history. *N. Engl. J. Med. 291:*925–929, 1974.
18. DeGroat, W. C., and Krier, J. The sacral parasympathetic reflex pathway regulating colonic motility & defaecation in the cat. *J. Physiol., 276:*481–500, 1978.
19. Denny-Brown, D., and Robertson, E. G. An investigation of the nervous control of defaecation. *Brain, 58:*256–310, 1935.
20. Devroede, G., Arhan, P., Duguay, C., et al. Traumatic constipation. *Gastroenterology, 77:* 1258–1267, 1979.
21. Devroede, G., and Lamarche, J. Functional importance of extrinsic parasympathetic innervation to the distal colon & rectum in man. *Gastroenterology, 66:*273–280, 1974.

22. Dietrick, R. B., and Russi, S. Tabulation and review of autopsy findings in fifty-five paraplegics. *J.A.M.A.*, 41–44, 1958.
23. Epstein, N., Hood, D. C., and Ransohoff, J. Gastrointestinal bleeding in patients with spinal cord trauma. *J. Neurosurg., 54:*16–20, 1981.
24. Ewe, K. Physiological basis of laxative action. *Pharmacology, 20:*(Suppl.1)2–20, 1980.
25. Ewe, K., Przybylski, P., et al. Intestinal secretion induced by the laxative bisacodyl. *Gastroenterology, 72:*1056, 1977.
26. Fealey, R. D., Szurszewski, J. H., Merritt, J. L., et al. The effect of traumatic spinal cord transection on human upper gastrointestinal motility. *Gastroenterology, 82:*1053, 1982.
27. Fischer, J. E. Panel report on nutritional support of patients with liver, renal & cardio-pulmonary diseases. *Am. J. Clin. Nutr., 34:*1235–1245, 1981.
28. Frenckner, B. Function of the anal sphincters in spinal man. *Gut, 16:*638–644, 1975.
29. Gershon, M. D. The enteric nervous system; an apparatus for intrinsic control of gastrointestinal motility. *Viewpoints on Digestive Diseases, 13(4):*0, 1981.
30. Gershon, M. D., and Erde, S. M. The nervous system of the gut. *Gastroenterology, 80:*1571–1594, 1981.
31. Glick, M. E., Meshkinpour, H., et al. Colonic dysfunction in patients with thoracic spinal cord injury. *Gastroenterology, 86:*287–294, 1984.
32. Gore, R. M., Mintzer, R. A., and Calenof, L. Gastrointestinal complications of spinal cord injury. *Spine, 6(6):*538–544, 1981.
33. Gowers, W. R. The automatic action of the sphincter ani. *Proc. R. Soc. Lond. 26:*77–84, 1877.
34. Guttman, L. Spinal cord injuries-comprehensive management and research. In: *Disturbances of Intestinal Function.* Blackwell Scientific Publications, London, 1973.
35. Hardcastle, J. D., and Wilkins, J. L. The action of sennosides & related compounds on the human colon & rectum. *Gut, 11:*1038–1042, 1970.
36. Harvey, R. F., Dowsett, et al. A radioimmunoassay for cholecystokinin-pancreozymin. *Lancet, 2:*826–827, 1973.
37. Harvey, R. F., and Read, A. E. Saline purgatives act by releasing cholecystokinin. *Lancet, 2:*185–187, 1973.
38. Kamada, T., Fusamoto, H., Kawano, S., et al. Gastrointestinal bleeding following head injury: a clinical study of 433 cases. *J. Trauma, 17(1):*0, 0000.
39. Kewalramani, S. Neurogenic gastroduodenal ulceration and bleeding associated with spinal cord injuries. *J. Trauma, 19(4):*0, 0000.
40. Kuhlemeier, K. V., Miller III, J. M., and Nepomuceno, C. S. *Paraplegia, 14:*195–201, 1976.
41. Masri, W. E., Cochrane, P., and Silver, J. R. Gastrointestinal bleeding in patients with acute spinal injuries. *Injury, 14:*162–167, 0000.
42. Meshkinpour, H., Nowroozi, F., and Glick, M. E. Colonic compliance in patients with spinal cord injury. *Arch. Phys. Med. Rehabil., 64:*0, 1983.
43. Miller, F., and Fenzi, T. C. Prolonged ileus with acute spinal cord injury responding to metaclopramide. *Paraplegia, 19:*43–45, 1981.
44. Miller, L. S., Staas, W. E., and Herbison, G. J. Abdominal problems in patients with spinal cord lesions. *Arch. Phys. Med. Rehabil., 56:*405–408, 1975.
45. Osteen, R. T., and Barsamian, E. M. Delayed gastric emptying after vagotomy and drainage in the spinal cord injury patient. *Paraplegia, 19:*46–49, 1981.
46. Peiffer, S. C., Blust, P., and Leyson, J. F. J. Nutritional assessment of the spinal cord injured patient. *Perspectives in Practice 78:*501–505, 1981.
47. Porter, N. The use of laxative in post-hemorrhoidectomy patients. *Brit. J. Clin. Pract., 29:*235–236, 1975.
48. Rachmilewitz, D., and Karmeli, F. Effect of bisocodyl & dioctyl sodium sulphasuccinate on rat intestinal prostaglandin E. 2, content sodium Na-K-ATPase and adenylcyclase activities. *Gastroenterology, 76:*1221A, 1979.
49. Sewing, K. F. Interaction of histamine H2 receptor antagonists with other drugs. In: *Proceedings International Symposium "Ranitidine: Therapeutic Advances".* Edited by Ni-

siewicz, and Wood. Excerpta Medical, 1984.

50. Stremple, J. F., Mori, H., and Lev, R. The stress ulcer syndrome. *Curr. Probl. Surg., 1:*64, 1973.

51. Surawicz, C. Saunders, et al. Effects of phenolphthalein on structure and function of intestinal mucosa. *Gastroenterology, 72:*1137, 1977.

52. Sutton, R. A., MacPhail, I., et al. Acute gastric dilatation as a relatively late complication of tetraplegia due to very high cervical cord injury. *Paraplegia, 19:*17–19, 1981.

53. Tanaka, M., Uchiyama, M., and Kitano, M. Gastroduodenal disease in chronic spinal cord injuries an endoscopic study. *Arch. Surg., 114:*0, 1979.

54. Tibbs, P. A., Young, A. B., Bivins, B. A., et al. Diagnosis of acute abdominal injuries in patients with spinal shock; value of diagnostic peritoneal lavage. *J. Trauma, 20(1):*55–57, 0000.

55. W. Grant Thompson, W. G. Laxatives: clinical pharmacology and rational use. *Drugs, 19:*49–58, 1980.

56. Thomson, The irritable gut. University Park Press, Baltimore, 1977.

57. Tuelove, S. C. Movements of the large intestine. *Physiol. Rev., 46:*457–512, 1966.

58. Wesselius, D., Casparis, A., et al. Treatment of chronic constipation with lactulose syrup. *Gut, 9:*84–86, 1968.

59. Wheatley, I. C., Hardy, K. J., and Dent, J. Anal pressure studies in spinal patients. *Gut, 18:*488–490, 1977.

60. Safety of stool softeners. *Medical Letter*, 1945–46, 1977.

6

Autonomic Dysfunction

RALPH F. BLOCH

It was already known by the ancient Egyptians of the 16th and possibly 30th century B.C. that spinal cord injury involved more than just motor and sensory loss as evidenced by the Edwin Smith papyrus (8). Hilton (46) presented a case report of a tetraplegic patient with autonomic dysfunction associated with micturition and defecation. Head and Riddoch (44) clearly described the association between events involving the neurogenic bladder and systemic manifestations, such as sweating, in a case series from World War I. The foundations for our present understanding were laid by Guttmann and Whitteridge (43). Since then, various investigators, chiefly among them Sir Ludwig Guttmann and his co-investigators, have continued to shed light on the various manifestations of altered autonomic control in spinal cord injured individuals.

Despite this long and distinguished history, we still don't have full grasp of the clinical and physiological complexities. We lack a clear and universally recognized taxonomy of autonomic dysfunctions in the tetraplegic. Our present understanding of the physiology of autonomic function in general, and in spinal man in particular, is limited. We still have to better define natural history and evaluate the therapeutic effectiveness of different treatment modalities. While autonomic dysfunction is most significant in the tetraplegic, high thoracic paraplegics also are at risk for generalized reactions. Patients with lesions below the midthoracic level are more likely to complain of local disturbances.

In this chapter we will first summarize relevant anatomical and physiological facts and concepts. We will then examine various syndromes in more detail.

The first manifestation of autonomic dysfunction in the clinical course of a tetraplegic is usually apneic bradyarrhythmia. The typical setting is the intensive care unit with the patient on a respirator. As the patient is being suctioned, he suddenly becomes bradycardic, or possibly develops sinus arrest, and goes into shock. Unfamiliarity with this syndrome has lead to inappropriate insertion of permanent pacemakers. As patients become more stable and are being mobilized, they start to develop orthostatic hypotension on sitting up. With the return of spasticity and automatic function of bowel and bladder, many tetraplegics start to show evidence of autonomic dysreflexia, i.e. hypertension, bradycardia, sweating, headaches, and other abnormalities in response to various noxious stimuli. Other areas we will discuss include the abnormal response to environmental temperature, changes in glucose homeostasis, and special considerations in the anesthetic management of the tetraplegic.

ANATOMY AND PHYSIOLOGY

The role of the autonomic nervous system was succinctly defined by Claude Bernard (6) as being responsible for the maintenance of a stable internal environment in the human body. The current standard reference is the textbook by Appenzeller (2).

The autonomic nervous system comprises all neurons outside the central nervous system that are not involved either with the acquisition of information from the external environment and the state of the locomotor system or with the control of striated muscle. Central nervous system pathways directly connected with these peripheral neurons also form part of the autonomic nervous system.

The autonomic nervous system has two major divisions: the sympathetic and the parasympathetic, each comprising both pre- and postganglionic fibers. The autonomic ganglia are anatomically well-defined agglomerates of the postganglionic cell bodies with their synaptic connections, serving as relay stations, lying outside the central nervous system. The preganglionic cell bodies usually lie in the brain or spinal cord. Most organs have both sympathetic and parasympathetic innervation. Some, however, such as sweat glands, piloerector muscles, and smooth muscle of some blood vessels, receive sympathetic innervation only.

Besides the well known efferent pathways, there are also afferent neurons running with the autonomic nervous system. In the parasympathetic division, the carotid sinus nerve and the depressor nerve, contained in the glossopharyngeal and vagus nerves, carrying afferent impulses from stretch and chemoreceptors in the walls of the carotid artery, heart, and aorta, are generally well known. Less well recognized is the presence of afferent fibers in the sympathetic pathways (75, 86).

The most central control of autonomic function is located in the hypothalamus (10, 36, 47). A hierarchical system of reflex loops centered along the neuraxis serves to control body temperature, sweating, other eccrine and some endocrine secretions, heartrate, cardiac contractility, and contraction of smooth muscle in airways, vessel walls, the skin, and the alimentary and urogenital systems. In this chapter we will ignore the autonomic innervation of the alimentary and genitourinary systems since these are covered elsewhere.

Pathways pass from the hypothalamus anterolaterally along the aqueduct of Sylvius, close to the red nucleus, and then laterally through the medulla. The parasympathetic division has its preganglionic neurons in the brainstem and the sacral cord. The parasympathetic preganglionic cells are situated in the Edinger-Westphal nucleus in the floor of the aqueduct, and the parasympathetic nuclei of the seventh, ninth, and tenth cranial nerves in the medulla. Autonomic fibers descend in the lateral white columns of the spinal cord. The sympathetic preganglionic neurons are situated in the intermediolateral grey columns of the spinal cord from T1 to L2. The parasympathetic preganglionic neurons of the sacral division also are situated in the intermediolateral grey matter, though they form a nucleus rather than a column.

There are three types of ganglia: para- and prevertebral ganglia, where sympathetic neurons synapse, and peripheral ganglia for parasympathetic synapses.

Myelinated preganglionic sympathetic fibers leave the cord through the ventral roots, passing a short distance through the ventral ramus. Through the white ramus communicans, they then reach the sympathetic ganglia and chain. Ascending sympathetic fibers in the neck synapse in three distinct cervical ganglia, i.e. the stellate, middle, and superior cervical ganglion. Unmyelinated postganglionic sympathetic fibers leave the ganglia through the grey rami communicantes, spreading out towards their target organs. Since all sympathetic outflow is below the cervical segments, complete cervical cord injuries effectively cause sympathetic deefferentiation. High thoracic lesions can still result in partial loss of sympathetic control of circulation and body temperature. Because of the sympathetic control of adrenal medulla, juxtaglomerular cells (20), and pineal gland (70) tetraplegia may also lead to major endocrine alterations. Corresponding clinical abnormalities remain to be studied.

Parasympathetic ganglia are situated within the target organs. The major parasympathetic supply to the body comes through the vagus, though the afferents from the carotid sinus and bodies seem to travel with the glossopharyngeus nerve. Since it leaves the central nervous system in the brainstem, vagal supply is spared in cervical injuries. Sacral parasympathetic supply to the urogenital and distal alimentary tract is commonly disturbed in most spinal cord injuries.

The transmitter in both sympathetic and parasympathetic ganglia is acetylcholine, which is also the common parasympathetic postganglionic transmitter. Sympathetic postganglionic action is mostly mediated by noradrenaline, though there are exceptions as in the innervation of sweat glands and vasodilator nerves to skeletal muscles, which release acetylcholine. Quite likely other neurotransmitters, such as dopamine (83) and ATP (9), will be shown to be involved as well.

Acetylcholine is hydrolyzed by acetylcholinesterase to choline and acetic acid. Norepinephrine, on the other hand, is inactivated mainly through reuptake by the nerve terminal, though it is also metabolized by the combined actions of monoamine oxidase (MAO) and catechol-O-methyl-transferase (COMT) (3).

APNEIC BRADYARRHYTHMIA

Apneic bradyarrhythmia is a syndrome of sudden shock and bradycardia, possibly proceeding to sinus arrest in response to tracheal suctioning.

A common setting for apneic bradyarrhythmia is in the tetraplegic on a respirator who is being suctioned for tracheal secretions. Within a few seconds, the heart rate may slow severely or stop all together, and the patient may go into shock. Restoration of ventilation is usually enough to reverse the episode (93).

In experimental spinal cord injury, the initial cardiovascular response is an acute rise in mean arterial and pulse pressure, and sinus tachycardia. This is shortly followed by sinus pauses, a shifting sinus pacemaker, nodal escape beats, brief runs of atrial fibrillation, multifocal premature ventricular contractions, ventricular tachycardia, and ST-T wave changes. Ectopic atrial and ventricular rhythm disturbances respond to atropinization. Control of tachycardia and ST-T changes requires both vagal and beta blockade (37, 38).

This immediate period of apparent sympathetic hyperactivity is followed by a reduction in plasma catecholamines (13, 19, 34, 65). This is associated with reduced cardiac contractility, increased venous capacity, and a tendency toward an increased incidence of pulmonary edema in response to plasma volume expansion (68).

The exact causes for these changes remain to be fully determined. The most basic explanation, sympathetic defferentation with vagal preponderance, is unlikely to completely explain all the phenomena described. Other mechanisms that must be taken into consideration are the vago-vagal reflex (32, 92), the specific role of hypoxia (1, 5, 28), the consequences of differential dysfunction of left and right stellate ganglia (63, 81, 89), and the role of endogenous opiate systems (48).

Incidence and natural history of apneic bradyarrhythmia have not been established. Current awareness is based on case reports and case series at best. An audit of autonomic drug prescription patterns (11) suggests that apneic bradyarrhthmia is not important after the patient leaves the intensive care unit. Apneic bradyarrhythmia in chronic tetraplegic patients does not appear to be a problem (35).

The management of apneic bradyarrhythmia is based on the careful avoidance of hypoxia and the use of prophylactic or symptomatic atropine. Transvenous pacemakers have been used episodically, but review of the literature has not shown that permanent pacemakers need be employed with an otherwise normal heart.

ORTHOSTATIC HYPOTENSION

Tetraplegic patients who suffer from orthostatic or postural hypotension faint and have abnormally low systolic and diastolic blood pressures when they first sit up rapidly, be it in bed or wheelchair. The symptoms quickly abate when the patient resumes the recumbent position (41).

The natural history of orthostatic hypotension is not well established. Tetraplegics rarely sit up in the first few weeks of their injury since spinal instability, associated injuries, and general homeostatic instability confine them to bed, often in an intensive care setting. Conversely, orthostatic hypotension uncommonly is clinically important in chronic tetraplegics once they assume regular activities, even though it is still demonstrable with appropriate blood pressure recording. Repeated postural challenge seems to reduce the severity of hypotensive episodes in the short term (17, 54). Review of temporal prescription profiles in tetraplegics suggests that drugs that tend to raise blood pressure and pulse rate are prescribed most commonly between the first and third month after the injury (11). Though orthostatic hypotension is recognized as a fairly common phenomenon in early tetraplegia, true incidence and prevalence are not known. Though chronic tetraplegics still show a hypotensive response to postural change, they rarely faint on sitting up. It has not yet been established whether this is due to a reduced fall in blood pressure, improved collateral cerebral circulation, or altered cerebrovascular autoregulation.

There are also major gaps in our understanding of the patho-physiology of orthostatic hypotension. Postural hypotension is by no means limited to subjects with tetraplegia. It has been described in patients subjected to prolonged immobilization (69), the elderly (55) patients with diabetic neuropathy (94), Guillain-Barre syndrome (52), Parkinsonism (4), and various rarer degenerative and congenital diseases of the nervous system, as well as such systemic disorders as amyloidosis and porphyria (56).

In normals, stable blood pressure is maintained by an increase in cardiac output or peripheral resistance in response to any fall in central arterial blood pressure, the so-called baroreceptor reflex (29). Cardiac output is determined by heartrate and stroke volume, which in turn depends on preload, cardiac contractility, and afterload. The preload, representing diastolic ventricular filling, is a function of intravascular blood volume and venous tone. Except for a component of heart rate, all these parameters are controlled by sympathetic pathways (21), that are deefferented in tetraplegics and quantitatively reduced in subjects with high thoracic lesions. In the acute period, release of catecholamines in response to postural change, as reflected in urinary excretion of methoxyhydroxymandelic acid, is reduced (87), while the serum dopamine-beta-hydroxylase level (57) appears to increase in response to tilting, suggesting that the neuronal synthesis of norepinephrine may still be responsive to gravitational stress, the release is not. In chronic tetraplegics, on the other hand, raised urinary MHMA levels after tilting might suggest recovery of some postural reflexes, possibly at a spinal level. These findings require further experimental confirmation (13).

The massive sympathetic discharge in response to gravitational challenge of normal subjects causes a sufficient vasomotor, inotropic and mild chronotropic response to maintain a stable blood pressure. As a result, there is no need for a change in fluid balance. In tetraplegic subjects, on the other hand, there is no significant sympathetic response to postural changes to prevent venous pooling in the dependent areas, and increase the pumping action of the heart and the peripheral vascular resistance. Prolonged bedrest causes reduced tissue turgor with resulting extravasation of fluid in the dependent areas and a reduction of the intravascular volume. As a consequence, there is a marked decrease in venous return and cardiac output. A compensatory attempt at increasing heartrate by reduced vagal tone is insufficient to maintain cardiac output. Associated with these neuroregulatory changes is a decrease of urinary output and a significant decrease in the urinary Na/K ratio. Since there is no consistent release of cortisol, these results suggest release of antidiuretic hormone and aldosterone in response to postural change. Urinary 17-hydroxy corticosteroids are, however, increased chronically in tetraplegics, suggesting a general stress response.

Differences in the severity of symptomatic orthostatic hypotension between acute and chronic tetraplegics may be due to the recovery of spinal postural reflexes, the adaptation of the renin-angiotensin system or changes in the sensitivity to cerebral perfusion pressure.

Since clinically significant orthostatic hypotension appears to be a self-limited disorder, management is directed mainly at symptomatic control during the immediate postacute period when patients first assume sitting posture. Modalities that have been evaluated in case studies and case series include pressure gradient stockings, abdominal binders, antigravity suits (49, 88), 5% inhaled carbon dioxide (23) and oral steroids. The exact place of these measures in the management of orthostatic hypotension in tetraplegics remains to be established by properly controlled studies.

AUTONOMIC DYSREFLEXIA

Autonomic dysreflexia (AD) is a paroxysmal syndrome of hypertension, bradycardia, hyperhidrosis, facial flushing, and headache in response to noxious visceral and other stimuli below the level of spinal cord injury in chronic tetraplegics and high thoracic paraplegics.

Symptoms of autonomic dysreflexia include headaches, sweating on forehead, and local flushing of face and neck. Other less common symptoms are piloerection, nasal obstruction, and paresthesia (58). Clinical signs include hypertension, tachycardia as well as bradycardia, hyperhidrosis above the level of the lesion, penile erection, and various eye signs, including mydriasis, conjunctival congestion, lid lag, and Horner's syndrome.

The dangers inherent in autonomic crises are mentioned in the literature (59, 60, 79, 82), including seizures, transient visual loss, aphasia, and subarachnoid hemorrhage. The reports are anecdotal and do not allow for estimating the true risk for these complications. With rapid intervention, the risk is probably low. It is unlikely that the arterial hypertension is entirely responsible for possible complications since much higher levels of blood pressure are reached in strenuous isometric exercise, such as competitive weight lifting, without commonly giving rise to either headache or neurological complications.

Dysreflexia can be triggered by bladder distension (7) and infection, defecation and distension of the rectum (76), cutaneous stimulation (16), spontaneous and induced musclespasm (15), range of motion exercises (67), administration of intrathecal neostigmine, electrical stimulation for the collection of semen for artificial insemination (31, 33, 42, 77), labor (39, 40, 95), and during surgery (61, 78). Lindan (62) reported that psychological stress could trigger autonomic dysreflexia. This is contradicted by the results of a careful experimental study (45).

The pathophysiology of autonomic dysreflexia is not yet fully understood (30). There is general consensus that plasma epinephrine levels do not rise during episodes of autonomic dysreflexia. The exact role of norepinephrine and dopamine beta-hydroxylase is more controversial. While some authors report a rise in these (71, 72), others (64) failed to find a change during and following autonomic dysreflexic episodes. Plasma renin activity appears to remain stable during autonomic dysreflexia (73). Three possible mechanisms can be hypothesized in the pathophysiology of autonomic dysreflexia: loss of supraspinal inhibitory control, denervation hypersensitivity of sympathetic spinal, ganglionic or peripheral receptor sites, and the formation of abnormal synaptic connections due to axonal sprouting. Experimental evidence currently available does not allow to choose between these possibilities. Measurement of sympathetic activity in man after spinal cord injury, using microelectrode recordings, suggests that: (a) the sympathetic resting activity below the level of the lesion is lower than in normals; (b) various visceral and somatic stimuli to structures caudal to the spinal cord lesion cause spontaneous neural activity; and (c) the duration of resulting vasoconstriction was prolonged, compared with normals (90). Any of these hypotheses explain how a spinal reflex, with visceral or somatic afferents and sympathetic efferents, can become excessive and cause an adrenergic storm.

As a consequence of sympathetic overactivity, cardiac output and peripheral resistance increase, resulting in a rise in peripheral blood pressure. In the absence of a normal baroreceptor loop, the system can only respond by increasing vagal tone. Heart rate response is variable since the sympathetic activity has a chronotropic effect while the vagal tone would tend to slow the heart (14).

The epidemiology of autonomic dysreflexia is based on retrospective studies. Kewalramani (58) reviewed charts of 40 patients with tetraplegia and diagnosed AD. Lindan (62), on the other hand, reviewed the charts of 444 patients successively admitted to a spinal cord injury service. The latter did not establish clearly defined criteria to diagnose AD. Kewalramani defined criteria as follows:

Bradycardia pulse rate <60/min.

Tachycardia pulse rate >100/min or >30 over basal rate.

Hypertension >40 torr over basal blood pressure. Basal values average over prior 5 days.

Unfortunately, these criteria have been neither validated nor are they widely accepted. Lindan found that 48% of 213 successive patients with a complete lesion at or above T6 developed AD over a nonspecified period. A suggested sex difference in the incidence of AD is statistically not significant. The incidence was, however, significantly higher with cervical injuries (60%) than in high thoracic lesions (20%). Autonomic dysreflexia was rarely detected before 2 months after injury and was present in most cases at 6 months. Of all patients who developed AD during the survey period, 92% had it at 1 year after injury. In the 103 subjects who developed autonomic dysreflexia, 9 demonstrated symptoms associated with malignant hypertension, such as transient neurological deficits, dyspnea, and nausea.

The therapeutic approach to autonomic dysreflexia has three components: (a) identification and removal of the trigger stimulus; (b) elevating the patient's torso to induce venous pooling in the legs and thereby decrease cardiac output; and (c) antihypertensive medication. Most rapid-acting antihypertensive drugs have been used at one time or another (Table 6.1). The use of many of these drugs has been discontinued. At present, prazosin is recommended when control of recurrent autonomic dysreflexia in otherwise mobile patients is desired. Hydralazine is the drug of choice to deal with a severe episode unresponsive to less intensive interventions when there is no access to invasive monitoring. The use of diazoxide or sodium

Table 6.1..
Drugs that have been used to treat autonomic dysreflexia.

Mecamylamine	2–10 mg t.i.d.
Guanethidine	5 mg t.i.d., tapered
Phenoxybenzamine	30 mg b.i.d.
Prazosin	0.5–1 mg t.i.d.
Hydralazine	10–20 mg I.M./I.V.
Trimethaphan*	1 mg/ml
Phentolamine	5 mg I.M.
Pentolinium	15–20 mg I.V.
Diazoxide*	1–3 mg/kg Q. 5–15 min
Sodium nitroprusside*	0.5–8.0 mg/kg/min

* These drugs should be titrated under controlled conditions.

nitroprusside is not recommended outside an intensive care unit where the drug infusion can be titrated against objective hemodynamic parameters. The latter two drugs, however, hardly ever become necessary. No data is currently available from controlled studies on the relative efficacy of the different medications. Most important is the awareness by physicians, nurses, patients, and family members of the need for rapid recognition and prompt intervention.

TEMPERATURE CONTROL

Heat prostration and hypothermia are likely to occur in spinal cord injured subjects. The true incidence and the clinical burden of such occurrences, however, is not known, despite a good understanding of physiological thermoregulation (22, 25, 26, 53).

Thermoregulation, like other physiological control systems, comprises afferent and efferent paths as well as control centers in the spinal cord and the hypothalamus. The system senses skin temperature peripherally and core temperature centrally. Temperature regulation is based on changing production and loss of heat. There theoretically are three mechanisms each to raise and lower body core temperature: (a) peripheral vasoconstriction; (b) shivering; and (c) biochemical changes to less efficient metabolic pathways to raise the temperature. To lower core temperature, the body may use: (a) peripheral vasodilation; (b) sweating; and (c) panting.

Not all of these are normally used by the adult human. Sweating and cutaneous vasomotor tone are under sympathetic control while shivering is mediated by somatic motor pathways.

Shivering does not occur below the level of a complete spinal cord injury. In normals, peripheral blood flow appears to remain at a fairly stable low level over an ambient temperature range from 20–30°C; in para- and quadriplegics, peripheral blood flow and ambient temperature seem to be linearly related over a comparable range. In normals, a rapid rise in blood flow appears between 30 to 40°C, which is not observed in the spinal cord injured (91). Sweating is increased above the level of injury but reduced below the injury in paraplegics (51) and almost absent in quadriplegics (24, 50). There also is an excessive rise in core temperature and a decreased ability to withstand hot and humid environment in quadriplegics. Quadriplegics also show a reduced systemic response to intense localized cold stress (84), with early quadriplegic patients intermediate between normals and subjects with a remote injury (12). In patients with lumbar paraplegia, partial control of sympathetic tone and skin temperature may exist (74). Given the neuroanatomy of the autonomic nervous system, this is not surprising since collateral paravertebral sympathetic pathways may exist at this level.

Despite these major changes in the ability of the spinal cord injured to modify heat production and loss, clinically significant disturbances of body temperature in these patients are uncommon. This is probably due to the protective effects of clothing. Consequently, tetraplegics should be advised against unprotected exposure to extreme temperatures.

Excessive sweating (hyperhidrosis) in patients with spinal cord injury can be associated with autonomic dysreflexia. It may, however, indicate the development of postraumatic syringomyelia (80).

ABNORMAL GLUCOSE HOMEOSTASIS

Another abnormal physiological observation in search of a clinical syndrome is the response to insulin hypoglycemia in tetraplegics. In these patients, iatrogenic hypoglycemia, induced by exogenous insulin, causes reduced systolic and diastolic blood pressures and a rise in heart rate. There is no associated rise in plasma adrenaline. There is a markedly reduced rise in blood lactate and a delayed trough in plasma-free fatty acids. Despite the more severe fall in blood glucose, tetraplegics do not show the neuroglycopenic symptoms exhibited by normal subjects (18, 66).

SPECIAL CONSIDERATIONS IN ANESTHESIA

Patients with acute spinal cord injuries often have other, associated injuries requiring surgery. Chronic patients commonly require urological procedures and repair of pressure sores. Like anybody else, they may undergo any number of elective and emergency operations. Since patients with injuries above T7 have abnormal sympathetic function, they deserve particular attention when undergoing anesthesia. There also may be an expectation by less experienced anesthesiologists that patients can tolerate noxious stimuli more easily in insentient areas, and that they therefore require less anesthetic attention.

Clinical problems involving anesthesia in spinal cord injured patients include apneic bradyarrhythmia (93), autonomic dysreflexia (61, 78), abnormal responses to volume deficiency and overload (85), respiratory management, and spasticity.

General anesthesia with halothane appears effective in preventing intraoperative autonomic dysreflexia (27). Based on anecdotal evidence, local nerve blocks and spinal anesthesia seem to reduce the incidence of serious spasticity and dysreflexic episodes. Further studies are required to clearly and prospectively evaluate the optimal anesthetic management of spinal cord patients, both in the acute and chronic period.

SUMMARY

The various clinical manifestations of altered autonomic function in spinal man not only present complex clinical challenges but also point towards important insights into basic physiology. Much basic research and systematic clinical studies are necessary to provide us with a better understanding of abnormal autonomic physiology and to give us the tools to more effectively manage these patients.

REFERENCES

1. Angell-James, J., and De Burgh, D. M. Cardiovascular responses in apneic asphyxia: role of arterial chemoreceptors and the modification of their effects by a pulmonary inflation reflex. J. Physiol. (Lond.), 201:87–104, 1969.
2. Appenzeller, O. The Autonomic Nervous System. North Holland Publishing Company, Amsterdam, 1970.
3. Axelrod, J., Weil-Malherbe, H., and Tomchick, R. The physiological disposition of H3-epinephrine and its metabolite metanephrine. J. Pharmacol. Exp. Ther., 127:251–256, 1959.
4. Barbeau, A., Gillo-Joffroy, L., Boucher, R., Nowaczynski, W., and Genest, J. Renin-aldosterone system in Parkinson's disease. Science, 165:291–292, 1969.
5. Berk, J. L., and Levy, M. N. Profound reflex bradycardia produced by transient hypoxia or hypercapnia in man. Eur. Surg. Res., 9:75–84, 1977.
6. Bernard, C. Lécons sur les phénomenes de la vie. Bailliére, Paris, 1878.
7. Braddom, R. L., and Johnson, E. W. Mecamylamine in control of hyperreflexia. Arch. Phys. Med. Rehabil., 50:448–453, 1969.
8. Breasted, J. H. Edwin Smith Surgical Papyrus. University of Chicago Press, Chicago, 1930.
9. Burnstock, G., Campbell, G., Satchell, D., and Smythe, A. Evidence that adenosine triphosphate or a related nucleotide is the transmitter substance released by non-adrenergic inhibitory nerves in the gut. Br. J. Pharmacol., 40:668–688, 1970.
10. Clark, G., Magoun, W. H., and Ranson, S. W. Hypothalamic regulation of body temperature. Publ. Inst. Neurol. N. W. Univ. Med. Sch., 11:61–80, 1939.
11. Claus-Walker, J., and Halstead, L. S. Autonomic drugs in spinal cord injury, a temporal presciption profile. Arch. Phys. Med. Rehabil., 59:363–367, 1978.
12. Claus-Walker, J., Halstead, L. S., Carter, R. E., Campos, R. J., Spencer, W. A., and Canzoneri, J. Physiological responses to cold stress in healthy subjects and in subjects with cervical cord injuries. Arch. Phys. Med. Rehabil., 55(11):485–490, 1974.
13. Claus-Walker, J., Vallbona, C., Carter, R. E., and Lipscomb, H. S. Resting and stimulated endocrine function in human subjects with cervical cord transection. J. Chron. Dis., 24:193–207, 1971.
14. Corbett, J. L., Debarge, O., Frankel, H. L., and Mathias, C. J. Cardiovascular responses in tetraplegic man to muscle spasm, bladder percussion, and head-up tilt. Clin. Exp. Pharmacol. Physiol., Suppl. 2:189–93, 1975.
15. Corbett, J. L., Frankel, H. L., and Harris, P. J. Cardiovascular changes associated with skeletal muscle spasm in tetraplegic man. J. Physiol. (Lond.), 215:381–393, 1971.
16. Corbett, J. L., Frankel, H. L., and Harris, P. J. Cardiovascular reflex responses to cutaneous and visceral stimuli in spinal man. J. Physiol. (Lond.), 215:395–409, 1971.
17. Corbett, J. L., Frankel, H. L., and Harris, P. J. Cardiovascular responses to tilting in tetraplegic man. J. Physiol., 215:411–431, 1971.
18. Corrall, R. J., Frier, B. M., McClemont, E. J. W., Taylor, S. J., and Christie, N. E. Recovery mechanisms from acute hypoglycemia in complete tetraplegia. Paraplegia, 17:314–318, 1979–1980.
19. DeBarge, O., Christensen, N. J., Corbett, J. L., Eidelman, B. H., Frankel, H. L., and Mathias, C. J. Plasma catecholamines in tetraplegics. Paraplegia, 12:44–49, 1978.
20. Donald, D. E. Studies on the release of renin by direct and reflex activation of renal sympathetic nerves. Physiologist, 22:39–42, 1979.
21. Donald, D. E., and Sheperd, J. T. Autonomic regulation of the peripheral circulation. Annu. Rev. Physiol., 42:429–439, 1980.

22. Downey, J. A., Chiodi, H. P., and Darling, R. C. Central temperature regulation in spinal man. *J. Appl. Physiol.*, 22:91–94, 1967.

23. Downey, J. A., Chiodi, H. P., and Miller, J. M., III. The effect of inhalation of 5% carbon dioxide in air on postural hypotension in quadriplegia. *Arch. Phys. Med. Rehabil.*, 47:422–426, 1966.

24. Downey, J. A., Huckaba, C. E., Kelley, P. S., Tam, H. S., Darling, R. C., and Cheh, H. Y. Sweating responses to central and peripheral heating in spinal man. *J. Appl. Physiol.*, 450(5):701–706, 1976.

25. Downey, J. A., Huckaba, C. E., Myers, S. J., and Darling, R. C. Thermoregulation in spinal man. *J. Appl. Physiol.*, 34:790–794, 1973.

26. Downey, J. A., Miller, J. M., and Darling, R. C. Thermoregulatory responses to deep and superficial cooling in spinal man. *J. Appl. Physiol.*, 27:209–212, 1969.

27. Drinker, A. S., and Helrich, M. Halothane in the paraplegic patient. *Anesthesiology*, 24:399–400, 1963.

28. Edelman, N. H., Richards, E. C., and Fishman, A. P. Abnormal ventilatory and circulatory responses to hypoxia in familial dysautonomia. *J. Clin. Invest.*, 46:1051, 1967.

29. Epstein, S. E., Beiser, G. D., Stampfer, M., and Braunwald, E. Role of the venous system in baroreceptor mediated reflexes in man. *J. Clin. Invest.*, 47:139–152, 1968.

30. Frankel, H. L., and Mathias, C. J. Cardiovascular aspects of autonomic dysreflexia since Guttmann and Whitteridge. *Paraplegia*, 17:46–51, 1979.

31. Frankel, H. L., and Mathias, C. J. Severe hypertension in patients with high spinal cord lesions undergoing electroejaculation-management with prostaglandin E2. *Paraplegia*, 18:293–300, 1980.

32. Frankel, H. L., Mathias, C. J., and Spalding, J. M. K. Mechanisms of reflex cardiac arrest in tetraplegic patients. *Lancet, Dec. 13*:1183–1185, 1975.

33. Frankel, H. L., Mathias, C. J., and Walsh, J. J. Blood pressure, plasma catecholamines and prostaglandins during artificial erection in male tetraplegics. *Paraplegia*, 12:205–211, 1974.

34. Frewin, D. B., Levitt, M., Myers, S. J., Co, C. G., and Downey, J. A. Catecholamine response in paraplegia. *Paraplegia*, 11:238–244, 1973.

35. Garner, S. H., Bloch, R., and Sutton, J. R. Diving reflex response in chronic quadriplegia. *Med. Sci. Sports. Exerc.*, 16:2, 1984.

36. Gebber, G. L., and L. R. Klevans. Central nervous system modulation of cardiovascular reflexes. *Fed. Proc.*, 31:1245, 1972.

37. Greenhoot, J. H., and Mauck, H. P. The effect of cervical cord injury on cardiac rhythm and conduction. *Am. Heart J.*, 83(5):659–661, 1972.

38. Greenhoot, J. H., Shiel, F. O., and Mauck, H. P. Experimental spinal cord injury. *Arch. Neurol.*, 26:524–529, 1972.

39. Guttmann, L. The paraplegic patient in pregnancy and labour. *Proc. R. Soc. Lond.*, 56:383–387, 1963.

40. Guttmann, L., Frankel, H. L., and Paeslack, V. Cardiac irregularities during labour in paraplegic women. *Paraplegia*, 3:144–151, 1965.

41. Guttmann, L., Munroe, A. F., Robinson, R., and Walsh, J. J. Effect of tilting on the cardiovascular responses and plasma catecholamine levels in spinal man. *Paraplegia*, 1:4–18, 1963.

42. Guttmann, L., and Walsh, J. J. Prostigmine assessment test of fertility in spinal man. *Paraplegia*, 9:39–51, 1971.

43. Guttmann, L., and Whitteridge, D. Effects of bladder distension on autonomic mechanisms after spinal cord injuries. *Brain*, 70:361–404, 1947.

44. Head, H., and Riddoch, G. The autonomic bladder, excessive sweating and some other reflex conditions in gross injuries of the spinal cord. *Brain*, 40:188–263, 1917.

45. Heidbreder, E., Ziegler, A., Heidland, A., Kirsten, R., and Grueninger, W. Circulatory

changes during mental stress in tetraplegic and paraplegic man. *Klin. Wochenschr., 60:*795–801, 1982.

46. Hilton, J. A course of lectures in pain and the therapeutic influence of mechanical and physiological rest in accidents and surgical diseases. *Lancet, Oct. 27:*401–404, 1860.

47. Hilton, S. M. Hypothalamic regulation of the cardiovascular system. *Brit. Med. Bull., 22:*243–248, 1966.

48. Holaday, J. W. Cardiovascular effects of endogenous opiate systems. *Annu. Rev. Pharmacol. Toxicol., 23:*541–594, 1983.

49. Huang, C. T., Kuhlemeier, K. V., Ratanaubol, U., McEachran, A. B., DeVivo, M. J., and Fine, P. R. Cardiopulmonary response in spinal cord patients: effect of pneumatic compressive devices. *Arch. Phys. Med. Rehabil., 64:*101–106, 1983.

50. Huckaba, C. E., Frewin, D. B., Downey, J. A., Tam, H. S., Darling, R. C., and Cheh, H. Y. Sweating responses of normal, paraplegic and anhidrotic subjects. *Arch. Phys. Med. Rehabil., 57(6):*268–274, 1976.

51. Jaeger-Denavit, O., Lacert, P., Pannier, S., and Grossiord, A. [Study of cutaneous blood flow as a function of local skin temperature in paraplegia and quadraplegia due to spinal cord lesions] Étude du débit sanguin cutané en fonction de la température cutanée locale chéz les paraplégiques et les tétraplégiques par lesion médullaire. *Rev. Eur. Étud. Clin. Biol., 17(5):*518–524, 1972.

52. Johnson, R. H. *Some aspects of the autonomic nervous system in man.* M.D. Thesis, University of Cambridge, 1966.

53. Johnson, R H. Temperature regulation in paraplegia. *Paraplegia, 9:*137–145, 1971.

54. Johnson, R. H., Smith, A. C., and Spalding, J. M. K. Blood pressure response to standing and to Valsalva's manoeuvre: independence of the two mechanisms in neurological diseases including cervical cord lesions. *Clin. Sci., 36:*77–86, 1969.

55. Johnson, R. H., Smith, A. C., Spalding, J. M. K., and Wollner, L. Effect of posture on blood pressure in elderly patients. *Lancet, 1:*731–733, 1965.

56. Johnson, R. H., and Spalding, J. M. K. *Disorders of the autonomic nervous system.* Blackwell Publishers Ltd., Oxford, 1974, pp 79–113.

57. Kamelhar, D. L., Steele, J. M., Jr., Schacht, R. G., Lowenstein, J., and Naftchi, N. E. Plasma renin and serum dopamine-beta-hydroxylase during orthostatic hypotension in quadriplegic man. *Arch. Phys. Med. Rehabil., 59:*212–216, 1978.

58. Kewalramani, L. S. Autonomic dysreflexia in traumatic myelopathy. *Am. J. Phys. Med., 59(1):*1–21, 1980.

59. Kurnick, N. B. Autonomic hyperreflexia and its control in patients with spinal cord lesions. *Ann. Intern. Med., 44:*678–86, 1956.

60. Kursh, E. D., Freehafer, A., and Persky, L. Complications of autonomic dysreflexia. *J. Urol., 118:*70–72, 1977.

61. Lambert, D. H., Deane, R. S., and Mazuzan, J. E. Anesthesia and the control of blood pressure in patients with spinal cord injury. *Anesth. Analg., 61(4):*344–348, 1982.

62. Lindan, R., Joiner, E., Freehafer, A. A., and Hazel, C. Incidence and clinical features of autonomic dysreflexia in patients with spinal cord injury. *Paraplegia, 18:*292, 1980.

63. Malliani, A., Schwartz, P. J., and Zanchetti, A. Neural mechanisms in life threatening arrhythmias. *Am. Heart J., 100(5):*705–714, 1980.

64. Manger, W. M., and Gifford, R. W. *Pheochromocytoma.* Springer Verlag, New York, 1977.

65. Mathias, C. J., Christensen, N. J., Frankel, H. L., and Spalding, J. M. K. Cardiovascular control in recently injured tetraplegics in spinal shock. *Q. J. Med., 190:*273–287, 1979.

66. Mathias, C. J., Frankel, H. L., Turner, R. C., and Christensen, N. J. Physiological responses to insulin hypoglycaemia in spinal man. *Paraplegia, 17:*319–326, 1979–1980.

67. McGarry, J., Woolsey, R. M., and Thompson, C. W. Autonomic hyperreflexia following passive stretching to the hip joint. *Phys. Ther., 62(1):*30–31, 1982.

68. Meyer, G. A., Berman, I. R., Doty, D. B., Moseley, R. V., and Gutierez, V. S. Hemodynamic

responses to acute quadriplegia with or without chest trauma. *J. Neurosurg., 34:*168–177, 1971.

69. Miller, P. B., Johnson, R. L., and Lamb, L. E. Effects of four weeks of absolute bedrest on circulating functions in man. *Aerospace Med., 35:*1194–1200, 1964.

70. Moore, R. Y., Heller, A., Wurtman, R. J., and Axelrod, J. Visual pathway mediating pineal response to environmental light. *Science, 155:*220–223, 1967.

71. Naftchi, N. E., Demeny, M., Lowman, E. W., and Tuckman, J. Hypertensive crises in quadriplegic patients—changes in cardiac output, blood volume, plasma dopamine-beta-hydroxylase activity and arterial prostaglandin PGE2. *Circulation, 57:*336–341, 1978.

72. Naftchi, N. E., Wooten, G. F., Lowman, E. W., and Axelrod, J. Relationship between serum dopamine-beta-hydroxylase activity, catecholamine metabolism and hemodynamic changes during paroxysmal hypertension in quadriplegia. *Circ. Res., 35:*850–861, 1974.

73. Nanninga, J. B., Rosen, J. S., and Kumlovsky, F. Effect of autonomic dysreflexia on plasma renin. *Urology, 7:*638–640, 1976.

74. Normell, L. A., and Wallin, B. G. Sympathetic skin nerve activity and skin temperature changes in man. *Acta Physiol. Scand., 91(3):*417–426, 1974.

75. Pick, J. *The Autonomic Nervous System.* J. B. Lippincott Company, Philadelphia, 1970.

76. Pollock, L. J., Boshes, B., Chor, H., Finkelman, I., Arieff, A. J. and Brown, M. Defects in regulatory mechanisms of autonomic function in injuries to spinal cord. *J. Neurophysiol., 14:*85–93, 1951.

77. Rossier, A. B., Ziegler, W. H., Duchosal, P. W., and Meylan, J. Sexual function and dysreflexia. *Paraplegia, 9:*51–59, 1971.

78. Schonwald, G., Fish, K. J., and Perkash, I. Cardiovascular complications during anesthesia in chronic spinal cord injured patients. *Anesthesiology, 55(5):*550–558, 1981.

79. Scott, M. B., and Morrow, J. W. Phenoxybenzamine in neurogenic bladder dysfunction after spinal cord injury. *J. Urol., 119:*483–484, 1978.

80. Stanworth, P. A. The significance of hyperhidrosis in patients with post-traumatic syringomyelia. *Paraplegia, 20(5):*282–287, 1982.

81. Talano, J. V., Euler, B. S., Walter, C. R., Behrooz, E., Loeb, H. S., and Rolf, M. G. Sinus node dysfunction. *Am. J. Med., 64:*773–781, 1978.

82. Thompson, C. E., and Whitham, A. C. Paroxysmal hypertension in spinal cord injuries. *N. Engl. J. Med., 239:*291–294, 1948.

83. Thorner, M. O. Dopamine is an important neurotransmitter in the autonomic nervous system. *Lancet, 1:*662, 1975.

84. Totel, G. L. Physiological responses to heat of resting man with impaired sweating capacity. *J. Appl. Physiol., 37:* , 1974.

85. Troll, G. F., and Dohrmann, G. J. Anaesthesia of the spinal cord-injured patient: cardiovascular problems and their management. *Paraplegia, 13:*162–171, 1975.

86. Uchida, Y. Afferent sympathetic nerve fibers with mechanoreceptors in the right heart. *Am. J. Physiol., 228:*223–230, 1975.

87. Vallbona, C., Lipscomb, H. S., and Carter, R. E. Endocrine Responses to orthostatic hypotension in quadriplegia. *Arch. Phys. Med. Rehabil., 47:*412–421, 1966.

88. Vallbona, C., Spencer, W. A., Cardus, D., and Dale, J. W. Control of orthostatic hypotension of quadriplegic subjects with a pressure suit. *Arch. Phys. Med. Rehabil., 44:*7–18, 1963.

89. Van Stee, E. W. Autonomic innervation of the heart. *Environ. Health Perspect., 26:*151–158, 1978.

90. Wallin, B. G., and Stjernberg, L. Sympathetic activity in man after spinal cord injury. *Brain, 107:*183–198, 1984.

91. Walther, O. E., Simon, E., and Jessen, C. Thermoregulatory adjustments of blood skin flow in chronically spinalized dogs. *Pflugers Arch., 322:*323–335, 1971.

92. Weiss, S., and Ferris, E. B. Adams-Stokes syndrome with transient complete heart block of vagovagal reflex origin. *Arch. Intern. Med., 54:*931–951, 1934.

93. Welply, N. C., Mathias, C. J., and Frankel, H. L. Circulatory reflexes in tetraplegic patients during artificial ventilation and general anesthesia. *Paraplegia, 13:*172–182, 1975.

94. Yamamoto, K. Autonomic involvement in polyneuritis and its related disorders. *Brain Nerve (Tokyo), 19:*1199–1208, 1967.

95. Young, B. K., Katz, M., and Klein, S. Pregnancy after spinal cord injury: altered maternal and fetal responses to labor. *Obstet. Gynecol., 62(1):*59–63, 1983.

7

Urinary Tract Infections in the Patient with a Neurogenic Bladder

MICHAEL R. ACHONG

Urinary tract infection and its complications have long been recognized as important causes for morbidity and mortality in patients with neurogenic bladders. During World War I, 80% of all paraplegics died from urinary tract infections or decubitus ulcers within weeks of injury (27) and only 10% were alive a year after their injuries (29). In the preantibiotic era, catheter-associated urinary tract infection could not be treated. Therefore it was the availability of antimicrobial drugs that rekindled interest in the use of some form of artificial drainage procedure. Thus during World War II, early suprapubic cystostomy became popular, and most patients were managed with either a chronic indwelling urethral catheter or transurethral resection of the bladder neck and prostate.

The main complications of urinary tract infection in patients with neurogenic bladders include bacteremia, recurrent and persistent infections, persistent asymptomatic bacteriuria especially in those with chronic indwelling urethral catheters, nephrolithiasis, hydronephrosis, pyelonephritis, and contiguous spread of infection resulting in periurethral abscesses and fistula formulation (55). All too frequently, the end result was renal failure, which has been implicated as a cause of death in up to half of the patients with spinal cord injury over the last 40 years (33). This situation resulted in the old adage that "the paraplegic patient is as old as his kidneys." The goal in recent years has been to maintain the neurogenic bladder patient catheter-free with sterile urine. These efforts, together with the availability of antimicrobial drugs, have resulted in a lower mortality from renal failure in more recent studies (33), although urinary tract infection is still a major cause for morbidity and mortality in paraplegic patients.

PATHOGENESIS

The normal urinary tract is sterile except for the distal urethra, which may be colonized with organisms similar to the normal skin flora such as staphylococci, streptococci, and diphtheroids. Several mechanisms normally combine to keep the urine sterile (26). The urethra provides a mechanical barrier that isolates the urinary tract from the bacterial flora of the perineum. Voiding, with the flushing action of the outflow of urine, is another major defense mechanism of the urinary tract. Other defense mechanisms, such as an antibacterial property inherent in the epithelial lining of the bladder, are less well identified.

Infection in the urinary tract most commonly occurs when microorganisms colonizing the perineum and the distal urethra ascend to the bladder, persist, and multiply in the urine. In patients with neurogenic bladders, many of the normal host defenses against urinary tract infection are impaired (39):

1. Incomplete emptying of the bladder results in large residual urine volumes (40).
2. Vesicoureteric reflux of urine facilitates the spread of infection from the bladder to the kidneys (2).
3. Nephrolithiasis and urinary tract infection may perpetuate each other. Bacteria such as Proteus may produce the enzyme urease that splits urea to form ammonium hydroxide, thereby producing an alkaline urine that favors the formation of stones composed of a chemically complex material called struvite (19). In turn, nephrolithiasis may be a focus for persistent urinary tract infection as bacteria trapped within a stone are secluded from host defense mechanisms and antimicrobial drugs in the urine.
4. Insertion of a urethral catheter bypasses the most effective single defense mechanism of the human host, the urethra. The risk of bacteriuria increases with the frequency of urethral catheterization (11), the length of time the urethral catheter remains in place (16), and the number of times the closed drainage system is disrupted by disconnections between the catheter and the collecting tube (54). Bacteriuria is an inevitable consequence of chronic indwelling urethral catheters (72).

MICROBIOLOGICAL ASPECTS

The microorganisms usually incriminated in urinary tract infections in patients with neurogenic bladders are the Gram-negative aerobic bacteria that are the normal commensal flora of the large bowel and the perineum. The organisms most frequently isolated include Escherichia coli, Proteus mirabilis, Klebsiella species, Enterobacter, Pseudomonas aeruginosa, and Gram-positive cocci such as Streptococcus fecalis. The prevalence of infection due to the particular bacterial species in patients with neurogenic bladder is greatly dependent upon whether the patient is at home or in the hospital, the bacterial flora predominating locally, the extent of systemic and topical antibiotics used, and the extent of catheterization. Antimicrobial therapy in the individual patient and the local prescribing patterns of antibiotics spares those species that are resistant to the drugs used and facilitates the emergence of multidrug resistant bacteria. Organisms such as Pseudomonas aeruginosa, Providencia stuartii, and Candida species are more likely to be found in patients with infections associated with urethral instrumentation and those who have received repeated courses of antimicrobial drugs. Another important association is that between infection caused by the Proteus species and the development of nephrolithiasis; once renal stones are formed, however, a variety of organisms may cause infection with the stone providing a nidus.

The influence of urethral catheterization on the types of bacteria causing urinary tract infection is of special importance for patients with neurogenic bladders. In a prospective study of bacteriuria in 60 patients undergoing *intermittent* urethral catheterization for neurogenic bladder (11), 23% maintained sterile urine, 18% experienced one episode of bacteriuria, and 59% had more than one episode. Several aspects of this study should be noted:

1. Bacteriuria was defined as the isolation of the same bacterial species in any amount on two successive days. The main organisms isolated were Escherichia coli, Klebsiella species, Enterobacter species, Pseudomonas aeruginosa, and Streptococcus fecalis.

2. No topical antibiotic or antiseptic solutions were instilled into the bladder after the urine was drained and prior to each catheter withdrawal.

3. The mean length of the period of surveillance of the program of intermittent catheterization was 13.5 weeks per patient.

Not surprisingly, the incidence of bacteriuria increased with the length of time the patient was on the program of intermittent catheterization as well as the number of catheterizations. In other studies of bacteriuria during intermittent urethral catheterization, Pearman (48) reported sterile urine throughout the treatment program in 50% of 36 patients, while Ott and Rossier (47) noted that 17% of their 42 patients maintained sterile urine. These results are difficult to compare because of differences in criteria used for the definition of bacteriuria, in the frequency of catheterizations and in the duration of the treatment program. Furthermore, Pearman (48) instilled a combination of kanamycin and colistin prior to each catheter withdrawal, while both Donovan and associates (11) and Ott and Rossier (47) did not instill antibiotic or antiseptic solutions into the bladder prior to catheter withdrawal.

A related but distinct issue is the influence of *chronic* indwelling urethral catheterization on bacteriuria. In a prospective study of 20 patients with chronic indwelling urethral catheters followed for an average of 30 weeks,

Warren and co-workers (72) found bacteriuria (defined in the study as 100,000 oranisms per ml of urine) in about 98% of the specimens cultured, and 77% were polymicrobial. The ability of certain bacterial species to persist in the urine varied considerably. Of the episodes of bacteriuria caused by Gram-positive cocci (such as coagulase-negative staphylococci, streptococci excluding Streptococcus fecalis, and diphtheroids), over 75% lasted less than a week. In constrast, the mean duration of episodes of bacteriuria due to Escherichia coli, Proteus mirabilis, and Pseudomonas aeruginosa were 4 to 6 weeks, while those due to Providencia stuartii averaged 10 weeks, and extended to 36 weeks. The persistence of Providencia species in the urine once they have gained access to the urinary tract or catheter probably explains why these organisms have become increasingly important as causes for infection associated with chronic indwelling urethral catheters, particularly in hospitalized patients (28).

CLINICAL DIAGNOSIS

Urinary tract infections are traditionally considered to be localized in the lower urinary tract or to also involve the kidneys. The typical clinical picture of cystitis and urethritis consists of one or several of these symptoms: increased frequency of urination, burning pain on urination, urgency, and suprapubic pain or tenderness. With acute pyelonephritis, the typical clinical picture consists of fever (>38°C), chills, pain, and tenderness in one or both costovertebral angles or flanks, all of which are often preceded by the symptoms of a lower urinary tract infection. Although these distinguishing features have been widely applied in clinical practice, there is actually a poor correlation between the symptoms and signs and the site of infection as determined by the bladder wash-out technique (15). Despite this criticism, distinction between upper and lower tract infections is still pursued on clinical grounds because of the therapeutic and prognostic implications. These distinguishing clinical features are probably even more inaccurate when applied to patients with neurogenic bladders who may have disturbed micturition as well as complete or partial loss of sensation. Lower tract infections in particular may be asymptomatic in patients with neurogenic bladder, and when symptoms do occur, they may be atypical and consist of increased spontaneous voiding and incomplete bladder emptying with larger residual volumes (39).

LABORATORY DIAGNOSIS

Various investigations are employed to answer these questions: does the patient have a urinary tract infection, and, if so, is the infection localized to the upper versus the lower urinary tract?

Does the Patient Have a Urinary Tract Infection?

The presence of pyuria is often sought as evidence of urinary tract infection. In the clinical studies of Kass (25), pyuria (defined as five or more white blood cells per high power field in the centrifuged urinary sediment) was noted in almost half the patients who had significant bacteriuria (defined as >100,000 organisms per ml of a midstream urine specimen) but in only 2% of those with lesser degrees of bacteriuria. He concluded that "pyuria is of value diagnostically only when it is clearly present" (25). However, measurement of pyuria by examination of the urinary sediment lacks precision as performed in most laboratories. The problem is that an unknown quantity of either a random voided urine specimen or midstream specimen of urine is centrifuged for a variable period, and an unknown dilution of the sediment is then examined under the microscope (63). The use of different criteria for pyuria affects the sensitivity of this test in the diagnosis of urinary tract infection (37). Stamm and colleagues (61) suggested that a more reliable procedure is to examine an unspun midstream specimen of urine in a hemacytometer chamber used to quantitate leukocyte counts. With that procedure, Stamm and his colleagues (61) defined pyuria as >8 leukocytes per ml of urine. However, a further detraction from the use of pyuria as a diagnostic test for urinary tract infection is that it is a nonspecific finding present in many conditions, including urethritis, interstitial nephritis from noninfectious causes, nephrolithiasis, and with contamination of urine with vaginal secretions in patients with vaginitis. In patients with a neurogenic bladder, it is even less clear whether particular degrees of pyuria are a sensitive and specific reflection of urinary tract infection.

The cornerstone of the laboratory diagnosis of urinary tract infection is quantitative urine culture. The growth of any number of potentially pathogenic organisms from a suprapubic needle aspirate of bladder urine is diagnostic of urinary infection. The classic studies of Kass (24, 25) and Sanford (57) introduced the concept of "significant bacteriuria," which described a midstream specimen of urine yielding more than 100,000 organisms per ml of urine as diagnostic of urinary tract infection. Two important provisos are often ignored when applying this concept: the urine specimen should be a properly collected midstream specimen of urine, and the specimens should be processed rapidly or stored in a refrigerator at 4°C. Kass and Sanford showed that over 95% of women with acute pyelonephritis have 100,000 or more bacteria per ml of urine and that this number of organisms, when found in two successive cultures, was 90% accurate in distinguishing bacteriuria. Smaller numbers of organisms reflect contamination of the specimen with organisms from the distal urethra and perineum. This criterion of "significant bacteriuria" has been applied indiscriminately to all sorts of situations including catheter specimens of urine (52). Several points are noteworthy:

1. Bacteriuria of more than 100,000 organisms per ml of urine is an insensitive diagnostic criterion when applied to *symptomatic* lower urinary tract infection (61). In acutely dysuric women, a recent study

suggests that the best diagnostic criterion of urinary tract infection is >100 bacteria per ml of urine (62).

2. There are no quantitative studies of bacteriuria in catheterized patients that are comparable to the classic studies of noncatheterized individuals. Cultures from the tips of urethral catheters withdrawn from patients do not predict the presence of bacteriuria as it is contaminated with bacteria from the distal urethra (20). In patients with indwelling urethral catheters sampling by catheter puncture is preferred over urine sampling from the catheter end as it does not disrupt the closed drainage system. Even so, samples of urine obtained by catheter puncture may yield bacteria on culture that are not present in urine samples obtained by simultaneous suprapubic bladder aspiration (6).

3. A variety of techniques of microscopic examination of urine have been shown to be reliable predictors of "significant bacteriuria" (66, 63), but the reliability of these procedures in diagnosis of urinary tract infection presumes that the classical definition of "significant bacteriuria" is an accurate criterion of symptomatic lower urinary tract infection.

Localization of the Site of Urinary Infection (34)

The definitive test for localization of the site of infection within the urinary tract is culture of urine obtained directly from both ureters via ureteric catheterization (60). The invasive nature of this technique and the need for a general anesthetic limit its use. However, it is the "gold standard" against which other tests are compared in the diagnosis of upper urinary tract infection. The bladder washout technique developed by Fairley and his colleagues (14, 15) compares favorably with the technique of direct urethral catheterization in detecting upper urinary tract infection. In this method, the urinary bladder is catheterized, an initial urine specimen obtained, then the bladder is irrigated with 0.2% neomycin solution followed by irrigation with sterile saline solution. After emptying the bladder, 3 10-minute aliquots of urethral urine are collected and cultured. A lower tract infection is suggested by the eradication of bacteriuria in the specimens obtained after the instillation of the neomycin solution. In upper tract infections, the urine specimens obtained after neomycin instillation will have a bacterial count exceeding the first bladder wash culture by a factor of 10 or more. In the one published study where the bladder washout test was applied to patients with neurogenic bladder, there was no comparison with direct ureteral catheterization (46) so that no conclusions could be made about its value in this group of patients.

Another noninvasive test that has been recently used to identify the site of urinary tract infection is the "antibody-coated bacteria assay" (65). A fluorescent technique is used to identify antibody-coated bacteria in the urine sediment. The premise is that the presence of these bacteria reflects upper urinary tract infection. The technique is not standardized, and different investigators have used different reagents and different criteria for judging the presence of coating (42). These factors may be responsible for the unreliable performance of the test when it is compared with "gold standards" of upper tract infection such as direct bilateral ureteral catheterization and Fairley's bladder washout technique. Not surprisingly, the antibody-coated bacteria test has been found to be unreliable in identifying upper urinary tract infection in patients with neurogenic bladders (41).

PREVENTION

Intermittent Urethral Catheterization

The main mechanisms by which infection can be prevented in the neurogenic urinary tract are: (a) establishment of a pattern of automatic reflex micturition; (b) minimization of residual volume of urine remaining in the bladder after voiding; and (c) avoidance of chronic indwelling urethral catheterization. About 30 years ago, Guttman and his colleagues (21) strongly advocated a strictly aseptic technique of intermittent urethral catheterization as the optimal way to manage urinary retention during the initial and early stages after spinal cord injury. Pearman (49) surveyed 99 patients with spinal cord injuries for an average of 36 months after their discharge from the hospital and found that 98.7% of the males and 91.7% of the females managed by intermittent catheterization during the initial period had remained catheter-free. In contrast, 52 (82.5%) of 63 patients with neurogenic bladder managed with indwelling urethral catheters during the initial period were catheter-free when surveyed for a period of 4 to 43 months from the time of the injury (35). Guttman's method of catheterization requires a highly trained and dedicated medical and nursing staff. Lapides and associates (32, 36) have recommended a less stringent aseptic technique of frequent intermittent urethral catheterization that has been described as "nonsterile" or "clean." There have been no direct comparisons of the two techniques of urethral catheterization, and a practical compromise is to apply Guttman's technique to the initial care of the patient in the hospital and then use Lapides' technique in outpatients.

In addition to intermittent urethral catheterization, various forms of antimicrobial drug prophylaxis have been advocated as useful concomitant measures. In general, the prophylactic use of antimicrobial drugs would most likely be effective if the following criteria are satisfied:

1. The infection is caused by a single microbial species.
2. The susceptibility of the infecting organisms to antimicrobial agents is constant.
3. The group of patients at risk is well-defined.
4. The period of time during which the patient is at risk is well defined and relatively short.

The situation in patients with neurogenic bladders undergoing intermittent catheterization hardly satisfies criteria 1., 2., and 4. above. Furthermore, any demonstrable efficacy of antimicrobial drug prophylaxis must be weighed against the well-documented disadvantages of chemoprophylaxis:

1. The promotion of multidrug resistant bacteria.
2. Adverse drug reactions.
3. Cost of antimicrobial drugs.
4. Relaxation of other measures to prevent infection.

The methodologic quality of the majority of studies of antimicrobial drug prophylaxis in urology is strikingly poor (5, 8). For its observations and conclusions to be accepted as reliable and valid, clinical trials of drug treatment should satisfy several methodologic standards (9):

1. Prospective design.
2. Use of concurrent controls.
3. Clear definition of disease or condition under study with stratification of patients according to its extent or severity.
4. Use of random allocation to treatment groups.
5. Inclusion of enough patients in the trial to show a clinically important difference between treatments if it should exist.
6. Use of double-blind technique and explicit definition of outcome.
7. Observation of adverse drug effects.

A few examples will illustrate the shortcomings of clinical trials. Pearman (50) has advocated the instillation of 50 mg of kanamycin and 10 mg of colistin in 25 ml of water into the bladder at the end of each catheterization in patients on a program of intermittent aseptic urethral catheterization. In that study, concurrent controls were not used as the patients seen during the period February 1976 to January 1977 had the antibiotic instillations into the bladder while those seen in the period February 1977 to January 1978 received no antibiotic instillations. Even so, the effect of such antibiotic instillations was not dramatic; the mean incidence of significant bacteriuria during intermittent catheterization was 1.43% for males receiving the instillations of antibiotics and 0.75% for males not receiving them. The comparable figures for females were 2.48% on antibiotics and 1.07% not on antibiotics. Based on a cross-over study of only 31 patients, Duffy and Smith (13) recommended that 200 mg of nitrofurantoin macrocrystals be given by mouth daily to all patients learning intermittent self-catheterization. Anderson (1) carried out a randomized prospective study of antimicrobial drug prophylaxis in 64 males with neurogenic bladders undergoing intermittent urethral catheterization. Patients were randomized to receive:

1. Sterile, intermittent catheterization only with no oral or bladder-instilled antibiotics (16 patients).
2. A 30 ml solution containing 4.8 mg neomycin plus 24,000 units polymyxin B instilled into the bladder after each catheterization (17 patients).

3. A single daily dose of 100 mg nitrofurantoin macrocrystals orally (15 patients).
4. The combination of the bladder instillations with the neomycin-polymyxin B solution and 100 mg nitrofurantoin macrocrystals orally (16 patients).

Infection was defined as a colony count $\geq$10,000 organisms per ml of urine, and patients were stratified into two groups being catherized at 4 and 8 hourly intervals. The infection rates (number of episodes of infection/number of catheterizations) for the various groups being catheterized at 4 hourly intervals were: group 1, 0.79%; group 2, 0.33%; group 3, 0.12%; and group 4, 0.14%. The comparable infection rates for the patients being catheterized at 8 hour intervals were: group 1, 2.6%; group 2, 1.5%; group 3, 1.2%; and group 4, 0.32%. Thus the oral daily dose of 100 mg of nitrofurantoin macrocrystals as well as the bladder instillation of the neomycin-polymyxin solution decreased the infection rate using the criteria of infection outlined by Anderson. This definition of infection was not as strict as that used by Donovan and his colleagues (11), who considered an infection as the isolation of the same bacterial species from the urine on two successive days, regardless of the quantitative estimate of bacteriuria. The infection rate reported in that study was 0.7% in patients who did not receive any bladder instillations of antibiotics although they routinely received ascorbic acid and, in some instances, methenamine mandelate as well. The dosages of these oral drugs were not clearly defined. Dubo and colleagues (12) recommended the prophylactic use of one regular strength tablet of trimethoprim sulfamethoxazole (containing 80 mg of trimethoprim and 400 mg of sulfamethoxazole) in patients on intermittent urethral catheterization but few details of outcome were given in their abstract.

The value of oral methenamine salts in patients having intermittent urethral catheterization, with or without concomitant so-called urinary acidifying agents, is unsettled. Given orally, acidic agents such as cranberry juice (10) and ascorbic acid (3, 22) have an inconsistent and at times transient effect on urine pH. For methenamine to be converted to formaldehyde, the metabolite responsible for its antibacterial activity, it must be exposed to an acid pH for at least 1 hour (43). Nahata et al (45) studied two patients having intermittent urethral catheterization and found that urinary formaldehyde concentrations were two to five times higher than in patients with chronic indwelling urethral catheters. The production of an alkaline urine by urea-splitting organisms such as Proteus species would mitigate against the efficacy of methenamine. Furthermore, the risks of long-term prophylactic or suppressive use of methenamine in patients with impaired renal function may be considerable as acidifying agents given concomitantly or the organic acids such as mandelic acid and hippuric acid may exacerbate the systemic metabolic acidosis associated with the underlying renal disease.

Chronic Indwelling Urethral Catheterization

Bacteriuria is an inevitable consequence of chronic indwelling urethral catheterization (72). Bacteriuria may be delayed or decreased by the use of a closed collecting system (30), one in which the continuity of catheter, collecting tube, and urine bag is maintained, and the lower end of the bag opened intermittently for emptying. Urine specimens for analysis or culture should be obtained by aspiration from the catheter itself or a special side port using a needle and syringe. When such a closed drainage system is used with indwelling urethral catheters, irrigation of the bladder and collecting systems with antimicrobial drugs is of no benefit in decreasing bacteriuria (69). Condom-catheter drainage of the urinary tract is sometimes used as an alternative to chronic indwelling urethral catheterization but it may also be complicated by urinary tract infection (23, 64).

There are no well-designed studies that support the prophylactic use of oral antimicrobial drugs in patients with chronic indwelling urethral catheters (70). Although widely used, oral methenamine is of no proven value in decreasing bacteriuria associated with chronic indwelling urethral catheterization (44, 68). The problem with methenamine in patients with chronic indwelling urethral catheterization is that the optimal generation of formaldehyde requires exposure of the drug to an acid milieu for at least 1 hour (43)—a situation not obtainable with continuous drainage of the urine from the bladder with a catheter. Other measures such as daily meatal care regimens (7), daily changes in the urine bag (56), or the addition of antiseptic solutions to the urine bag (17) are of no benefit in situations where standards of catheter care and closed drainage are maintained. It cannot be overemphasized that bacteriuria associated with chronic indwelling urethral catheterization is best avoided by avoiding catheterization altogether.

Bacteriuria in patients with chronic indwelling urethral catheters may serve as a reservoir for transmission of multiple antibiotic-resistant bacteria between hospitalized patients (58). Transmission of bacteria from patient to patient via the hands of hospital personnel is an important mode of spread for organisms that cause nosocomial bacteriuria. Guidelines for the prevention of catheter-associated urinary tract infections include (67):

1. Strict Aseptic ("nontouch") technique on insertion.
2. Meticulous hand-washing by health personnel before and after any handling of the catheter or its drainage system.
3. Maintenance of a closed collecting system.
4. The collecting bag should be emptied regularly and positioned below the level of the bladder so as to minimize retrograde intraluminal spread of bacteria from collecting bag to bladder.
5. Use of separate receptacles to drain each patient's urine collection bag.
6. Particularly during epidemics of catheter-associated infection, pa-

tients with urethral catheters should be separated geographically and different personnel should be assigned to their care.

TREATMENT

Symptomatic Infections

Treatment is usually initiated after appropriate urine and blood specimens are obtained but before microbiological results are available. The important decisions with regard to treatment are:

1. *The choice of drug.* This depends on the efficacy of the particular drug or drugs in eradicating urinary tract infection, its risk of adverse effects, its cost, and the convenience of the available formulations. Sulfonamides and ampicillin or amoxicillin are frequently used as first-line antimicrobial drugs in otherwise healthy adults, although there is increasing prevalence of resistance to these drugs even by the commonly encountered Escherichia coli. This would seem more likely in patients with neurogenic bladders because they have probably had previous urinary tract infections and would have been exposed to multiple courses of antibiotics that facilitate the emergence of multidrug resistant bacteria. It is important for the clinician to be aware of the patterns of bacterial sensitivity to drugs in his own setting and to apply this knowledge in choosing an antibiotic before microbiological results are available. Patients with suspected pyelonephritis may have an associated bacteremia, and parenteral therapy may be necessary initially. A rational initial choice of treatment is the combination of ampicillin with an aminoglycoside such as tobramycin because this would afford coverage against a wide range of Gram-negative aerobic bacilli as well as Streptococcus fecalis (53). Urinary antiseptics such as nalidixic acid and methenamine have no place in the treatment of upper urinary tract infections because they do not yield sufficiently high serum concentrations to be effective against renal parenchymal infection and any accompanying bacteremia.

2. *The dosage.* This is of particular importance in patients with impaired renal function. Drugs that are normally eliminated mainly by the kidneys and carry the risk of dose-related adverse effects have to be used in decreased dosages if accumulation and the associated toxicity are to be avoided. Nitrofurantoin is best avoided in patients with renal impairment because it is not only ineffective but carries a higher risk of peripheral neuropathy (18). The dosage of aminoglycoside antibiotics such as gentamicin and tobramycin may have to be markedly decreased if drug accumulation and its associated risk of nephrotoxicity and ototoxicity are to be avoided. Patients with severe renal impairment can be safely treated with

modest decreases in dosage of ampicillin or trimethoprim sulfamethoxazole (4).

3. *Duration of treatment.* There has been much recent interest in the optimal duration of therapy for urinary tract infections (31). Upper tract infections are usually treated for about 2 weeks, the first 3 days or so being with parenteral drugs until systemic toxicity from the infection subsides. Several studies of lower tract infections in otherwise healthy young women indicate that single, large oral doses of antibiotics such as 3 g of ampicillin or amoxicillin and 4 regular strength tablets of co-trimoxazole (160 mg TMP, 800 mg SMX) are curative in a large number of patients (59). These observations should not be extrapolated to patients with neurogenic bladders until the appropriate clinical trials are done and document the efficacy of this approach in this particular group of patients.

Patients With Indwelling Urethral Catheters

The acquisition of urinary tract infection during chronic indwelling urethral catheterization has been associated with nearly a threefold increase in mortality among hospitalized patients (51), but the reason for this association is not yet clear. However, treatment is not recommended for bacteriuria in asymptomatic patients with chronic indwelling urethral catheters because such therapy will never eradicate bacteriuria as long as the catheter remains in place (72) and will merely facilitate the emergence of multidrug resistant bacteria. A drug to which the infecting organism is susceptible should be chosen for symptomatic infections and should only be continued until the symptoms are alleviated without attempting to eradicate the organism from the urinary tract.

Recurrent Infections

These are divided into:

1. Reinfection as a result of reentry of new organisms from the perineal area into the urinary tract at a variable interval after eradication of a prior infection. Most reinfections occur 1 to 3 months after stopping therapy, and the infection is usually confined to the lower urinary tract. This type of recurrent infection is not a failure of treatment but a new infection possibly related to a defect in host defense mechanisms such as large residual urine volumes remaining in the bladder after voiding.

2. Persistence as persistently positive urine cultures appear throughout therapy due to inadequate antibacterial effect.

3. Relapse as recurrence of infection with the same organism after initially negative urine cultures. This usually occurs within 1 to 2 weeks of stopping therapy. It is a failure of therapy that may reflect

a persistent upper tract infection or the presence of a calculus or other anomaly to account for persistence of organisms in the urinary tract. Chronic bacterial prostatitis may be the cause for relapsing urinary tract infection in men, particularly when no genitourinary tract anomalies can be identified (38).

The main value to the above differentiation is that prolonged, continuous prophylactic or suppressive therapy with small doses of antimicrobial drugs may be useful in preventing reinfection while attention should be given to prolonged courses of treatment for upper tract infection in relapse. Many antimicrobial agents diffuse poorly from serum into prostatic fluid, and this may explain relapses of urinary tract infection due to chronic bacterial prostatitis. For these patients, Meares (38) recommends one double strength tablet of trimethoprim sulfamethoxazole (which contains 160 mg of trimethoprim and 800 mg of sulfamethoxazole) twice daily for 12 weeks.

REFERENCES

1. Anderson, R. U. Prophylaxis of bacteriuria during intermittent catheterization of the acute neurogenic bladder. *J. Urol., 123:*364–366, 1980.
2. Bailey, R. R. The relationship of vesico-ureteric reflux to urinary tract infection and chronic pyelonephritis—reflux nephropathy. *Clin. Nephrol., 1:*132–141, 1973.
3. Barton, C. H., Sterling, M. L., Thomas, R., Vaziri, N. D., Byrne, C., and Ryan, G. Ineffectiveness of intravenous ascorbic acid as an acidifying agent in man. *Arch. Intern. Med., 141:*211–212, 1981.
4. Bennett, W. M., and Craven, R. Urinary tract infections in patients with severe renal disease. *J.A.M.A., 236:*946–948, 1976.
5. Berger, S. A., and Nagar, H. Antimicrobial prophylaxis in urology. *J. Urol., 120:*319–322, 1978.
6. Bergqvist, D., Bronnestam, R., Hedelin, H., and Stahl, A. The relevance of urinary sampling methods in patients with indwelling Foley catheters. *Br. J. Urol., 52:*92–95, 1980.
7. Burke, J. P., Garibaldi, R. A., Britt, M. R., Jacobson, J. A., Conti, M., and Alling, D. W. Prevention of catheter-associated urinary tract infections. Efficacy of daily meatal care regimens. *Am. J. Med., 70:*655–658, 1981.
8. Chodak, G. W., and Plaut, M. E. Systemic antibiotics for prophylaxis in urologic surgery: a critical review. *J. Urol., 121:*695–699, 1979.
9. Department of Clinical Epidemiology and Biostatistics, McMaster University Health Sciences Center. How to read clinical journals. V To distinguish useful from useless or even harmful therapy. *Can. Med. Assoc. J., 124:*1156–1162, 1981.
10. Der Marderosian, A. H. Cranberry Juice. *Drug Ther. 7:*151–160, 1977.
11. Donovan, W. H., Stolov, W. C., Clowers, D. E., and Clowers, M. R. Bacteriuria during intermittent catheterization following spinal cord injury. *Arch. Phys. Med. Rehabil. 59:*351–357, 1978.
12. Dubo, H., Ramsey, E., Harding, G., and Ronald, A. Intermittent catheterization and low dose trimethoprim-sulphamethoxazole (TMP-SMX) prophylaxis in bladder management of acute spinal cord injury patients. *Ann. Roy. Coll. Phys. Surg. Can., 14:*225 (Abstract No. 266), 1981.
13. Duffy, L., Smith, A. D. Nitrofurantoin macrocrystals prevent bacteriuria in intermittent self-catheterization. *Urol., 20:*47–49, 1982.
14. Fairley, K. F., Bond, A. G., Brown, R. B., and Habersberger, P. Simple test to determine the site of urinary tract infection. *Lancet, ii:*427–428, 1967.

15. Fairley, K. F., Grounds, A. D., Carson, N. E., Laird, E. C., Gutch, R. C., McCallum, P. H. G., Leighton, P., Sleeman, R. L., and O'Keefe, C. M. Site of infection in acute urinary tract infection in general practice. *Lancet, ii:*615–618, 1971.
16. Garibaldi, R. A., Burke, J. P., and Dickman, M. L. Factors predisposing to bacteriuria during indwelling urethral catheterization. *N. Engl. J. Med., 291:*215–219, 1974.
17. Gillespie, W. A., Simpson, R. A., Jones, J. E., Nashef, L., Teasdale, C., and Speller, D. C. E. Does the addition of disinfectant to urine drainage bags prevent infection in catheterized patients? *Lancet i:*1037–1039, 1983.
18. Gleckman, R., Alvarez, S., and Joubert, D. W. Drug therapy reviews: nitrofurantoin. *Am. J. Hosp. Pharm., 36:*342–351, 1979.
19. Griffith, D. P. Infection-induced renal calculi. *Kidney Int., 21:*422–430, 1982.
20. Gross, P. A., Harkavy, L. M., Borden, G. E., and Kerstein, M. Positive Foley catheter tip culture—fact or fancy. *J.A.M.A., 228:*72–73, 1974.
21. Guttman, L., and Frankel, H. The value of intermittent catheterization in the early management of traumatic paraplegia and tetraplegia. *Paraplegia, 4:*63–84, 1966.
22. Hetey, S. K., Kleinberg, M. L., Parker, W. D., and Johnson, E. W. Effect of ascorbic acid on urine pH in patients with injured spinal cords. *Am. J. Hosp. Pharm., 37:*235–237, 1980.
23. Hirsh, D. D., Fainstein, V., and Musher, D. M. Do condom catheter collecting systems cause urinary tract infection? *J.A.M.A., 242:*340–341, 1979.
24. Kass, E. H. Chemotherapeutic and antibiotic drugs in the management of infections of the urinary tract. *Am. J. Med., 18:*764–781, 1955.
25. Kass, E. H. Asymptomatic infections of the urinary tract. *Trans. Assoc. Am. Phys., 69:*56–64, 1956.
26. Kaye, D. Host defense mechanisms in the urinary tract. *Urol. Clin. North Am., 2:*407–422, 1975.
27. Kennedy, R. H. The new viewpoint toward spinal cord injuries. *Ann. Surg., 124:*1057–1065, 1946.
28. Klastersky, J., Bogaerts, A., Noterman, J., Van Laer, E., Daneau, D., and Mouawad, E. Infections caused by Providence bacilli. *Scand. J. Infect. Dis., 6:*153–160, 1974.
29. Kuhn, W. G., Jr. The care and rehabilitation of patients with injuries to the spinal cord and cauda equina. A preliminary report on 113 cases. *J. Neurosurg., 4:*40–68, 1947.
30. Kunin, C. M., and McCormack, R. C. Prevention of catheter-induced urinary tract infections by sterile closed drainage. *N. Engl. J. Med., 274:*1155–1161, 1974.
31. Kunin, C. M. Duration of treatment of urinary tract infections. *Am. J. Med., 71:*849–854, 1981.
32. Lapides, J., Diokno, A. C., Gould, F. R., and Louis, B. S. Further observations on self-catheterization. *J. Urol., 116:*169–171, 1976.
33. Le, C. T., and Price, M. Survival from spinal cord injury. *J. Chronic Dis., 35:*487–492, 1982.
34. Lorentz, W. B. Localization of urinary tract infection. *Urol. Clin. North Am., 6:*519–527, 1979.
35. Marosszeky, J. E., Farnsworth, R. H., and Jones, R. F. The indwelling urethral catheter in patients with acute spinal cord trauma. *Med. J. Aust., 2:*62–66, 1973.
36. Maynard, F. M., and Diokno, A. C. Clean intermittent catheterization for spinal cord injury patients. *J. Urol., 128:*177–180, 1982.
37. McGuckin, M., Cohen, L., Macgregor, R. R. Significance of pyuria in urinary sediment. *J. Urol., 120:*452–454, 1978.
38. Meares, E. M. Prostatitis. *Kidney Int., 20:*289–298, 1981.
39. Merritt, J. L. Urinary tract infections, causes and management, with particular reference to the patient with spinal cord injury: a review. *Arch. Phys. Med. Rehabil., 57:*365–373, 1976.
40. Merritt, J. L. Residual urine volume: correlate of urinary tract infection in patients with spinal cord injury. *Arch. Phys. Med. Rehabil., 62:*558–561, 1981.

41. Merritt, J. L., and Keys, T. F. Limitations of the antibody-coated bacteria test in patients with neurogenic bladders. *J.A.M.A., 247*:1723–1725, 1982.

42. Mundt, K. A., Polk, B. F. Identification of site of urinary tract infections by antibody-coated bacteria assay. *Lancet, ii*:1172–1175, 1979.

43. Musher, D. M., and Griffith, D. P. Generation of formaldehyde from methenamine: effect of pH and concentration, and antibacterial effect. *Antimicrob. Agents Chemother., 6*:708–711, 1974.

44. Nahata, M. C., Cummins, B. A., McLeod, D. C., Schondelmeyer, S. W., and Butter, R. Effect of urinary acidifiers or formaldehyde concentration and efficacy with methenamine therapy. *Eur. J. Clin. Pharmacol., 22*:281–284, 1982.

45. Nahata, M. C., Cummins, B. A., McLeod, D. C., and Weichers, D. O. Urinary formaldehyde concentration after methenamine therapy in patients on intermittent catheterization. *J. Fam. Pract., 16*:398–402, 1983.

46. Naso, F., and Ditunno, J. F., Jr. The Fairley test: an aid in the diagnosis of pyelonephritis in paraplegia. *Arch. Phys. Med. Rehabil., 55*:279–281, 1974.

47. Ott, R., and Rossier, A. B. Importance of intermittent catheterization in bladder re-education of acute traumatic spinal cord lesions. *Proc. Veterans. Adm. Spinal Cord Inj. Conf., 18*:139–148, 1971.

48. Pearman, J. W. Prevention of urinary tract infection following spinal cord injury. *Paraplegia, 9*:95–104, 1971.

49. Pearman, J. W. Urological follow-up of 99 spinal cord injured patients initially managed by intermittent catheterization. *Br. J. Urol., 48*:297–310, 1976.

50. Pearman, J. W The value of kanamycin-colistin bladder instillations in reducing bacteriuria during intermittent catheterization of patients with acute spinal cord injury. *Br. J. Urol., 51*:367–374, 1979.

51. Platt, R., Polk, B. F., Murdock, B., and Rosner, B. Mortality associated with nosocomial urinary tract infection. *N. Engl. J. Med., 307*:637–642, 1982.

52. Platt, R. Quantitative definition of bacteriuria. *Am. J. Med., Supplement to July 28 issue*:44–52, 1983.

53. Platt, R. Diagnosis and empiric therapy of urinary tract infection in the seriously ill patient. *Rev. Infect. Dis., (Suppl.), 5*:S65–S73, 1983.

54. Platt, R., Polk, B. F., Murdock, B., and Rosner, B. Reduction of mortality associated with nosocomial urinary tract infection. *Lancet, 1*:893–897, 1983.

55. Price, M., Kottke, F. J., and Olson, M. E. Renal function in patients with spinal cord injury: the eighth year of a ten-year continuing study. *Arch. Phys. Med. Rehabil., 56*:76–79, 1975.

56. Reid, R. J., Webster, O., Pead, P. J., and Maskell, R. Comparison of urine bag-changing regimens in elderly catheterized patients. *Lancet, ii*:754–756, 1968.

57. Sanford, J. P., Favour, C. D., Mayo, F. H., and Harrison, J. H. Evaluation of the "positive" urine culture: an approach to the differentiation of significant bacteria from contaminants. *Am. J. Med., 20*:88–93, 1956.

58. Schaberg, D. R., Weinstein, R. A., and Stamm, W. E. Epidemics of nosocomial urinary tract infection caused by multiply resistant Gram-negative bacilli: epidemiology and control. *J. Infect. Dis., 133*:363–366, 1976.

59. Souney, P., and Polk, B. F. Single-dose antimicrobial therapy for urinary tract infections in women. *Rev. Infect. Dis., 4*:29–34, 1982.

60. Stamey, T. A., Govan, D. E., and Palmer, J. M. The localization and treatment of urinary tract infections: the role of bactericidal urine levels as opposed to serum levels. *Medicine, 44*:1–36, 1965.

61. Stamm, W. E., Wagner, K. F., Amsel, R., Alexander, E. R., Turck, M., Counts, G. W., and Holmes, K. K. Cause of the acute urethral syndrome in women. *N. Engl. J. Med., 303*:409–415, 1980.

62. Stamm, W. E., Counts, G. W., Running, K. R., Fihn, S., Turck, M., and Holmes, K. K. Diagnosis of coliform infection in acutely dysuric women. *N. Engl. J. Med., 307:*463–468, 1982.

63. Stamm, W. E. Measurements of pyuria and its relation to bacteriuria. *Am. J. Med., Supplement to July 28 issue:* 53–58, 1983.

64. Storer, S. L., and Fleming, W. C. Recurrent bacteriuria in complete spinal cord injury patients on external condom drainage. *Arch. Phys. Med. Rehabil., 61:*178–181, 1980.

65. Thomas, V. L., and Forland, M. Antibody-coated bacteria in urinary tract infections. *Kidney Int., 21:*1–7, 1982.

66. Tilton, R. E., and Tilton, R. C. Automated direct antimicrobial susceptibility testing of microscopically screened urine samples. *J. Clin. Microbiol., 11:*157–164, 1980.

67. Turck, M., and Stamm, W. Nosocomial infection of the urinary tract. *Am. J. Med., 70:*651–654, 1981.

68. Vainrub, B., and Musher, D. M. Lack of effect of methenamine in suppression of, or prophylaxis against, chronic urinary infection. *Antimicrob. Agents Chemother., 12:*625–629, 1977.

69. Warren, J. W., Platt, R., Thomas, R. J., Rosner, B., and Kass, E. H. Antibiotic irrigation and catheter-associated urinary tract infections. *N. Engl. J. Med., 299:*570–573, 1978.

70. Warren, J. W., Muncie, H. L., Jr., Bergqvist, E. J., and Hoopes, J. M. Sequelae and management of urinary infection in the patient requiring chronic catheterization. *J. Urol., 125:*1–8, 1981.

71. Warren, J. W., Anthony, W. C., Hoopes, J. M., and Muncie, H. L., Jr. Cephalexin for susceptible bacteriuria in afebrile long-term catheterized patients. *J.A.M.A., 248:*454–458, 1982.

72. Warren, J. W., Tenney, J. H., Hoopes, J. M., Muncie, H. L., and Anthony, W. C. A prospective microbiologic study of bacteriuria in patients with chronic indwelling urethral catheters. *J. Infect. Dis., 146:*719–723, 1982.

73. Washington, J. A., II, White, C. M., Laganiere, M., and Smith, L. H. Detection of significant bacteriuria by microscopic examination of urine. *Lab. Med., 12:*294–296, 1981.

8

Pain in Spinal Cord Injured Patients

ELDON TUNKS

THE IMPORTANCE OF PAIN AFTER A SPINAL CORD INJURY

In the early part of the century, spinal cord injury (SCI) was tantamount to a terminal diagnosis for many patients. Although it was recognized that pain often was associated with such injuries, the problem of pain was overshadowed by the catastrophic significance of other consequences of spinal cord injury—unsuspected visceral emergencies, sepsis, bedsores—especially in the absence of rehabilitation programs. With the advent of World War II, earlier and better evacuation of the wounded, large hospitals for injured veterans, and improved vital support techniques allowed for the development of rehabilitation methods, and patients with various spinal cord injuries have since come to be able to expect a practically normal life span (23). Rehabilitation techniques and technology have made it possible for the severely disabled to enjoy a great measure of reintegration into their families and normal society, but with such advances also come problems (5, 7, 18, 23, 35). Whereas pain might be treated with sedation and analgesics in a "terminal patient," persistent pain may pose obstacles to the resumption of normal living or impair the quality of life. In this chapter, we will review the problem of pain associated with spinal cord injury and discuss the evolving understanding of pain mechanisms and the available treatments.

How Common Is It?

Kennedy reported in 1946 that one-third to one-half of spinal cord injured patients will have some form of unpleasant sensory disturbance, such as root pains or causalgia. He added that such pain tends to decrease with time, but that in less than 10% of cases, it may be both severe and persistent enough to warrant surgical intervention (23). Similarly, Loyal Davis reported in 1947 on a series of 471 spinal cord injured patients, mostly war veterans. Although 90% of these patients had pain at some time following injury, 27% were experiencing pain sufficient to interfere with their function

(7). Botterell (1953) reported in 125 cases of spinal injury that 6% had no pain, 64% had a degree of pain that was not disabling, and 30% had pain of such a disabling degree that one-third required surgical relief. Botterell did not believe that such pain tended to diminish with time (5).

It should be noted that there are a variety of pain syndromes associated with spinal cord injury and that the time course of the onset and duration of such pain varies from case to case, anywhere from time of injury itself to more than a decade after spinal cord injury (5, 22, 36, 39). For example, in Kaplan's study of 52 paraplegics and quadriplegics in an average follow-up of 6 years duration pain was found to be present during the initial hospitalization in 19. During subsequent follow-up, it disappeared in 3 of the initial pain cases, but subsequently developed in an additional 13 others so that eventually over 50% were suffering some degree of pain, although it moderately or severely interfered with function in only 5% (22). In a follow-up of 200 SCI cases using a questionnaire, Nepomuceno found that 80% of the total group reported "abnormal sensations," which 48% called painful, 25% called extremely painful, and 44% reported painful enough to interfere with their functioning. The onset was within 6 months of the SCI for 65% of those reporting abnormal sensations, from 7 months to 4 years for 25%, and after 4 years for 4%. An unknown time of onset of pain occurred in 6%. Pain increased with time for 41% (39). In comparing studies, the impression is that about one-third of patients can be expected to have some degree of pain dating from the time of injury (5, 22, 35), and that more than half of the patients might be expected to have at least some degree of pain by the time they come to discharge. Whether or not the patient spontaneously complains of pain will depend on a variety of factors including severity of the pain itself, morale, the success of rehabilitation, and the way the question is asked.

Clinical Features of Pain After Spinal Injuries

In discussion of pain associated with spinal injury, it is necessary to consider the mechanism, level, and nature of the lesion.

When the mechanism of the injury involves trauma, in the weeks after the acute injury one must expect pain from soft tissue damage—ligaments, muscle insertions, joint capsule, and periosteum for example, may all serve as important local sources of pain. Structural damage to the spine will likely be an important contributor to discomfort because of fractures or damage to articular facets. Pain is an important concomitant of instability at the site of injury, and its presence is an important indicator of the need for further stabilization or surgical fusion.

The level of the injury determines not only what is damaged but also what is spared—both of these variables are essential to understanding the clinical pain syndrome that may present. For example, lumbar level lesions, because of damage to the cauda equina, are very apt to produce a burning dysesthetic pain but are also likely to preserve visceral sensations that might be associated with an abdominal emergency. The patient with a higher cord injury may also suffer dysesthetic pain in the lower extremities and may suffer abdominal pains in the absence of visceral disease, or a lack of abdominal pains in the presence of a surgical emergency. This will be discussed later in the chapter.

There are four dimensions of the nature of the lesion that condition the development of a pain syndrome: (a) completeness of the lesion; (b) type of cord injury; (c) specific neurological structures damaged, and (d) evolution of secondary pathological changes at the level of the lesion and in the central nervous system.

Whether the spinal cord lesion is complete or incomplete probably has little effect on whether pain will appear (although some have observed that a partial injury to the cauda equina may be more likely to lead to a burning dysesthesia in the lower extremities (5)). However, the diagnostic significance of pain rising below the level of the lesion is affected by the completeness of the lesion. Specifically, a patient with visceral disease and an incomplete thoracic lesion might experience pain in the abdomen earlier than another patient who has a complete lesion at the same level (6).

Depending on the cause of damage, very different neuropathological consequences may occur. Cord compression or contusion resulting from spinal fracture and displacement characteristically leads to major damage at the center of the cord, and there may be damage to segmental nerve roots and dorsal root ganglia in the vicinity. Metastatic tumors or vascular injuries tend to produce wedge-shaped lesions in the cord (21). Penetrating or transecting injuries may produce a combination of the above. Because the production of pain is dependent on the three factors of interrupted sensory pathways, interference with inhibitory mechanisms, and local disturbance of cell assemblies where "modulation" of input and inhibition takes place, different patterns of lesion to the cord may produce very different effects, depending on the structures that are injured (25, 26, 41). The cord being totally transected, as opposed to suffering a penetrating and partial wound, does not offer, therefore, any protection against developing pain, and painful dysesthesias are noted both in cases of spinal cord transection (30) and postcordotomy (25, 26, 54).

The neurological structure injured determines the probability of pain, its severity, and its type. For example, cervical cord injuries are less frequently associated with problems of severe pain than are injuries to the cauda equina (5, 7, 8). Botterell found that severe pain occurred in 15% of his cervical cord-injured patients but in 51% of those with lesions to the cauda equina. Similarly, Loyal Davis reported a 10% incidence of pain related to cervical cord injury, 25% in those with thoracic injuries, and a 42% incidence with lesions to the lumbar enlargement or cauda equina. Most authors agree that where there is injury to the lower thoracic and lumbar regions pain syndromes are apt to be most severe (5, 8, 39). Cord injuries may also be associated with injury to segmental nerve roots, and it is possible that the hyperalgesia that may be encountered at a sensory level margin may in some cases be due to damage to the segmental root or dorsal root ganglion (for possible mechanisms see references 1 and 20).

Subsequent to spinal cord injury there is an evolution of pathological changes likely both at the lesion and elsewhere in the central nervous system. At the level of the lesion, damage to the cord and its coverings may lead to adhesions. These may compromise the delicate vascular supply to the cord or may act as mechanical irritants tethering cord and roots during attempted movement. There is at least a theoretical reason to believe that if there is trauma to a nerve root, even if continuity is not interrupted, the site of injury may develop abnormal properties leading to the experience of pain (20). After cord transection, proximal cord function may be altered so as to precipitate pain of central nervous system origin. Whether this occurs in the distal end of the proximal cord (36, 42) or at higher levels of the nervous system (26, 30) is a matter of some dispute. In the central nervous system itself changes may occur after injury distant from the original level of the lesion. As a result of denervation, changes in neural connectivity, or neuronal hypersensitivity, pain may be generated at higher levels of the CNS (26, 30, 41). Although rare, syrinx formation long after injury may lead to a worsening neurological status and onset of new pain (49).

We will return to the above variables later in this chapter.

The Complexity of Spinal Cord Function in Health and Disease

The description of the classical sensory and motor tracts and pathways in the spinal cord as described in standard neurological textbooks is a useful approximation when applied to clinical diagnosis and prediction of deficits soon after injury. However, much research is demonstrating that spinal cord function is actually very complex. For example, while it is correct that the anterolateral columns of the spinal cord carry nociception ("pain signals") from the opposite body side, it is likely that there are both ipsilateral and contralateral alternate pathways for sensation that become particularly important when the cord is disrupted or injured. Similarly, the zone of dorsal root entry to the cord is likely the site of interaction of sensory input, local modulation by interneurons, and inhibition by neural influences that descend from higher in the central nervous system (30, 37, 41). For example, Noordenbos and Wall described a case in which the spinal cord had been cleanly cut at T3 except for part of one anterolateral quadrant. Predictably, temperature and pinprick could be identified only on the contralateral side. However, localization of touch and pressure, sensation of pain, and detection of Von Frey hair stimuli could be identified on both sides, and passive movement could be detected on the side in which the anterolateral quadrant was preserved (41). Experimental work with monkeys also seems to indicate that pain subsequent to spinal cord injury probably depends on disruption or preservation of both afferent and efferent tracts (25). It is not just within the spinal cord that pain mechanisms might be sought. A number of authors have implicated the sympathetic nervous system in the pain syndromes that may arise after cord injury (14, 24, 30, 51). The concept put forward is that afferent (sensory) signals arising below the level of cord lesion may be able to bypass the lesion by traveling the same route taken by the sympathetic supply along the vascular tree, thereafter entering the central nervous system at higher levels (14, 43). These hypotheses will be discussed in more detail below.

Pain Locations

Pain after spinal cord injury is likely experienced at multiple sites. Patients who experience injuries at the cervical level are most likely to experience pain in the upper extremities but may frequently experience additional pain in the legs, buttocks, or trunk. Thoracic injuries may produce pain in the trunk or abdomen near the level of injury, but also in the legs more frequently than is usually encountered in the case of cervical injuries. Lower thoracic and lumbar injuries often lead to a diffuse burning pain in the lower limbs, but pain at or above the level of the lesion in the trunk is not unusual. Patients with injuries to the cauda equina are the most likely to experience perineal dysesthesia or phantom visceral pains that might be described as abdominal cramps or a burning in the bladder (5, 39).

PAIN AT OR ABOVE THE LEVEL OF LESION

Spinal cord injured patients are as likely as anyone else to suffer from other painful medical disorders such as headaches, neuralgias, or pains related to infections. Depending on the level of the lesion, pain could occur in any part of the upper body and should not be overlooked simply because the patient has a spinal injury and a previous history of pain (32).

The patient may also experience pain related to the spinal injury itself, as discussed in the previous section. The pain of spinal fracture will likely be experienced at the level of injury as a dull aching discomfort, worse with movement, and probably associated with some tenderness of the paravertebral muscles near the injury. Such pain settles with immobilization and simple analgesics. Should this pain return some weeks later after immobilization has been discontinued, one would have to suspect that stability is not yet complete. Besides fracture pain, discomfort could be generated at damaged apophyseal joints so that movements of the spine near the site of injury may provoke discomfort, necessitating surgical fusion (8, 32).

Just as a workman or athlete might develop a myofascial pain syndrome because of repeated strain of a limb or muscle group, patients with spinal cord injuries who must learn to practice use of wheelchairs and transfers may be subject to similar pain syndromes. In a questionnaire survey of spinal cord injured patients living in the community, Nichols found that over 50% of respondents reported having shoulder pain. The authors suspected that this pain could be due to such factors as wheelchair usage, transfers, or other muscular strains since it appeared that this shoulder pain tended to become more common with time postinjury (40). Furthermore, in anyone who has had a musculoskeletal injury, it is reasonable to expect that a certain number will go on to have a more or less persistent myofascial syndrome in the region of the injury, showing tenderness for example, in the paraspinal muscles or in the typical "fibrositis points" of the shoulder girdle and neck (47). Pain in SCI patients is frequently associated with complaint of spasticity and muscle cramp (22). The typical description is of a dull aching discomfort, and specific treatments may be offered for the spasticity. Not only may spasticity aggravate pain, but pain may aggravate spasticity so that specific treatment for the discomfort (such as electrical nerve stimulation or minor analgesics) may have to be offered. Because of disturbed sensory function, and the possible presence of central pain syndromes and phantom sensations, it may be difficult for some patients to separate out such discomforts.

In quadriplegic patients a particularly important syndrome is the painful shoulder due to immobility. Excruciating pain may develop in the shoulders and elbows of a patient who has been bedridden for too long (48). This pain may serve as a further disincentive for the patient to participate in physiotherapy or to get himself mobile. This problem of "periarthritis" or "adhesive capsulitis" is best managed by prevention, beginning an active rehabilitation approach early on. (An innovative approach to the problem was suggested in a report of 15 cases of quadriplegia treated by positioning the patients' arms in abduction (48). Whether or not such innovative methods may be chosen, the essential is early activation.)

Although pains such as these are not unusual, their appearance should never be taken for granted. For example, the new appearance of shoulder pain in a quadriplegic patient may be due to other causes as well, such as the rupture of a viscus or other intraabdominal disease (6). Examination and diagnosis is always necessary.

A rare late sequela of spinal cord injury is the development of a posttraumatic syringomyelia. Shannon analyzed data on 13 patients, 6 with complete cord injuries and 7 with incomplete. These developed the signs of syringomyelia in periods ranging from 2 to 21 years postinjury. They all had in common new neurological signs, with a new pain complaint the most important and common symptom. Because the syrinx has a tendency to dissect upward within the spinal cord perhaps several segmental levels, the patient may experience the symptoms of pain or paresthesias, aggravated on the Valsalva maneuver, and the signs of dissociate sensory loss, weakness, and possibly Horner's syndrome all above the level of the original lesion. In cases with incomplete cord injury there may also be sensory or motor loss below the original lesion level. In Shannon's series pain was successfully alleviated either by syringostomy or by cord section through the syrinx in cases with complete lesions (49).

PAIN ASSOCIATED WITH NERVE ROOT LESIONS

As mentioned earlier, at the time of spinal cord injury nerve roots and dorsal root ganglia may become injured, torn, or caught in arachnoiditis with the result of radicular pain at the level of the lesion (18, 22). Such pain may have various characteristics, in some cases being constant, diffuse, and burning, notwithstanding the fact that the body part in which it is experienced feels numb, and the pain is not improved by touching or rubbing it. It may be worse with prolonged sitting, agitation, or fatigue, and also may be the cause of emotional upset and agitation. In cases where there has been some preservation of sensation there may be an additional quality of hyperalgesia. This means that although the sensory thresholds may be impaired, stimulation in the painful area tends to provoke a marked exacerbation of a burning or painful pins-and-needles sensation, radiating widely within the damaged dermatome(s). This sort of pain is definitely most common in injuries to the cauda equina where it occurs in a majority of patients. Thoracic injuries may also be associated with root pain, but it occurs only occasionally in those with cervical cord injuries (7). Its onset may be any where from a few days to several weeks after injury. Although the symptoms may abate with time, there are occasional cases in which the problem goes on for months or years.

A number of hypotheses have been advanced to attempt to explain this sort of pain. Howe, on the basis of animal experiments, advanced two hypotheses. Even very minimal traction on a dorsal root ganglion is capable of producing prolonged sensory fiber discharge that could be the concomitant of the radicular pain such as is found in adhesive arachnoiditis. It is also noted that damage to a peripheral nerve trunk could create a zone of irritability within the segment of damaged nerve so that subsequent minor stimulation at that point might provoke long after-discharges, which presumably could be interpreted as pain (20). A neurochemical mechanism for such a phenomenon was put forward by Wall and Gutnick. They created experimental neuromas in animals and then observed the effect of adding noradrenaline, which produced a marked and prolonged discharge in the fine sensory fibers that presumably subserve the perception of pain. These discharges could furthermore be blocked by addition of an alpha-adrenergic blocker or by electrical stimulation of the injured nerve (52). Studies such as these would suggest that some radicular pain may result from the interaction of peripheral sympathetic nervous influences and injured nerve roots. Unfortunately in practice, the results of sympathetic block are equivocal at best in relieving the burning dysesthesias associated with cauda equina injury or radicular pain at the segment of cord injury. The other possible mechanism is that there is disturbed sensory input to the cord because of root injury; since normal sensory function depends on a balance between fiber systems afferent to the cord and descending inhibitory influences, pain is released due to disturbed CNS mechanisms (30, 36).

Possible treatment for radicular pain, which includes electrical nerve stimulation, psychotropic medication, or surgery, will be discussed later.

HYPERALGESIC BORDER REACTIONS

After trauma to dorsal roots or to sensory nerves, a painful condition may arise, characterized by a painful band of hypersensitivity (hyperalgesia) extending along the edge of the damaged dermatome between the area of impaired sensation and the adjacent normal dermatome (1, 36). This hyperalgesia is in addition to any spontaneous pain that may also be experienced in the region of the affected dermatome. Similarly, patients who have spinal cord injury may experience a band of hyperalgesia at the marginal zone between the damaged and the preserved sensation (5, 8, 17, 22, 29, 30, 32). Even light touch or the pressure of clothing or bed clothes at this region may provoke marked discomfort. The symptom may be accompanied by the signs of muscular irritability or tension, and by sweating or vasodilation at and below the level of the hyperalgesia. The neurological mechanism responsible for this hyperalgesia after spinal injury is not really understood. Some have proposed that pain may be generated in the damaged spinal cord just proximal to the lesion (36, 42). Neuroma formation on the damaged spinal cord has been blamed as well, although without proof (28). Denervation may also disturb higher levels of the central nervous system with the result that pain would be generated at more central levels of the CNS (26, 30).

CENTRAL PAIN SYNDROMES

Before discussing pain of central nervous system origin, it must be pointed out that the designation "central pain" is for the convenience of the physician. As far as the patient is concerned, the pain is simply felt more or less diffusely and intensely. The patient may have difficulty in describing the components that cause his pain: whether there is a painful spasm or a spasm-like pain, or whether he feels painful visceral sensations or pains akin to visceral discomforts. After listening to the history and carrying out an examination, the diagnostician arrives at a judgment as to the probable central, visceral, or peripheral origins of the pain.

The general descriptions of the pain discussed here will be grouped under: (a) burning diffuse pain, (b) phantom limb discomforts, and (c) visceral-like pains.

Burning Pains

The same sort of diffuse burning pain that may be associated with root lesions may be encountered in lesions to other levels of the spinal cord. Although such burning pain is most common with lesions in the lumbar levels, it may be found with spinal cord lesions at thoracic or cervical levels as well. The typical complaint is of a diffuse tingling and burning pain experienced in the area of loss of normal sensation (7). This diffuse and constant pain is unrelieved by rubbing or touching the affected part, and may at times also be described as a painful pins-and-needles sensation, a crushing, or a pulling sensation. Alternatively, the patient may experience episodic stabbing pains radiating through the anesthetic areas "like a knife, stabbing, twisting, and withdrawing all at the same time." Such pains do not have clearly demarcated boundaries, and may be felt diffusely in the soles, legs, and the abdominal wall, and in the case of lumbar injuries, perhaps in the perineum (7, 22, 32, 36, 39, 42). If the patient has an incomplete spinal lesion and some degree of preservation of sensation below the level of the lesion, sensory perception may take on an unpleasant quality, usually of the sorts mentioned here. The burning dysesthetic pain syndromes, either persistent or intermittent, are the most common of the central pain syndromes encountered in spinal cord injury.

Onset of central pain may be any time from immediately after the injury to months or even years postinjury. A few cases with early onset of such pain tend to improve in subsequent years (42), but the consensus is that most pain problems persist, although it is the minority of patients who have an intolerable degree of suffering. It is the opinion of the author that the degree of suffering from such pain does not depend simply on the lesion, but also on the success of rehabilitation, the level of physical activity, and morale and psychosocial factors. This may account for the fact that pain for some people is a problem early in the rehabilitation but with time becomes much less prominent and may no longer be complained of. Whereas it is true that central pain syndromes may also occur months or years after the original injury, the appearance of such pain must not be taken for granted; any new appearance of pain requires an appropriate diagnostic workup to rule out disease below the level of the lesion or further cord pathology.

A number of factors may contribute to exacerbations of central pain syndromes; these include visceral diseases or disturbances, movement, smoking or alcohol, emotional factors, fatigue, and even weather changes (5, 7, 8). One-third of patients, particularly those with higher cord injuries, may experience an increase in their central pain syndrome with having a full bladder or fecal impaction. For example, a quadriplegic may experience headache, flushed face, nausea, and an increased sense of burning below the level of lesion when he has a full bladder. Urinary tract infection is even more likely to produce an aggravation of central pain, which would likely be associated with a rise in temperature, pulse rate, and blood pressure. Modern nursing care usually prevents the problem of bedsores, but skin lesions, particularly infected ones, may trigger a marked increase in the patient's burning pain. Some patients experience an increase in their pain when they have a fever due to any cause. Other lesions such as the fracture of an osteoporotic limb or osteomyelitis might also occur, and might remain undetected except for an increase in the central pain problem, swelling, and warmth of the injured part.

Some patients may experience an increase in their central pain problem while being moved or when they make voluntary efforts to move a paralyzed limb.

Emotional causes are very important. States such as fatigue, anxiety, or depression, or a disturbed mental state that might be associated with social or family problems may all contribute to an increased complaint of pain and probably increased pain itself.

In all of this, it is important to understand that the central pain syndrome is a product of disturbed information processing in the central nervous system. Deprived of its normal input, inhibition, and modulation mechanisms, numerous extraneous environmental and physical factors may trigger pain. Because of the possibility that increased pain may be related to occult disease, the clinician must be vigilant.

Phantom Sensations

There is no clear distinction between the diffuse, poorly localized dysesthesias and the painful phantoms suffered by patients with spinal cord injury; usually these discomforts are experienced simultaneously. However, instead of a diffuse and poorly localized discomfort, the patient may particularly experience awareness of pain of a specific body part within the region of anesthesia. For example, burning may be felt in the soles of the feet, or specific cramp-like sensations in the limbs, or patients may feel as if their legs are distorted and twisted into painful positions, when in reality they are not. Phantom pains may occur immediately after spinal cord lesions but occasionally may develop after an interval, perhaps with waxing of other dysesthetic pain. Phantom pain is affected by the same bodily disease and environmental factors that influence the burning dysesthesias. Such things as passive movement of an anesthetic body part or transcutaneous electrical stimulation may also bring about unexpected changes of position or awareness of a phantom.

Painful Visceral-Like Sensations

Just as a patient may experience phantom pain in the limbs, there may be unpleasant sensations experienced in the abdomen, described in such terms as a burning feeling in the bladder, a feeling as if the bladder were filled and painful, or painful bowel awareness resembling fecal urgency (5, 18). These phantom visceral pains are easily confused with the distorted sensations arising from the abdomen but altered by spinal cord injury. The latter problem is discussed below.

Possible Mechanisms of Central Pain

The various central pain syndromes discussed above are not necessarily due to identical mechanisms, although they may be related in some ways. For example, it is reasonable to surmise that visceral-like sensations may arise partly because of sensory fibers from the viscera travelling through the vascular adventitia and joining the sympathetic chain and thereafter the spinal cord above the level of the lesion (7, 14, 24, 43). The visceral sensations might be particularly disagreeable because of the lack of modulation of such sensory input due to the traumatic deafferentation, and the visceral sensations might be further modified by the lack of the normal parietal sensory component, the latter being interrupted by the spinal cord lesion.

One might further suppose that the burning dysesthesias that are poorly localized may arise largely because of postdeafferentation changes at higher levels of the nervous system, as will be discussed below. Phantom sensations and painful phantoms could result from "mnemonic traces" of the body image being distorted by loss of normal proprioceptive input after deafferentation.

When discussing possible mechanisms of central pain, Pollock recorded his observations in 1951 on several patients with spinal cord injuries. He noted that although there was a complete transection of the cord, a burning sensation was felt below the level of lesion, and this sensation persisted even after limb amputation. Noting also that anesthetic applied to the segment of the cord below the lesion did not abolish the pain, he concluded that such pain was not originating in the limbs nor in peripheral sympathetic fibers. He observed that when anesthetic was applied to the cord segment just proximal to the spinal cord lesion, both dysesthetic burning and also phantom sensations disappeared (42). Botterell reported similar observations in 1953 (5). He proposed that pain in complete cord lesions might result from disturbance of function of the central nervous system following the lesion, and he hypothesized that such pain "is independent of peripheral stimuli, either interoceptive or exteroceptive, arising below the level of injury ... Pain can be explained by escape of thalamic function, due to interruption of ascending spinal pathways, with resulting loss of the inhibitory effect of the normal afferent impulses" (5). The idea that painful disturbance may arise in the segments of cord just above the lesion might gain further support from the work of Nashold, who reported his technique of "dorsal-root entry zone coagulations" (DREZ coagulations) at the level of and just above the cord lesion for the relief of the intractable pain following SCI (36). Taking the existence of painful neuromas after peripheral nerve injury as an analogy, some have proposed that these pain syndromes are due to the development of neuromas in the region of the damaged cord (42). Mathews in fact observed that minute neuromas have been described involving the nerves that travel with the blood vessels supplying the cord in the case of syringomyelia and traumatic transection. He further observed that these neuromas may increase in size with time and hypothesized that they may have some bearing on pain syndromes that develop some time after cord injury (28).

On the other hand, Melzack and Loeser surveyed the literature on "phantom body pain in paraplegics" and "central pain syndromes." They cited the evidence that pain may persist although there is complete cord transection or even cordectomy with segments of the cord removed. Because sympathetic block with anesthetics fails to relieve such pain, and spinal cord resections above the levels of the original lesion also fail to stop phantom pain, and because such pains may even exist in high spinal cord injury, they hypothesized that there may exist "central pattern-generating mechanisms" depending on a disturbed balance of input and inhibition in higher brain centers after deafferentation (30). Levitt performed a left-sided cordotomy in six macaques; this procedure led to the development of a painful deafferentation syndrome (characterized by self-mutilation of the right hind limb) in all monkeys after a lapse of a few days. After the deafferentation syndrome had developed, another cordotomy was performed at a different segmental level on the right side of the cord (ipsilateral to the painful limb). Not only did this second cordotomy fail to relieve the deafferentation syndrome produced by the first lesion but it also led to the appearance of a deafferentation syndrome in the left hind leg in four of the six monkeys. The syndrome was bilaterally symmetrical despite the fact that the lesions on the two sides of the cord were at different segmental levels. Levitt cited evidence that the deafferentation syndrome can be prevented by simultaneous or prior lesioning of the CNS at the following locations: spinal cord hemisection at the same segmental level ipsilateral to the deafferentation syndrome (contralateral to the first lesion), the ipsilateral deep cerebellar nuclei, the contralateral precentral gyrus, or the contralateral bulbar pyramid. However, such CNS lesioning after the deafferentation syndrome is developed does not alleviate the syndrome. Levitt interpreted the findings as evidence that the postcordotomy experimental pain syndrome depended on development of supraspinal CNS abnormalities triggered by deafferentation (26). The interpretation that pain syndromes after cord injury depend on central mechanisms might be seen to gain support from the common observation in rehabilitation units that the pain tends to become less severe as the patient becomes more generally active (8); presumably, the sensory and kinesthetic input associated with activity might alleviate the disturbances originally caused by the deafferentation from the injured spinal cord.

The mechanism of phantom sensations and painful phantoms after cord injury might also be traced to function of the spinal cord just above the level of the lesion. Pollock observed that when anesthetic was applied to the end of the proximal segment of injured cord, both the dysesthetic pain and also the phantom body awareness disappeared (42). Mihic and Pinkert report an interesting case study in which spinal anesthesia induced the sudden onset of painful phantom in the lower legs. The patient felt as if the legs were twisted into an uncomfortable position, and this sensation persisted for the duration of the anesthetic (33). The above reports suggest that phantom sensations, or painful phantoms, may arise for reasons other than the development of denervation hypersensitivity or plasticity changes in the rostral CNS after cord injury (processes that may take some period of time to fully develop). Instead, such phantom sensations may occur because of disturbance of the "mnemonic traces" in the nervous system that govern the body image, as a result of a sudden loss of the normal peripheral proprioceptive and sensory input. Because, however, there is often a clinical association between dysesthetic and diffuse pain and painful body awareness below the level of the lesion, these various early and late neural mechanisms may be linked or may in some way influence each other.

NORMAL VERSUS ABNORMAL VISCERAL SENSATION

Normal individuals are able to distinguish many different visceral states in health and disease. The cues available include common visceral sensations such as bowel or bladder fullness, reflex visceral events such as the production of nausea or changed patterns of elimination, and body wall ("parietal") sensations. Thus, an individual can distinguish normal visceral sensations related to the need for elimination or to satiety after eating, as examples. These normal sensations can also be distinguished from those that might herald disease; for example, people who become ill are able to describe the difference between the deep epigastric and retrosternal discomfort of gastritis from the burning of cystitis or from the radiating pain of renal colic.

Before discussing the case of visceral events in spinal cord injured patients, we will briefly review some of the mechanisms of normal visceral sensations (43). The adequate stimuli for the production of visceral-related pain include distension or spasm of the muscular wall of a hollow viscus, traction on ligaments or mesentery within the abdomen, ischemia, or inflammation. The sensory innervation to the viscera is served by small diameter fibers with large overlapping sensory fields. These fibers travel through the abdominal ligaments and mesentery and through the vascular adventitia, joining the sympathetic chain and eventually the spinal cord. Whereas sensory input from the body wall to the spinal cord is more clearly segmentally localized, sensory input from the viscera via the sympathetic system is much more diffuse and multisynaptic. The body wall and the visceral sensory afferents eventually converge on second-order nociceptive transmission cells, whence the "pain fibers" are projected mainly through the lateral spinothalamic tracts on the opposite side of the cord. Fibers from the parietal (body wall) peritoneum, on the other hand, travel with the rest of the body wall sensory supply and therefore have a more strictly segmental input to the cord than the sensory fibers from the viscera. In addition, sensory supply to the peritoneum of the diaphragm is through the phrenic nerve, which arises from C3 to C5 and travels up through the mediastinum. For this reason, patients with high spinal cord injuries likely will have preservation of this diaphragmatic sensibility; this may be very important diagnostically.

Considering the above and taking for example the case of a normal individual developing appendicitis, pain may be first felt as a vague periumbilical discomfort while the inflammation is still confined to the vicinity of the appendix. Nausea, malaise, and changes in bowel function may be experienced reflexly. Movement of the inflamed viscera may be felt as rebound tenderness, an important diagnostic sign. All of this constitutes a good early-warning system for the normal individual. When the inflammation from the appendix spreads to the parietal peritoneum, the pain may be felt to localize to the body wall in the right upper quadrant, with accompanying muscle spasm and hyperalgesia of the skin. In another example, a patient with a ruptured viscus is likely to develop severe rebound tenderness immediately, with abdominal muscle spasm and hyperalgesia of the abdominal wall and pain referred to the shoulder because of irritation of the diaphragmatic peritoneum supplied by the phrenic nerve.

After spinal cord injury, this wealth of visceral sensory information may be lost to various degrees depending on the level and the completeness of the lesion. Because the parietal peritoneum innervation is shared by body wall innervation, this will be most affected by the level of the lesion. Much visceral sensation also travels with the spinothalamic tract; this is seen in the fact that visceral sensibility to pain may be impaired or lost totally after spinal cord injury. But because of the more diffuse multisynaptic visceral sensory input to the spinal cord, there may be some degree of preservation of common visceral sensations. Reflex changes associated with visceral events may be the only warning system with some patients. Due to the lack of inhibition of muscular tone below the level of the lesion, increases in spasticity and tone may be additional cues to visceral events. It is important to underline the importance of the phrenic nerve innervation of the diaphragm—pain referred to the left shoulder or to both shoulders must be taken very seriously as a possible indicator of a ruptured viscus or other serious intraabdominal pathology.

Perception of Visceral Events After SCI

Patients with lesions below the thoracic level may have fairly good preservation of visceral sensation. Those with higher cord lesions usually retain the capacity to perceive vague feelings of abdominal fullness or discomfort in the periumbilical region. Quadriplegia may rob the patient of most or all of these common visceral sensations, and the only indication the patient may have of a full bladder about to empty will perhaps be sudden onset of a throbbing headache, red face, blocked nose, and sweating. Visceral events such as fecal impaction or urinary retention may be accompanied by such autonomic signs as headache, nausea, chills, weakness, and pilomotor erections (7, 22, 32).

Pain Associated With Visceral Disease in Patients After SCI

Any discussion of spinal cord injury and pain must include the diagnostic issues that arise because of impairment of normal painful sensation. This subject has received extensive attention in reviews elsewhere (4, 6, 7, 22, 32, 34, 42). Pollock documented numerous patients with lesions to the spinal cord who were unable to experience pain associated with such conditions as cystitis, epididymitis, nephrolithiasis, or passage of bladder stones, orchiectomy, ureteral catheterization, or genitourinary surgery (42). Charney studied 24 patients with spinal cord injuries from C4 to L3 levels who also had surgical diseases of the abdomen. The patients with complete lesions between the C3 and T6 levels usually demonstrated early vague abdominal pains and autonomic hyperreflexia. If parietal peritoneum were involved, they might localize the pain to the dermatome. Patients with incomplete lesions were generally able to localize their pain earlier, and patients with lesions below the T7 level usually localized their pain earlier than those patients with higher level lesions, but all groups experienced distress later than would be expected with normals (6). Berly and Wilmot studied the incidence of acute abdominal pathology in 945 spinal cord injured patients during the first month of injury; the incidence of such problems was 4.66%. Most were accounted for by peptic ulcerations and complications, particularly in patients with complete lesions above T_5. There was a lesser but significant incidence of pancreatitis, fecal impaction, and other pathologies (4). This points out the necessity to be particularly vigilant during the first few months after injury. A series of typical scenarios follows.

A patient with spinal cord lesion may not reliably experience pain or abdominal tenderness. For example, a patient with quadriplegia complains of loss of appetite and nausea. A sudden rise in blood pressure and pulse is found and temperature is elevated to 39°. There is some vomiting and reflex spinal sweating, but without pain in the abdomen or tenderness to palpation. However, there appears to be more abdominal muscle spasm than before, with increased spasticity. The patient complains of headache. Rectal examination reveals soft stools. An x-ray of the abdomen shows distended air-filled bowel, but not apparently more so than noted on previous examination. White blood count is found to be elevated. Urinalysis is positive for many pus cells, with heavy growth of E-Coli bacilli. The patient responds to treatment for urinary tract infection.

Pain may be confused with other pathologies. A paraplegic with mid-thoracic lesion complains of upper abdominal discomfort. His temperature is 38.5°. He reports that the usual burning sensation in the legs has increased in severity. He is vaguely tender in the epigastrium and upper abdomen. On examination there appears to be more distension of the abdomen than usual, with the colon apparently full of feces. Rectal examination confirms presence of hard feces. White blood count is 20,000 with leukocytosis. Urinalysis is normal. An x-ray of the abdomen shows dilated loops of bowel and presence of feces. Enema produces evacuation with good results. However, abdominal discomfort continues with persistence of fever and rigors. Pain is now felt between the shoulder blades as well. Cholangiogram demonstrates cholelithiasis.

Pain may be felt above the level of the lesion. A quadriplegic with a lesion at C_5 complains of a vague abdominal pain. His temperature, pulse rate, and blood pressure are found to be elevated and there is reflex spinal sweating. White blood count is 22,000. The patient feels very nauseated, and soon after the initial complaint begins to experience pain in the left shoulder, and then in both shoulders. Abdominal x-ray shows air under the diaphragm. He is found to have a perforated peptic ulcer.

Another C_5 quadriplegic begins to complain of nausea, anorexia, weakness, and pain in the neck. Temperature is slightly elevated to 38° C. Pulse and blood pressure are slightly elevated, and pulse irregularity is noted. Electrocardiogram shows evidence of myocardial infarction, which is confirmed by serum enzymes.

When examining a patient suspected of having visceral problems, the level of the lesion and whether it is complete must be taken into account. The previous history of the patient, medications taken in the recent past, changes in the type of pain being experienced, or spasticity changes must be noted. Changes in temperature, pulse rate, blood pressure, or sweating may all provide valuable cues. Abdominal tenderness may be found, but its absence does not rule out pathology. Masses must be sought, and rectal examination is necessary. There may be a new hyperalgesia or an increase in previously existing border-zone hyperalgesia. Complete blood count, differential blood count, urinalysis, microscopic urine examination, and urine culture should be ordered. X-ray examinations relevant include chest x-ray, x-ray of the abdomen, and in some cases, intravenous pyelogram. Further examinations depend on the findings.

There are other possible causes for abdominal pain in spinal cord injured patients. As mentioned in the section on "Central Pain Syndromes," phantom pain may sometimes be experienced in the abdomen. Sometimes a nonabdominal lesion may be present. For example, an infected skin lesion over the sacrum could provoke fever and an increase in pain of central origin felt, for example, in the legs and abdomen. Musculoskeletal or radicular pain may be referred from the spine to the abdomen. Ashby reported on 73 patients (not cord injured) who were experiencing abdominal pains. Local tenderness and spasm was often found in the lower thoracic region. Many of the patients had previously had spinal problems. Pain was aggravated by movement and was alleviated by intercostal nerve block (2). Pain may also be referred to the abdomen by myofascial (referred pain) mechanisms, or there may be tenderness in abdominal muscle insertions (10, 47). The point of the above comments is that in the case of a low spinal cord or cauda equina lesion, there are numerous possible causes of pain in the abdomen, including visceral, central pain phenomena, local, or referred pain.

TREATMENT OF PAIN ASSOCIATED WITH SCI

Pharmacological Treatments

Analgesics

Simple antipyretic analgesics such as acetaminophen or ASA, with or without codeine, may be effective, especially for the acute pain experienced during the first few weeks following injury. The antiinflammatory action may also be desired, in which case it may be preferable to use analgesics containing ASA or other more potent antiinflammatory drugs such as naproxen for a short time. During this time, benzodiazepines may also be desirable to reduce muscle spasm. Analgesics should be given on a fixed-time schedule for the two following reasons: (a) a more stable blood level can be obtained if the analgesic is given at a specific frequency compatible with the biological half-life of that drug. This permits a more consistent pain control, and, where the antiinflammatory component is desired, better suppression of inflammation; and (b) PRN scheduling of analgesics has a tendency to create a behavioral sequence in which the complaint of pain becomes the necessary ticket to receive attention. For some patients this could set the basis for development of inappropriate illness behavior. As the pain and inflammation from the soft tissue and fracture injuries subside, analgesics can be gradually decreased and withdrawn. In particular, the prolonged use of codeine or other opiate or sedative medication should be avoided because these can lead to a chronic use problem that is hard to break, and there can be a tendency to eventual escalation of doses. This is discussed further below.

In the longer term, some patients may develop arthritic changes at the level of fracture for which antipyretic analgesics may be warranted and effective. One should remember the tendency of almost all drugs of this type to produce peptic ulceration, which unfortunately may not be detected by the patient with a spinal cord lesion. Therefore, for more prolonged treatment of this sort of discomfort, acetaminophen or enteric-coated ASA may be a better choice. Spinal cord patients are as likely as anyone else to suffer from painful conditions like headaches. The majority of headache patients, including those with vascular headaches, obtain substantial relief from modest doses of simple antipyretic analgesics taken at the first sign of headache onset. For such episodic use, enteric-coated ASA would be less appropriate; a single dose of 600 mg of ASA or an equivalent dose of acetaminophen is best.

As mentioned above, one should be cautious about prolonged use of opiate analgesics (7). There are many reasons for such caution, not the least of which is that the majority of painful syndromes experienced by spinal cord patients do not respond very well to opiates. For example, patients with pain associated with nerve root lesions, hyperalgesic border reactions, or diffuse burning dysesthesias obtain marginal relief from opiates and no more than might be expected from an equivalent amount of a nonopiate sedative. It is interesting to note the report of Levitt and Levitt, who experimentally induced dysesthesias by cordotomy in macaque monkeys (25, 26). They observed that opiates did not seem to alleviate the dysesthetic syndrome (25). Because opiates may not be very effective in reducing pains of neurological origin, there may be an easy tendency to escalate the dose in attempt to improve the analgesia. However, this may be detrimental, not only because of induction of tolerance but also because of the negative psychological effects—producing apathy, poor energy, and loss of appetite. Spinal cord patients often have problems with their bowel control and opiates may complicate the matter further. Because the quality of sensory function of SCI patients is already impaired, the use of centrally acting analgesics (opiates) could at times be dangerous due to masking other occult disease. Opiates also have a short-acting anxiolytic and depression-relieving effect in patients who experience emotional distress—patients with emotional problems may slip into a medication-dependency problem, asking for medication for motives of emotional distress more than for analgesia. However, at some times opiates might still be necessary. For example, after an orthopaedic procedure, which some SCI patients may require, potent analgesia is indicated. In such a case, it is preferable to use an adequately potent opiate in the immediate postoperative period. For such purposes, morphine is superior to the shorter-acting meperidine and should be given in adequate doses on a fixed-time schedule, succeeded a few days later by oral doses of antipyretic analgesic combined with codeine, which is later tapered according to a definite schedule.

Psychotropic Drugs

For over two decades, tricyclic compounds related to the major tranquilizers and antidepressants have been recognized as having some analgesic properties (31). Research has found these drugs to be particularly indicated in the painful syndromes that may follow neurological injury (38, 50). Unfortunately, only anecdotal reports exist in the literature at this time regarding the effectiveness of such drugs in the treatment of pain associated with SCI (17, 29), and the impression from these is that a minority of patients obtain satisfactory relief from troublesome central pain syndromes by using such drugs or combinations of them. However, considering the persistent and difficult nature of pains of neurological origin, even this is encouraging. The author would recommend that, if use of psychotropic drugs is contemplated, they should be started by using a single drug at low dosages, only very carefully increasing the dose or adding drugs. A sample regime might start a patient on 25 mg of amitriptyline at night. Considering the long half-life of the drug, the dose should not be increased any more frequently than weekly. At intervals of from 7 to 14 days, the doses may be raised by increments of 25 mg to a final dose of from 50 to 150 mg, all taken as one nighttime dosage, unless there appears to be some contraindication to it. Our experience is that the levels necessary for pain control are less than the levels that would usually be necessary for antidepressant effect. The patient must be monitored for adverse anticholinergic effects on bowel or bladder, excessive sedation, or adverse psychological effects. If the patient is elderly, a much smaller dosage will be tolerated. If there is insufficient analgesia after 2 weeks of maximum dosage of amitriptyline, perphenazine might be added at an initial dosage of 2 mg, gradually increasing to a maximum dosage of 6 mg if necessary. Unless the patient obtains decided improvement with a minimum of adverse effects, the psychotropic medication should not be continued. (Some laboratories are able to render serum levels that may sometimes be useful in determining if dosages are within the therapeutically effective range.) Psychotropic drugs may exert part of their helpful effect by reducing anxiety or depression and therefore reducing the psychological influences on the pain syndrome. It may be, however, that there may also be specific neuropharmacological effects on specific nervous pathways subserving pain sensation (31, 38, 50). In using these drugs, one must be aware of their numerous potentially adverse effects. Phenothiazines are sympatholytic, and most tricyclic antidepressants have anticholinergic properties that may change bowel and bladder function. Tricyclic antidepressants can produce paralytic ileus and, in susceptible patients, may have a negative inotropic effect on the heart or cause arrhythmias. Lethargy and other unpleasant mental effects can impair the patient's participation in his rehabilitation program.

The author's opinion is that psychotropic drugs should be reserved for pain of apparently neurological origin if that pain is sufficiently severe to interfere with function in the rehabilitation program. They should be introduced, used only with careful supervision, and only as long as their benefits are clearly demonstrable.

Other Drugs

Since central pain syndromes may be aggravated by spasticity, it is sometimes helpful to introduce muscle relaxants. Benzodiazepines are a logical choice, although they are not strongly potent for this application. Dantrolene sodium is an effective muscle relaxant, but the patient must be observed for possible toxicity. Baclofen may reduce spasticity and relieve some pains of neurological origin.

Anticonvulsants such as carbamazepine, valproate sodium, or phenytoin sometimes have a role in alleviation of neuralgias and some dysesthetic pains. They might be particularly indicated in cases of intermittent stabbing pains of neurological origin. However, as with the psychotropic drugs, only a minority of patients will report benefit from these medications, and therefore the patient must be reviewed.

It is possible that there will be a future development of new pharmacological agents with specific benefit for pain associated with spinal cord injury. For example, Dunn and Davis reported a small survey of 10 SCI patients who were using marijuana—about half the patients reported a helpful decrease in phantom pain, spasticity, and headache pain (11). It is conceivable that these pharmacological effects may be refined in the future to produce effective drugs for controlling spasticity and pain.

Electroanalgesia

It has long been known that pain may be attenuated by stimulation of certain sensory fiber systems; in particular, electrical stimulation of large diameter sensory fibers or the extensions of this system in the spinal cord has been found to have notable analgesic effect. Electrical nerve stimulation of certain locations within the brain or brainstem is also known to relieve pain. The discussion here confines itself to electrical dorsal column stimulation of the spinal cord (DCS) and electrical stimulation at the cutaneous level (transcutaneous electrical nerve stimulation, or TENS) since there is data only regarding the last two methods in the literature on SCI.

Electrical stimulation of the dorsal columns of the spinal cord was described by Shealy in 1970 with initial enthusiasm because of obvious success of the method. This enthusiasm was however muted after longer follow-up demonstrated that only some painful conditions responded well, and that the therapeutic effect steadily declined with time, even with the initially successful patients. Thus Long in 1975 followed up a series of patients who had received DCS for a variety of painful conditions. (Although most of the patients had pain due to neurological injury, only one of the original group had pain associated with central cord injury—in this case with burning dysesthesia, and this patient received no benefit at all from DCS, even initially.) The stimulation method included the implantation of the electrodes over the dorsal columns of the spinal cord. At the time of the surgical implantation of the electrode, 13 of the total 69 patients were failing to obtain benefit. After a year, 45 of the 55 who could be traced reported that they no longer experienced pain relief. Subsequently nine patients had their stimulators reimplanted at a higher level but this did not lead to any additional improvement (27). In 1980, Richardson reported a comparison of DCS in 10 patients with paraplegia and 10 with pain due to other causes. Of the 10 paraplegic patients with intractable pain, all had initial percutaneous placement of electrodes over the dorsal columns. Because of initial good results, five of these patients went on to have surgical implantation of permanent electrodes. The types of pain encountered in the paraplegic group included three cases of "visceral pain", one case of "radicular pain," and six cases of "central pain." After a year, only one patient was still obtaining significant pain relief using the original stimulator, and in a further five patients, therapeutic benefit had lasted only a few months. Another patient was pain free while using conus medullaris electrical stimulation for micturition, and another had stopped having dysesthesia while using almost constant percutaneous epidural stimulation—the latter patient had also improved neurologically and his stimulator had subsequently been removed. These disappointing results contrasted with the results in nine patients without paraplegia who were suffering neuroma or stump pain; only three of these nine failed to show some relief a year after starting percutaneous DCS or implantation of dorsal column stimulator (45).

There is not much data regarding the application of TENS for treatment of pain associated with spinal cord injuries. The scattered reports that exist suggest that TENS may occasionally be of benefit, especially with regard to either musculoskeletal or radicular pain at the level of injury. Pain within the zone of denervation is less likely to respond. As an example, Davis and Lentini reported on the use of TENS in 31 patients with spinal cord injury. They reported 11 successes and 2 partial successes. Good results were most likely obtained with pain originating at the site of injury or radicular pain at the level of injury. Unfortunately, radicular pain below the lesion level or central phantom pain were successfully or partially successfully treated in only one out of four of these cases. According to their report (9), rather large electrodes were used, and it is possible that because of using the large electrodes, effective levels of peripheral nerve stimulation were not reached. Furthermore, the authors did not clearly indicate the placement of the electrodes, whether over "trigger points," painful zones, or peripheral nerves, nor did they report the parameters of the stimulation. This makes it difficult to determine if these results are apt to be representative of TENS in the treatment of pain from spinal cord injury.

Hachen used electrical nerve stimulation in 39 patients, 7 quadriplegics and 32 paraplegics, with lesions to the thoracic spine or cauda equina. The TENS was applied in long 6-hour sessions over the first week. (Stimulus parameters included use of rectangular wave forms, pulse duration of 1 to 10 microseconds, and frequency of 40 to 100 cycles/sec, and placements are not indicated in their report.) After the first week of these prolonged TENS treatments, 19 patients (49%) reported complete or almost complete relief, 16 patients (41%) had slight to moderate relief, and 4 patients (10%) had none. In the succeeding 3 months, electrical nerve stimulators were consigned to the patients who applied them according to "variable stimulus parameters," presumably as the patients themselves wished. At 3 months of follow-up, 11 (28%) were still obtaining complete or almost complete relief, 19 (49%) were obtaining slight to moderate relief, and 9 (23%) had no relief (16). From this report, one does not know if the loss of therapeutic effect was due to the loss of therapeutic efficacy of the TENS itself or whether it was due perhaps to changes in electrode placement or stimulation parameters. Banerjee reported personal experience with five cases of SCI who were successfully treated with short periods of electrical nerve stimulation within the painful region but below the level of spinal cord injury. Stimulation amplitude was enough to produce evident muscle contractions. No follow-up data were given in that case report (3). Richardson observed that TENS was beneficial in relieving the pain associated with the extensive soft-tissue injuries in 75% of 20 patients (46).

The impressions from these reports are that TENS may be effective in some cases, particularly with pain originating at the level of injury, but that the results may be less satisfactory below the level of injury. Because TENS is noninvasive and poses little risk to the patient, it is worth attempting. Two cautions should however be observed. Apart from applying electrodes over the cardiac area (which should be avoided in any case), one must be wary that electrodes placed in an anesthetic area could possibly lead to burning of the skin if they are somehow accidentally dislodged or if the electroconductive medium should dry during prolonged application. To be considered also is the observation of Florante who noted that in recent quadriplegics TENS might aggravate bladder dysfunction if there is detrusor-sphincter dyssynergia. To be safe, one should do residual urine volume studies before and after commencing treatment, and there should be urine culture follow-up in the case of continued TENS use (12).

In terms of practical guidelines, the authors suggest that TENS might be usefully applied either over the segments in which radicular pain is experienced or over musculoskeletal trigger points for pain at or above the level of the lesion. Applications below the level of the lesion is not recommended; if done, it must include due safeguards. Electrodes must not be overly large since these may fail to deliver a sufficient current density for adequate stimulation beneath the electrode. Longer pulse widths of 100 to 250 microseconds would permit effective stimulation at lower stimulation intensities and may therefore reduce skin irritation. If good results do not follow traditional applications of about one-half hour, longer duration stimulations could be tried. Several days of TENS application ought to be completed before it is decided if TENS is going to be effective since it often occurs that results will improve during the first several days of treatment (55).

Anesthesiological Treatment

Whereas the treatment of peripheral nerve injuries by various techniques of sympathetic block may be quite effective in many cases, anesthesiological treatment of pain associated with spinal cord injury is much less so. In particular, pain that arises below the level of the lesion is likely to be resistant to sympathetic blocks (7, 30), and even amputations or resections of part of the spinal cord are unlikely to affect the pain.

Although causalgia and dysesthesias associated with peripheral nerve damage usually respond well to sympathetic blocks, radicular pain at the level of spinal injury or dysesthetic pain at the border of anesthesia of the spinal cord lesion level rarely show benefit from anesthesiological procedures.

One might consider injection of steroid or anesthetic into damaged apophyseal joints or rhizotomy of the nerve of Lushka that supplies these joints (8), but the author is not of the opinion that such procedures make a great deal of difference in the musculoskeletal pain syndromes experienced by most SCI patients. A better approach is to ensure stability of the spinal column by conservative or surgical means, and to treat pain associated with soft tissue injuries with antiinflammatory analgesics, codeine in the few weeks after injury, and perhaps electrical nerve stimulation that might be helpful either early or late after the injury.

Surgical Treatments

As suggested above, surgical intervention may be necessary, particularly in the weeks and the few months following the injury, to deal with structural problems resulting from injury to the spine (8). For example, fusion may be indicated to deal with instability or pain arising from damaged apophyseal joints. In the case of nerve root compression, laminectomy or diskectomy may be required.

With respect to pain arising below the level of the lesion, surgical interventions aimed at relieving pain must still be regarded as being somewhat experimental, although there is long-standing literature on the issue. In 1947, Loyal Davis recorded that 18 patients with pain associated with SCI had a total of 23 cordotomies, and that 1 had been relieved of burning pain and 4 of root pain. The remaining 13 had had no relief. Furthermore, six patients suffered complications from the cordotomies (7). In 1950,

Munro reported that 39 of a total of 72 patients had obtained some pain relief as a result of surgical procedures. Specifically, 28 out of 50 patients obtained benefit from exploratory laminectomy with neurolysis of the cauda equina. Only 1 out of 4 benefitted from lumbar sympathectomy and 10 out of 18 from cordotomy. That author was of the opinion that the failures in the cordotomized patients could be partly explained by inadequate surgical procedures, such as placing the surgical lesion too low, having insufficient cooperation from the patient, or placing the surgical lesion incorrectly. He thought that if an anterolateral cordotomy were properly performed at a high enough level, radicular pain and pain related to cauda equina injury would be likely to respond favorably (35). On the other hand, cordotomy (sectioning the lateral spinothalamic tract) has not enjoyed in general much success for long-term pain control. For example, White observed that unilateral thoracic cordotomy in humans leads to a 21% incidence of intractable contralateral painful paresthesias on subsequent follow-up (54). Work by Levitt and Levitt with cordotomy in macaque monkeys has also demonstrated the possibility that variously placed spinal cord lesions, including lesions that transect the contralateral cord, may produce painful dysesthesias (25, 26). However, the latter authors also noticed that "the release of the deafferentation syndrome which usually resulted from anterolateral cordotomy [in macaque monkeys] was prevented by a simultaneous ipsilateral lesion which included the lateral funiculus as well as the anterior quadrant at the same level." This might suggest that the return of pain or the onset of postcordotomy dysesthesia might be due to the presence of alternate pathways in the spinal cord capable of carrying pain-related signals. This may fit with the observations of Botterell who noted in 1953 that bilateral spinal tractotomy (between T1 and T5 in six cases) produced excellent results in three and further partial benefits in another two patients. The follow-up was from 2 to 8 years (5). One would, however, want to consider such operative measures with caution, especially in the case of partial cord lesions where residual nervous function below the lesion might be even further impaired.

A new and yet unproven technique has been suggested by Nashold. He had earlier reported that surgical coagulations of the "dorsal root entry-zone" (DREZ) of the spinal cord could relieve the persistent burning pain resulting from brachial plexus avulsion lesions (37). DREZ coagulations are carried out in the following way. At each side of the cord from one or two segments above the level of the lesion down to the lesion level or slightly below it, lesions are placed so as to obliterate dorsal root fiber entry along with the substantia gelatinosa of Rolando. Central pain syndromes in 13 patients following damage to the spinal cord (3 cases) or to the cauda equina or conus medullaris (10 cases) were treated with DREZ coagulations, and after a follow-up of from 5 to 38 months, seven patients were pain free, and all but two had at least 50% pain relief. Three patients, however, had suffered major complications that included further loss of motor function or of reflex bladder control (36). Several mechanisms were suggested as possibly explaining this result. Those authors had noted pain relief in a previous patient who had had one centimeter of his proximal injured cord resected, and noting also the relief by DREZ coagulations, proposed that some central pain syndromes following spinal cord injury may originate in the cord segment that is deafferented and lies in the segment just rostral to the spinal cord lesion. They proposed that DREZ coagulation may interrupt the ascending pain pathways in the dorsal or dorsolateral columns (25). They considered the possibility also that DREZ coagulations may destroy epileptiform "pain-generating centers" that may lie in the deafferented cord. Finally, they suggested that these lesions may somehow affect pain mechanisms that rely on an interaction between sensory input and CNS inhibition (36).

What is clear from all of this is that surgical intervention may be important in the period immediately following spinal injury to deal with structural problems, to improve stability, and possibly to deal with nerve root or spinal cord compression. Surgical procedures to the cord itself to deal with long-standing pain of spinal cord origin are less successful but with further study may eventually hold some promise.

Psychological Treatments

Helping the patient deal with psychological and psychosocial adjustment issues is an inseparable part of the rehabilitation process. Psychotherapeutic methods are therefore not directed in an isolated fashion to the pain alone but consider the whole context of pain, suffering, adjustment, and relationships. The following comments should however be made with respect to pain as one of the many psychological issues that patients will have to face after their injuries and during their long processes of rehabilitation.

Staff familiar with the rehabilitation environment are well aware that fluctuations in pain are sometimes indications of psychological distress, and that pain problems and pain complaints may well diminish with reductions in the psychological and psychosocial difficulties (5, 44). At times, the process of rehabilitation may be complicated in occasional individuals who have prior histories of personality disorders or medication or alcohol abuse. Where such preexisting disorders present themselves as excessive complaints of pain and inappropriate medication-taking behavior, the rehabilitation team may have to include specific psychological management in the total rehabilitation plan. More rarely, frank psychiatric illness may coexist or suddenly present, requiring psychotherapeutic or psychopharmacological intervention. Pain, or the aggravation of preexisting pain, may often be associated with agitated depression. Other mental disorders such as schizophrenia or organic brain syndrome with confusion might confuse the symptomatic picture of a hospitalized patient, but these mental disorders themselves are not particularly likely to include psychogenic pain. Expert psychiatric consultation and specific psychological treatment such as psychotherapy or psychotropic drugs might be required in the more difficult cases. Further details on this topic can be found in other references (19, 29).

Whereas some patients may need very specific psychotherapeutic or psychopharmacological treatment, all patients require supportive relationships and supportive psychotherapy from the professional staff. This must include the qualities of being able to listen carefully and to listen for covert messages in patients who are hesitant to express themselves. The matter of respecting an individual's need for a sense of control and autonomy is always an issue in patients with spinal cord injury. Because patients with SCi frequently experience a marked loss of self-esteem and are bewildered by the change in self-image, it is crucial that staff at all times show a respectful and an empathic attitude toward the patients. With regard to the pain problem in particular, it is prudent to not raise the issue of pain in daily conversation with the patient unless the patient himself wishes to do so. Multiple prescriptions or hasty prescription of medication should be avoided. If analgesics are to be used, the doses should be clearly specified and indications made as to when they should be given. Rather than simply writing "p.r.n.," it is best, if possible, to provide medications on a fixed-time basis, according to the biological half-life of that particular drug. The need for analgesics, sedatives, or psychotropic drugs must be reviewed as the patient's condition changes rather than perpetuating medication use to the detriment of the patient or lack of benefit. These rules will help avoid development of behavioral problems and power struggles around medication taking. Above all, problems such as pain are best dealt with by helping the patient see the whole context of his rehabilitation. The patient may be encouraged to know that with increased activity as rehabilitation progresses, the usual pattern is for pain to decrease or to become more tolerable and manageable (29).

Specific psychological methods that may be useful in treating pain include general relaxation and hypnosis. The latter techniques are well-known and have been practiced for many years. The general experience with hypnosis is that about 10% of patients obtain very good pain relief with this method. Those who do not benefit specifically by being able to achieve hypnotic analgesia may yet benefit from the techniques of relaxation that are usually part of the hypnotic therapeutic exercise. Relaxation-based therapies are probably more generally applicable, and although they are less dramatic than hypnosis, they are known by a larger cross section of rehabilitation staff and can be carried out by personnel other than psychologists and psychiatrists; these have the advantage of enhancing the patient's sense of self-control. Grzesiak published an anecdotal report noting the benefits of relaxation training and the psychological technique of "selective inattention" for control of pain associated with SCI (15). Treatments of this sort can be carried out individually or with groups of patients, and to be effective probably require a series of from 4 to 10 sessions, at a frequency of two or three sessions per week. It is quite unnecessary for the relaxation exercises to be complex (using for example the contraction-relaxation technique). It is usually sufficient to encourage the patient to "tune in" to his own breathing and to practice progressive muscle relaxation or the sensations associated with "quieting" his own thoughts and responses voluntarily, encouraging the patient in the meantime to use pleasant imagery or simply focus on relaxed thoughts and feelings.

Treating Pain in a Total Rehabilitation Context

The total program of rehabilitation involves the coordination of expert and support resources to facilitate each patient's reacquisition of function wherever possible, and new acquisition of different skills that will permit his reintegration and adaptation to his psychosocial and vocational environment. Inasmuch as pain interferes with the quality of life and obstructs this learning, it is an appropriate object of treatment but never in isolation from the total rehabilitation program (18). All rehabilitation programming should be seen as a whole; this is not just for the sake of coordinating the rehabilitation treatment plan but is also because of the need to fully engage the patient in knowledgeable participation in his own rehabilitation. All components of the rehabilitation plan should further the general rehabilitation motives. For example, it may be possible to relieve a patient's pain totally by prescription of high doses of psychotropic medications at the cost of complicating already-compromised visceral function, reducing motivation or clarity of thought, but it is not a good trade-off in terms of the general rehabilitation goals.

There is no place in rehabilitation for specialists who operate in isolation from each other or from the rehabilitation team. Therefore, professionals engaged in pain treatment must integrate their operations with the overall rehabilitation treatment plan, monitoring its progress also in terms of the patient's progress. If perhaps a specialty pain clinic is involved or specialists who do not have their usual working base within the rehabilitation setting, attention must be given to integrating interventions into the overall treatment. There must be also a clearly-identified physician in charge of care or a "case manager" who is aware of all of the particular elements of that patient's program. Remember too that the patient and his family are also part of the team. Objectives of treatment are not simply prescribed but are negotiated with the patient and his family.

Given that such conditions are met, one may reassure the patient that the persistent pain problem associated with his injury will have a tendency to diminish as rehabilitation progresses and as his self-initiated activity and mobility increase (8, 29, 32). Beyond the problem of pain as a sensation, the problems of living with pain and disability will also be dealt with across the whole rehabilitation trajectory. The patient may rebuild his future on his coping skills, his sense of psychological integrity, and his sense of personal security and confidence in his relationships in the contexts of his friends, family, and his vocational partners.

OPINIONS, AND THE STATE OF THE SCIENTIFIC EVIDENCE

The author has reviewed here the available relevant literature on the subjects of pain and pain treatment in patients with spinal cord injury, distilling hopefully a helpful clinical perspective. Several of the papers cited (7, 18, 19, 29, 32) represent the opinions of experienced and respected clinicians, drawing on their personal clinical experiences (and some with references to other published reports). Other papers are reports of examinations or follow-up of series of SCI patients (5, 7, 22, 42), or clinical impressions without citing the exact figures (23); the number of patients studied ranges from 44 to 471, with the period of observation or follow-up being from a few months to (probably) 8 years or more, with one paper reporting a continuing follow-up of 2 years (35). Two papers made an attempt to compare civilian versus veteran groups of SCI, one reporting on 228 veterans and 314 civilians (35) and another paper reporting on 416 veterans and 55 civilians (7); otherwise, there were no control or comparison groups used. Two papers analyzed data from a questionnaire follow-up (39, 44), and although 200 patients responded, this represented only 56% of the patients on the survey list. Enough data can be drawn from papers such as these to begin to build a composite picture of the clinical features of pain associated with SCI, short and long-term complications, and outcomes of general rehabilitation programs. To provide more exact answers, there is a need for future studies that employ validated measures of pain and disability, and that examine, with control groups, clinical outcomes with respect to specific SCI complications or specific treatment methods.

The purposes of differential diagnosis are served well by papers that describe complications and their clinical presentations and diagnoses in detail (6, 34, 49). Two such studies cited in this chapter included a detailed study of 13 cases of posttraumatic syringomyelia (49) and a comparative case study of 24 SCI cases who presented with surgical disease of the abdomen (6). Simple case studies can also be illuminating in this regard (34). However, such an important problem as "shoulder pain in SCI patients" is a matter of universal recognition but ubiquitous conjecture as to mechanisms or treatment (apart from the well-known fact that such pain diminishes as the patient is activated). One study used two mailings of a questionnaire, obtaining an overall follow-up rate of 79.5% (554 out of 697 patients), finding a high incidence of this problem in SCI individuals living in the community (40). Drawing on other research regarding the incidence of neck and shoulder pain in the general population, the authors found that

SCI individuals were at increased risk for shoulder pain. Although this is important as a statement of prevalence of the problem, it would be difficult on the basis of a questionnaire to establish the biological mechanisms or responsible factors leading to the development of such a syndrome. The other interesting report of the positioning technique for the prevention of shoulder pain in acute quadriplegics is based on only a handful of cases (48)—the results of their longer-term controlled study will be awaited with interest.

Four papers that bear on the possible mechanisms of pain after SCI are based on animal studies (1, 20, 25, 26). Another is an excellent and detailed individual case study (41) and another a case report (33). Melzack and Loeser based their hypotheses on a skillful review and discussion of the literature (30), a style adopted in other such papers as well (14, 24). Theoretical papers regarding the mechanisms of pain after SCI are generally good in quality but meager in quantity.

It is noteworthy that this chapter cannot draw on any well-controlled studies regarding treatment methods. The closest thing to such a study compares the results of dorsal column stimulation in 10 patients with SCI and in 9 patients with posttraumatic or postamputation pain, examining the results at 1 year as well (45). Even without control groups, follow-up studies are essential, especially if they do not confirm earlier favorable impressions, as in the followup of dorsal column stimulation procedures or cordotomy (27, 54) in which the long-term results have proven to be disappointing. (These two papers did not deal specifically with SCI, but included some cases of SCI, arachnoiditis, or plexus lesions.) An uncontrolled trial of intercostal nerve block in 73 patients with "abdominal pain of spinal origin" (but not SCI origin) was cited (2) along with two brief case reports (10, 47). Available also were reports of uncontrolled trials of a relaxation technique, dorsal root entry zone coagulations, and psychotropic drugs (15, 17, 36, 38). Although transcutaneous electrical nerve stimulation has attracted much interest in recent years, reports regarding its use in spinal cord injury pain are limited to a few case reports or uncontrolled trials (3, 9, 16, 17, 46). Two of these gave some information regarding stimulation parameters (16, 46), but one that followed up the patients after 3 months noted a loss of efficacy and possibly unstated changes in the stimulation parameters so that it would be hard to interpret the experimental outcome. Another study may have used an inadequate method (electrodes too large) (9). Uncontrolled trials or case reports give data on which clinical trials of specific methods may later be based, and provide some indicators regarding safety or possible complications of procedures. At this time, however, we must not fool ourselves: we have many impressions but few facts regarding treatment of SCI pain. To be more certain, we need well-controlled trials using standardized and reliable evaluation tools.

The author submits this critique of the state of the literature, not to discount the findings, practical experience, or considered opinions contained in this chapter, but in the hope that the ample opportunities for future research and discovery in the field of spinal cord injury pain will not be overlooked.

REFERENCES

1. Albe-Fessard, D., Nashold, B. S., Jr., Lombard, M. C., Yamaguchi, Y., and Boureau, F. Rat after dorsal rhizotomy: A possible animal model for chronic pain. In: *Advances in Pain Research and Therapy: Vol. 3.* Edited by Bonica, J. J., Albe-Fessard, D., and Liebeskind, J. C. Raven Press, New York, 1979, pp. 761–766.
2. Ashby, E. C. Abdominal pain of spinal origin: value of intercostal block. *Ann. R. Coll. Surg. Engl.*, *59:* 242–246, 1977.
3. Banerjee, T. Transcutaneous nerve stimulation for pain after spinal injury (letters to editor). *N. Engl. J. Med.*, *291:* 796, 1974.
4. Berlly, M. H., and Wilmot, C. B. Acute abdominal emergencies during the first four weeks after spinal cord injury. *Arch. Phys. Med. Rehabil.*, *65:* 687–690, 1984.
5. Botterell, E. H., Callaghan, J. C., and Jousse, A. T. Pain in paraplegia: clinical management and surgical treatment. *Proc. R. Soc. Med.*, *47:* 281–288, 1953.
6. Charney, K. J., Juler, G. L., and Comarr, A. E. General surgery problems in patients with spinal cord injuries. *Arch. Surg.*, *110:* 1083–1088, 1975.
7. Davis, L., and Martin, J. Studies upon spinal cord injuries: the nature and treatment of pain. *J. Neurosurg.*, *4:* 483–491, 1947.
8. Davis, R. Pain and suffering following spinal cord injury. *Clin. Orthop.*, *112:* 76–80, 1975.
9. Davis, R., and Lentini, R. Transcutaneous nerve stimulation for treatment of pain in patients with spinal cord injury. *Surg. Neurol.*, *4:* 100–101, 1975.
10. Diamond, A. W., and Roberts, H. J. Abdominal pain of spinal origin (letter to the editor). *Lancet, 2(8130):* 195, 1977.
11. Dunn, M., and Davis, R. The perceived effects of marijuana on spinal cord injured males. *Paraplegia, 12:* 175, 1974.
12. Florante, J., Leyson, J., Stefaniwsky, L., and Martin, B. F. Effects of transcutaneous nerve stimulation on the vesicourethral function in spinal cord injury patients. *J. Urol., 121:* 635–639, 1979.
13. Gilbert, R. W., Kim, J. H., and Posner, J. B. Epidural spinal cord compression from metastatic tumor: diagnosis and treatment. *Ann. Neurol.*, *3:* 40–51, 1978.
14. Gross, D. Pain and autonomic nervous system. In: *Advances in Neurology: Vol. 4.* Edited by Bonica, J. J. Raven Press, New York, 1974, pp. 93–103.
15. Grzesiak, R. C. Relaxation techniques in treatment of chronic pain. *Arch. Phys. Med. Rehabil., 58:* 270–272, 1977.
16. Hachen, H. J. Psychological, neurophysiological, and therapeutic aspects of chronic pain: preliminary results with transcutaneous electrical stimulation. *Paraplegia, 15:* 353–367, 1977–1978.
17. Heilporn, A. Two therapeutic experiments on stubborn pain in spinal cord lesions: coupling melitracen-flupenthixol and the transcutaneous nerve stimulation. *Paraplegia, 15:* 368–372, 1977–1978.
18. Heyl, H. L. Some practical aspects in the rehabilitation of paraplegics. *J. Neurosurg., 13:* 184–189, 1956.
19. Hohmann, G. W. Psychological aspects of treatment and rehabilitation of the spinal cord injured person. *Clin. Orthop., 112:* 81–88, 1975.
20. Howe, J. F., Loeser, J. D., and Calvin, W. H. Mechanosensitivity of dorsal root ganglia

and chronically injured axons: a physiological basis for the radicular pain of nerve root compression. *Pain, 3:* 25–41, 1977.

21. Kakulas, B. A., Harper, C. G., Shibasaki, K., and Bedbrook, G. M. Vertebral metastases and spinal cord compression. *Clin. Exp. Neurol., 15:* 98–113, 1978.

22. Kaplan, L. I., Grynbaum, B. B., Lloyd, K. E., and Rusk, H. A. Pain and spasticity in patients with spinal cord dysfunction: results of a follow-up study. *J.A.M.A., 182:* 918–925, 1962.

23. Kennedy, R. H. A new viewpoint toward spinal cord injuries. *Ann. Surg., 124:* 1057–1065, 1946.

24. Lawrence, R. M. Phantom pain: a new hypothesis. *Med. Hypotheses, 6:* 245–248, 1980.

25. Levitt, M., and Levitt, J. H. The deafferentation syndrome in monkeys: dysesthesias of spinal origin. *Pain, 10:* 129–147, 1981.

26. Levitt, M. The bilaterally symmetrical deafferentation syndrome in macaques after bilateral spinal lesions: evidence for dysesthesias resulting from brain foci and considerations of spinal pain pathways. *Pain, 16:* 167–184, 1983.

27. Long, D. M., and Erickson, D. E. Stimulation of the posterior columns of the spinal cord for relief of intractable pain. *Surg. Neurol., 4:* 134–141, 1975.

28. Mathews, G. J., and Osterholm, J. L. Painful traumatic neuromas. *Surg. Clin. North Am., 51(5):* 1313–1324, 1972.

29. Maury, M. About pain and its treatment in paraplegics. *Paraplegia, 15:* 349–352, 1977–1978.

30. Melzack, R., and Loeser, J. D. Phantom body pain in paraplegics: evidence for a central "pattern generating mechanism" for pain. *Pain, 4:* 195–210, 1978.

31. Merskey, H., and Hester, R. A. The treatment of chronic pain with psychotropic drugs. *Postgrad. Med. J., 48:*594–598, 1972.

32. Michaelis, L. S. The problem of pain in paraplegia and tetraplegia. *Bull. N.Y. Acad. Med., 461:* 88–96, 1970.

33. Mihic, D. N., and Pinkert, E. Phantom limb pain during peridural anaesthesia. *Pain, 11:* 269–272, 1981.

34. Miller, L. S., Staas, W. E., and Herbison, G. J. Abdominal problems in patients with spinal cord lesions. *Arch. Phys. Med. Rehabil., 56:* 405–408, 1975.

35. Munro, D. Two-year end-results in the total rehabilitation of veterans with spinal-cord and cauda-equina injuries. *N. Engl. J. Med., 242:* 1–16, 1950.

36. Nashold, B. S., and Bullitt, E. Dorsal root entry zone lesions to control central pain in paraplegics. *J. Neurosurg., 55:* 414–419, 1981.

37. Nashold, B. S., Urban, B., and Zorub, D. S. Phantom relief by focal destruction of substantia gelatinosa of Rolando. In: *Advances in Pain Research and Therapy: Vol. 1.* Edited by Bonica, J. J., and Albe-Fessard, D. G. Raven Press, New York, 1976, pp. 959–963.

38. Nathan, P. W. Chlorprothixine in post-herpetic neuralgia and other severe chronic pains. *Pain, 5:* 367–371, 1978.

39. Nepomuceno, C., Fine, P. R., Richards, J. S., Gowens, H., Stover, S. L., Rantanuabol, U., and Houston, R. Pain in patients with spinal cord injury. *Arch. Phys. Med. Rehabil., 60:* 605–609, 1979.

40. Nichols, P. J. R., Norman, P. A., and Ennis, J. R. Wheelchair user's shoulder? Shoulder pain in patients with spinal cord lesions. *Scand. J. Rehabil. Med., 11:* 29–32, 1979.

41. Noordenbos, W., and Wall, P. D. Diverse sensory functions with an almost totally divided spinal cord. A case of spinal cord transection with preservation of part of one anterolateral quadrant. *Pain, 2:* 185–195, 1976.

42. Pollock, L. J., Brown, M., Boshes, B., Finkelman, I., Chor, H., Arieff, A. J., and Finkel, J. R. Pain below the level of injury of the spinal cord. *AMA Arch. Neurol. Psychiat., 65:* 319–322, 1951.

43. Procacci, P., and Zoppi, M. Pathophysiology and clinical aspects of visceral and referred pain. In: *Advances in Pain Research and Therapy: Vol. 5.* Edited by Bonica, J. J., Lindblom, U., and Iggo, A. Raven Press, New York, 1983, pp. 643–658.
44. Richards, J. S., Meredith, R. L., Nepomuceno, C., Fine, P. R., and Bennett, G. Psychosocial aspects of chronic pain in spinal cord injury. *Pain, 8:* 355–366, 1980.
45. Richardson, R. R., Meyer, P. R., and Cerullo, L. J. Neurostimulation in the modulation of intractable paraplegic and traumatic neuroma pains. *Pain, 8:* 75–84, 1980.
46. Richardson, R. R., Meyer, P. R., and Cerullo, L. J. Transcutaneous electrical neurostimulation in musculoskeletal pain of acute spinal cord injuries. *Spine, 5:* 42–45, 1980.
47. Schwartz, R. G., Gall, N. G., and Grant, A. E. Abdominal pain in quadriparesis: myofascial syndrome as unsuspected cause. *Arch. Phys. Med. Rehabil., 65:* 44–46, 1984.
48. Scott, J. A., and Donovan, W. H. The prevention of shoulder pain and contracture in the acute tetraplegia patient. *Paraplegia, 19:* 313–319, 1981.
49. Shannon, N., Symon, L., Logue, V., Cull, D., Kang, J., and Kendall, B. Clinical features, investigation and treatment of post-traumatic syringomyelia. *J. Neurol. Neurosurg. Psychiatry, 44:* 35–42, 1981.
50. Taub, A. Relief of post-herpetic neuralgia with psychotropic drugs. *J. Neurosurg., 39:* 235–239, 1973.
51. Wainapel, S. F. Reflex sympathetic dystrophy following traumatic myelopathy. *Pain, 18:* 345–349, 1984.
52. Wall, P. D., and Gutnick, M. Ongoing activity in peripheral nerves: the physiology and pharmacology of impulses originating in a neuroma. *Exp. Neurol., 43:* 580–593, 1974.
53. Ward, N. G., Bloom, V. L., and Friedel, R. O. The effectiveness of tricyclic antidepressants in the treatment of coexisting pain and depression. *Pain, 7:* 331–341, 1979.
54. White, J. C. Cordotomy: assessment of its effectiveness and suggestions for improvement. *Clin. Neurosurg., 13:* 1–19, 1966.
55. Zoppi, M. La terapia non farmacologia del dolore. In: *Fisiopatologia e Terapia Medica del Dolore.* Edited by Teodori, U., Maresca, M., Pagni, C. A., Pepeu, G., Procacci, P., and Zoppi, M. Edizioni Luigi Pozzi, Rome, 1982, pp. 81–104.

9

Thrombosis Prevention and Treatment in Spinal Cord Injured Patients

A. G. G. TURPIE

INCIDENCE AND SIGNIFICANCE

Deep vein thrombosis and pulmonary embolism are among the most common and serious complications occurring in hospitalized patients. In the United States it has been estimated that pulmonary embolism occurs in more than 500,000 patients each year, leading to a fatal outcome in as many as 200,000. Almost all pulmonary emboli arise from venous thrombi in the deep veins of the legs or pelvis. In patients who are immobilized or who have undergone surgery, most venous thrombi arise in the veins of the calf and in many instances remain localized and asymptomatic. However, if untreated, extension into the popliteal, femoral, or iliac veins occurs in approximately 20%, which may give rise to significant obstruction to venous return or to the occurrence of pulmonary embolism (24, 90, 110). The incidence of venous thrombosis diagnosed by objective methods in selected populations of hospitalized patients is shown in Table 9.1. In patients with spinal cord injuries, venous thrombosis has been reported to occur in 15% to 60%, depending upon the severity of the injury, the presence of lower limb paralysis, and the presence of other associated risk factors (20, 36, 51, 127, 147, 151, 152). The reported incidence of fatal pulmonary embolism ranged from 2% to 16% of patients within 2 to 3 months of spinal cord injury (108, 119, 136, 138, 139).

Because of the frequency and significance of venous thromboembolism in hospitalized patients in general and in spinal cord injury patients in particular, it is important for clinicians to have a knowledge of the process of thrombosis and the awareness of advances in the development of diagnostic methods and approaches for the prevention and treatment of the condition.

Table 9.1.
Frequency of Venous Thrombosis as Detected by Objective Tests

Category	Incidence (%)
Elective Surgery	
Gynecological	7–45
Major abdominal	14–33
Thoracic	26–65
Retropubic prostatectomy	24–51
Transurethral prostatectomy	7–10
Hip replacement	48–54
Emergency Surgery	
Hip fracture	48–74
Childbirth	3
Medical	
Myocardial infarction	23–38
Stroke	21–60
Spinal Cord Injury	15–60

THROMBOGENESIS

The formation of a hemostatic plug after blood vessel injury is a vital homeostatic mechanism in man. The sequence by which blood is transformed from a fluid state into a solid hemostatic plug is a multistage process involving the interaction of platelets, blood vessel wall, and the blood coagulation mechanism. Thrombosis, in contrast, involves formation of an intravascular plug that may be one of two types depending upon the predominating constituents and their organization. Thrombi that form in situations of rapid flow, such as in the arterial circulation, consist predominantly of closely aggregated platelets stabilized by fibrin meshwork. Thrombi that occur in veins where blood flow is slow or stasis exists are composed mostly of red cells enmeshed within a fibrin lattice work with platelets dispersed regularly throughout the structure. Venous thrombi often begin at valve cusps and grow by extension into the lumen, propagating in an antegrade and retrograde direction, often extending into the branches and tributaries (133, 134, 135). Numerous factors are involved in the initial propagation, interruption, and dissolution of venous thrombi.

Blood Vessel Wall

The endothelial cell lining of vessels provides a nonthrombogenic surface in contact with blood. The reason endothelial cells are nonthrombogenic is not precisely known, but several factors may be important. Endothelial cells synthesize prostacyclin that partially inhibits platelet aggregation and thereby thrombus formation. The endothelial cell is a source of plasminogen activator and heparin-like molecules that, while probably not synthesized by the cells, are adsorbed by them. These substances could serve to inhibit thrombus formation. When the vessel is damaged, there is loss of endothelium, and the exposed subendothelial structures interact with blood producing rapid adherence of platelets at the site of endothelial damage and activation of blood coagulation (142).

Blood Platelets

A variety of stimuli provoke a number of responses in platelets contributing to thrombosis. When exposed to subendothelial structures, notably collagen in the basement membranes, platelets adhere rapidly. This stimulates the release of adenosine diphosphate as well as a number of other substances including phospholipids, which are involved in blood coagulation, platelet specific proteins such as betathromboglobulin and platelet factor 4, the products of arachidonic acid metabolism such as prostaglandin, thromboxane A_2, a potent platelet aggregating agent, and a number of other vasoactive amines that may produce vasospasm (5, 12).

Leukocytes

The role of white cells in the thrombotic process is incompletely understood, but evidence indicates that white cells at the site of blood vessel damage release certain materials such as tissue thromboplastins that may stimulate blood coagulation locally. They are also a source of lysozymes that contribute to the dissolution of thrombotic material (29, 146).

Coagulation Factors

At the site of damage to a blood vessel wall the coagulation system is activated by tissue factor derived from several sources (41, 72). Tissue factor triggers the extrinsic system of thromboplastin formation by reacting with factor VII. Simultaneously collagen activates factor XII, which initiates the intrinsic pathway of thromboplastin formation. Collagen activation involves sequential activation of coagulation factors XII, XI, IX, VIII, and X in a cascade fashion. The product of both extrinsic and intrinsic pathways is activated factor X, which with factor V (calcium and phospholipids derived from platelets) converts prothrombin to thrombin. Thrombin is a proteolytic enzyme that converts fibrinogen to fibrin, which constitutes the solid phase of thrombus.

Blood Flow

The development of stasis in a vessel is an important predisposing factor for thrombosis because it prevents mixing of the activated factors with their natural inhibitors. Anoxia and local trauma, such as prolonged and unrelieved mechanical pressure, may also occur, giving rise to endothelial damage (155).

Inhibitory Mechanism

Several mechanisms inhibit the development of thrombosis or serve to arrest its progress. These include protease inhibitors in plasma that chemically react with and inhibit serine proteases, including the activated coagulation factors. These inhibitors are antithrombin III, alpha$_2$-macroglobulin, alpha$_1$-antitrypsin, and C$_1$-esterase. Of these, antithrombin III, also known as heparin cofactor, appears to be the most important since its interaction with serine protease is the most rapid and it also inhibits activated factors XII, XI, IX, and X in addition to thrombin (97, 101, 102). Two recently described inhibitors, protein C and heparin cofactor II, may also play important roles inhibiting the genesis and growth of thrombi (62, 67, 145).

Liver function may also be considered an inhibitory pathway for thrombogenesis since activated clotting factors are cleared by passage through the liver.

Fibrinolytic Enzyme System

The fibrinolytic enzyme system is the most important mechanism for the dissolution of thrombi (33, 35, 98). Plasminogen, an inactive plasma protein, is converted to a potent enzyme plasmin by tissue activator released into the circulation. It serves to maintain the patency of the vascular tree. Plasminogen may also be activated by exogenous substances such as urokinase and streptokinase. Plasmin has a potent proteolytic effect on both fibrin and fibrinogen, and digests both of these molecules resulting in the formation of fibrinogen degradation products, some of which have anticoagulant properties. Potent inhibitors of plasmin in the circulation are alpha$_2$-macroglobulin, alpha$_1$-antitrypsin, and probably antithrombin III. Of these, alpha$_2$-macroglobulin and alpha$_1$-antitrypsin have the greatest antiplasmin effect (4).

RISK FACTORS FOR THROMBOSIS

A number of clinical circumstances increase the risk of deep vein thrombosis in hospitalized patients including those with spinal cord injury. These include increasing age, obesity, malignant disease, heart disease, the use of oral contraceptives, or a history of prior venous thromboembolism. Several of these risk factors may coexist and multiply the risk (37, 137).

Trauma

Trauma is a potent thrombogenic stimulus. The precise mechanism has not been established but possibly involves damage to blood vessel walls with release of tissue thromboplastin into the circulation, thereby activating coagulation. In addition, the stasis produced in the area of trauma favors thrombosis. The risk of thromboembolism is related to the severity, site, and extent of the trauma. Direct trauma to the leg, such as occurs during orthopedic surgery, carries a particularly high risk, and more than 50% of patients undergoing hip surgery develop venous thrombosis. Similarly, the incidence is approximately as high for knee surgery. In surgical trauma, the risk is directly associated with the duration of the procedure and the extent of the tissue damage.

Increasing Age

The incidence of deep vein thrombosis and pulmonary embolism increases directly with age, being infrequent before the fifth decade and rising sharply each decade thereafter. The precise mechanism of this clinical risk factor has not been elucidated, although it has been suggested that dilatation of veins occurs in the elderly thus favoring venous stasis.

Malignancy

The presence of malignant disease increases the risk of venous thrombosis by two or three times following surgery or trauma. The mechanism is the production of a procoagulant material by tumors that activate factor X (56). Tissue thromboplastin-like materials are present in some malignant tissues. In addition, some patients with malignant disease have reduced plasma fibrinolytic activity.

Immobilization

Immobilization is an important risk factor in thrombosis (54). Whether the effect is entirely due to stasis is uncertain, but the loss of pumping action of the calf muscles, dilatation of veins occurring with prolonged immobility, and stasis of blood in superficial or communicating veins of the legs are probably important factors (23). This is likely to be one of the major factors in the genesis of venous thrombi in spinal cord injuries with para- or quadriplegia.

Varicose Veins

Most but not all surveys have identified the presence of varicose veins as increasing the risk of thrombosis by approximately twofold. Whether this is due to the loss of endothelial cells, the decrease in production of fibrinolytic activity, or because of stasis is unknown.

Obesity

Most series have identified a high frequency of deep vein thrombosis in obese patients compared with normal individuals. In obese patients, there is impairment of fibrinolytic activity and possibly stasis in the deep veins of the legs that may contribute to their increased risk (3, 58).

Hormonal Alterations

Although there is some association between administration of estrogen-containing preparations and the occurrence of deep vein thrombosis, a causative effect has not clearly been documented (46, 55).

Blood Groups

Those in blood group O have been reported to have a lower frequency of venous thromboembolism than those with other blood groups, specifically group A. This mechanism is not known, but it has been suggested that a genetic predisposition to thrombosis may be operative (86).

DIAGNOSIS OF VENOUS THROMBOSIS

In diagnosing venous thromboembolic disease, accurate objective methods that are sensitive and specific are essential for the proper management of the disease and for the assessment of prevention methods. In the past decade, several methods of diagnosing venous thromboembolism have been evaluated prospectively, and accurate, noninvasive tests now are available that may be universally applied.

Clinical Diagnosis

Thrombosis in a leg vein may produce the characteristic manifestations of inflammation and swelling from interference with venous return. In some situations, as in classical phlegmasia cerula dolens, the clinical recognition is reliable in most instances. However, in the majority of patients with venous thrombosis, the signs and symptoms are often minimal and usually nonspecific (8, 39). In symptomatic patients with clinical presentations consistent with deep vein thrombosis, only 50% will have the disease when venography is carried out. On the other hand, fewer than half the cases of venous thrombosis involving major proximal veins are recognizable clinically. Because clinical diagnosis is insensitive and nonspecific, it is important for optimal care of patients that the diagnosis be established by objective methods. These methods include venography, impedance plethysmography, [125]Iodine-labelled fibrinogen leg scanning, and Doppler ultrasound (73, 78).

Venography

Venography is currently regarded as the definitive test for the diagnosis of venous thrombosis and is the reference method for evaluating all other techniques (118).

Venography involves injection of approximately 75 to 150 ml of radiopaque contrast medium into a dorsal vein of the foot. If adequate filling of the major deep veins is achieved, the presence of venous thrombosis can be reliably diagnosed by identification of a constant filling defect, the abrupt termination of a column of contrast media at a constant site, and the nonfilling of the deep system despite adequate venographic technique. Thrombosis is also implied by the presence of collateral vessels. If the iliac vessels or vena cava are not outlined by ascending venography, venography by direct puncture of the femoral veins may be required.

The complications of venography are extravasation of contrast media at the injection site, pain in the legs during injection, and rarely, hypersensitivity reactions. The occurrence of deep vein thrombosis following venography is rare. Complications may be minimized by flushing the venous system with isotonic saline after the examination and elevation of the legs to empty the veins of contrast medium.

Impedance Plethysmography (IPG)

Several plethysmographic techniques have been used for the diagnosis of venous thrombosis, and of these, electric impedance has been the most thoroughly evaluated. The technique is based on the fact that blood volume changes produced by venous occlusion in the thighs results in changes in electrical resistance in the calf. These changes in blood volume and electrical resistance are reduced in patients with obstruction to venous outflow due to thrombosis in the popliteal or more proximal veins (156, 157). Impedance plethysmography is performed with the patient supine and the leg elevated to 30° to 35°. Venous outflow from the leg is impeded with a pneumatic cuff applied to the midthigh and inflated to 40 to 45 mm/Hg. The changes in electrical resistance in the calf, resulting from alterations in blood volume distal to the cuff, are detected by calf electrodes and recorded on an ECG strip. The accuracy of the test is influenced by the degree of venous filling obtained during cuff occlusion and can be enhanced by repeating the test sequentially. There have been several studies to evaluate the use of impedance plethysmography for the diagnosis of venous thrombosis in patients with clinically suspected venous thrombosis (78, 79, 80, 81). Results indicate that IPG is highly sensitive to symptomatic proximal vein thrombosis. When used as a screening test in high-risk patients other than those with hip surgery, IPG is not reliable as most thrombi in these patients involve the calf, and involvement of the proximal vessels is often not totally occlusive in the early stages. Thus IPG would likely fail to detect the majority of calf vein thrombi and nearly 25% of those in the proximal veins. The routine use of IPG as a screening procedure therefore, cannot be recommended since alternative methods such as leg scanning are more reliable.

False positive IPG's may occur in conditions that interfere with venous return among such as congestive heart failure, constrictive pericarditis, or obstruction of the veins by external compression such as tumors. The test may not be technically possible in uncooperative patients and in those who cannot be properly positioned or relaxed. This would prove a problem in spinal cord injury patients on Stryker frames. The IPG may be negative when proximal vein thrombosis is associated with well-developed collaterals or when small nonocclusive thrombi are present.

The IPG is most useful when used as a diagnostic test in patients with suspected proximal vein thrombosis in whom a positive test may be regarded as sufficiently specific to justify treatment with anticoagulant drugs.

^{125}Iodine-labelled Fibrinogen Leg Scanning

The diagnosis of venous thrombosis using fibrinogen leg scanning depends upon incorporation of radioiodine-labelled fibrinogen into a thrombus which is detected by measuring an increase in surface radioactivity with a gamma ray detector. Leg scanning depends upon the deposition of radioiodine-labelled fibrinogen into or around an established thrombus or may be used as a screening procedure in high-risk cases to detect the earliest deposition of fibrin on the blood vessel wall (22, 49, 88).

To perform the test, 100 μC of ^{125}iodine-labelled fibrinogen are injected intravenously, and counts of radioactivity are made on the surface of the leg at several points over the major veins. The test is repeated daily for 7 to 10 days following a single injection of fibrinogen. The uptake by the thyroid gland of ^{125}iodine is prevented by the oral administration of potassium iodide. Venous thrombosis is suspected when there is increased radioactivity of more than 20% at any point on the leg compared with readings at adjacent points on the same leg or of a corresponding point in the opposite leg. The diagnosis of venous thrombosis can be made if the readings remain positive for more than 24 hours. The test is insensitive to thrombi in the pelvic veins and may be unreliable in the upper thigh because of the close proximity of the bladder, which contains excreted iodide, and because of the presence of large veins and arteries in the pelvic area that increase the background count (73). If patients have indwelling catheters or external collecting devices, the tubing and leg bags must be positioned away from the detector.

As a screening test in high-risk patients, the fibrinogen leg scan is highly sensitive to calf vein thrombi detecting more than 95%, but it is insensitive to thrombi in the pelvic veins. When used as a diagnostic test, it is relatively insensitive, being positive in approximately 70% of cases. It may become abnormal from 4 to 6 hours after the injection of labelled fibrinogen, but in other instances, 72 hours may pass before sufficient deposition within the thrombus occurs to give positive results (7).

Leg scanning is a safe procedure with few complications; the most common reaction is sensitivity to iodine, but this is seldom serious. Leg scanning has been used most extensively for evaluation of prophylactic methods where it has proven to be extremely useful. In practice, the use for screening in high-risk patients is reliable, but with the introduction of effective means of prophylaxis, is seldom cost effective. When prophylaxis is not totally effective, combining the use of prophylaxis with leg scanning that allows the detection of treatment failures has proven valuable.

Doppler Ultrasound

Doppler ultrasound flow meter examination is a noninvasive technique for the diagnosis of venous thrombosis depending upon the detection of changes in the velocity of blood flow in the veins. The Doppler ultrasound flow velocity detector contains a crystal that directs an ultrasonic beam percutaneously to an underlying vein where it is reflected from passing blood cells. If the column of blood in the vein is stationary, the frequency of the reflected beam is identical to the incident beam and no beat frequency is recorded. On the other hand, if the column of blood is moving, then the beam is reflected at a changed frequency proportional to the velocity of the flow. The frequency difference between the incident and the reflected ultrasound beam received by a second crystal in the probe is amplified to an audible signal or flow sound. This may be used to detect thrombosis at various levels in the leg in the femoral, popliteal, and posterior tibial regions (48, 82, 144). The position of the vein is determined by locating the sounds produced from the adjacent artery. The flow of venous blood is characterized by low frequency and respiratory variation that is augmented by various maneuvers such as movement of the ankle and manual compression of the calf. Thrombosis modifies the presence and characteristics of the sound during these maneuvers (7).

Doppler ultrasound has been compared to venography in patients with clinically suspected deep vein thrombosis and has been shown to be highly sensitive to iliac, femoral, and popliteal thrombi. The sensitivity in a number of studies exceeds 85%, and there is a low incidence of falsely positive results. The sensitivity to calf vein thrombi is low and in most series is less than 60%. The test has not been sufficiently evaluated as a screening test for surveillance in high-risk patients. The major limitations of Doppler ultrasound are that it requires considerable expertise to perform and the interpretation is subjective (7).

Several other approaches to the diagnosis of deep vein thrombosis have been evaluated, but none have been sufficiently refined to be suitable substitutes for the more established methods. These include isotope venography, isotope scan venography, thermography, and a variety of blood tests (14, 26, 50, 64, 70, 71, 87, 111).

CLINICAL DIAGNOSIS OF PULMONARY EMBOLISM

Prior to the use of heparin, the mortality rate from untreated symptomatic pulmonary embolism was as high as 30%. Since the introduction of heparin for the treatment of pulmonary embolism, the mortality rate is below 1%. This emphasizes the need for prompt recognition of the disease. However, the clinical diagnosis of pulmonary embolism, as with venous thrombosis, lacks sensitivity and specificity. There have been a number of studies demonstrating that only one-third of patients with clinical signs compatible with major pulmonary embolism have the diagnosis confirmed by angiography, and similarly pulmonary embolism is often undiagnosed, either because its presentation is atypical or because it is clinically silent (122). Clinical manifestations vary widely and are based largely on the size of the embolus and preexisting conditions of the heart and lungs. With massive pulmonary embolism, symptoms range from sudden and severe dyspnea, which may be associated with cardiopulmonary collapse, to minimal or only fleeting symptoms of dyspnea and apprehension. With submassive embolism, symptoms are seldom dramatic unless there is underlying cardiopulmonary disease. Usually there is dyspnea that might be quite transient. In a few patients, symptoms of pulmonary infarction consisting of pleuritic chest pain, cough, and hemoptysis occur. The symptoms are neither sufficiently sensitive nor specific to be reliable in the detection and quantification of pulmonary embolism. For this reason, a high index of suspicion must be maintained in all instances in which embolism is suspected, and objective methods of diagnosis should be employed. Frequently, especially in patients who have spinal cord injuries, the manifestations of pulmonary embolism are either lacking or sufficiently subtle as to remain undetected. Some suggestive symptoms in these patients, such as unexplained pyrexia, tachycardia, tachypnea, or change in cardiac rhythm, should raise the suspicion of pulmonary embolism.

Pulmonary angiography is the only specific diagnostic test for pulmonary embolism, but it is not universally available and may not be required in some patients with suspected embolism where other less-invasive tests are sufficiently diagnostic.

There are a number of screening tests that should be done to evaluate patients with symptoms and signs compatible with pulmonary embolism. These include chest x-ray, electrocardiogram, and radioisotope lung scan. Of these, the chest x-ray and lung scan are the most helpful since pulmonary embolism can be excluded if both are negative. The diagnosis of pulmonary embolism may be made with a high degree of certainty if the lung scan findings are "high probability." However, if the lung scan is "low probability" or "nonspecific," the patient may require pulmonary angiography.

Pulmonary Angiography

Pulmonary angiography is the most definitive method for the diagnosis of pulmonary embolism. Angiography is performed by injecting sufficient contrast medium through a catheter selectively placed in the right or left main pulmonary artery, or in the lobar arteries, segmental branches and the first two subdivisions. Abnormalities in the pulmonary angiogram that are consistent with a diagnosis of embolism are an intraluminal filling defect or the abrupt cutoff of a lobar, segmental or subsegmental artery. Areas of oligemia, asymmetry of flow, pruning of peripheral pulmonary arteries, or delayed emptying of pulmonary veins are unreliable signs of embolism.

Chest X-Ray

Chest x-ray is an essential diagnostic procedure if pulmonary embolism is suspected. A number of abnormalities in the chest film have been described in pulmonary embolism, but none of these are specific. However, the chest x-ray will identify other intrathoracic causes that may be responsible for the symptoms such as pneumonia, pneumothorax, or pulmonary hemorrhage. In pulmonary embolism, the chest film may appear normal or there may be pulmonary infiltrates, atelectasis, elevation of the diaphragm, pleural effusion, or altered vascular marking. In addition, a chest x-ray is necessary for proper interpretation of the lung scan.

Electrocardiogram

Changes in the electrocardiogram are nonspecific for the diagnosis of pulmonary embolism. Even in patients with massive pulmonary embolism, abnormalities of the ECG occur in only one-half of the cases. The most common change seen is T-wave inversion, but other more characteristic patterns of acute right ventricular strain occur. These include right axis deviation or right bundle branch block. Various arrhythmias, especially supraventricular in type, may develop in association with pulmonary embolism, but all are nonspecific.

Isotope Lung Scanning

Combined radioisotope perfusion and ventilation lung scanning has been considered the most valuable test for the diagnosis of pulmonary embolism (16, 44). This test is performed by intravenously injecting particles 10 to 15 mu in diameter labelled with gamma-emitting isotopes, which are distributed throughout the lungs in a manner corresponding to the blood flow. With pulmonary arterial obstruction, a perfusion defect in the involved area of lung can be detected by a gamma camera or rectilinear scanner. A minimum of four views (anterior, posterior, right and left lateral) and preferably six (right and left oblique) are required for proper evaluation. Ventilation scan involves the administration, by inhalation, of isotopes such as [133]xenon. The regional distribution of radioactive gas in the lung is compared with the pulmonary perfusion scan. This identifies areas that are being ventilated but not perfused, which should occur with pulmonary embolism. The limitation of scanning is that a number of pulmonary diseases alter perfusion and produce false positive scans. These include chronic obstructive disease of the airways, bronchospastic disease, pneumonia, congestive heart failure, and pleural effusion. The correct approach to the diagnosis of pulmonary embolism using lung scanning remains controversial because opinions differ about the specificity of ventilation perfusion lung scanning. Published data regarding the clinical use of ventilation perfusion scanning are taken largely from retrospective studies or from nonconsecutive patient series. In a recent study, it was found that patients with large perfusion defects with ventilation mismatch had a high probability of pulmonary embolism using angiography as the confirmatory test. Based on the results of this study, clinical recommendations can be made that ventilation scanning is helpful in patients with large perfusion defects because it markedly increases the probability of pulmonary embolism if a mismatch is found. However, the presence of a ventilation perfusion match does not rule out the possibility of pulmonary embolism, and the presence of small perfusion defects with a ventilation mismatch indicates neither a high nor low probability of pulmonary embolism (77).

Other Diagnostic Tests

There are a number of auxiliary investigations including arterial blood gases, tests of intravascular fibrin formation and degradation, and other nonspecific enzyme tests that are available. The use of ascending venography may be helpful in clinical decision making because venographically demonstrated venous thrombosis is present in some patients with suspected pulmonary embolism. However, a normal venogram does not exclude a diagnosis of pulmonary embolism.

Antithrombotic Therapy

Knowledge of thrombogenesis and the clinical risk factors for venous thromboembolism allow identification of approaches to antithrombotic therapy. Thus, approaches for prevention of venous thromboembolism include the use of methods to prevent damage to blood vessel walls, particularly the endothelial cells, to prevent stasis, to prevent stimulation of platelets, to inhibit the activation of blood coagulation, or to increase the fibrolytic enzyme activity of the blood. Once the process of thrombosis has started, methods are required to arrest the growth of thrombi and begin inhibition of blood coagulation by therapeutic anticoagulation.

Mechanical methods to prevent stasis in the deep veins of the legs are numerous and include simple means such as elevation of the legs, passive or active exercises during periods of immobilization, and more sophisticated techniques such as electrical stimulation of the calf muscles or use of intermittent compression devices such as external pneumatic compression of the legs. A novel method of increasing venous return is the use of the drug dihydroergotamine, which causes venoconstriction, thereby inhibiting stasis. Interference in platelet function by drugs including aspirin, hydroxychloroquine, dipyridamole, sulfinpyrazone, and dextran has been shown to be antithrombotic in a variety of conditions.

The coagulation system can be inhibited in a number of ways. Heparin is known to inhibit serine proteases, particularly activated coagulation factors XII, XI, X, IX, and thrombin (95, 124, 125). The effect of heparin has been demonstrated to occur through the antithrombin III molecule. Heparin complexes with antithrombin III produce a change in the steric configuration of antithrombin III. Antithrombin III is a naturally occurring inhibitor of thrombin reaction, and when it is combined with heparin, its inhibitory effect is greatly increased (34). It has been shown that various factors require different amounts of heparin/antithrombin III complex for their inhibition. Thus, formed thrombin requires relatively large amounts of heparin to inhibit its effect in contrast to factor Xa, which is more sensitive. Inhibition of factor Xa prevents the conversion of prothrombin to thrombin, and thus small amounts of heparin that inhibit factor X activation can produce thrombosis prophylaxis. Once a thrombus has formed and thrombin is present, however, larger amounts of heparin are required to arrest thrombosis. Oral anticoagulants (25), of which the coumadin derivatives are the best known, exert an effect by acting in the liver as competitive inhibitors of vitamin K, resulting in alteration of the liver's synthesis of vitamin K-dependent clotting factors, including factors II, VII, IX, and X. As as a result of this, the liver produces dysfunctional zymogens that are antigenically identical to normal clotting factors but lack coagulant activity because of failure of carboxylation of several glutamic acid residues, and therefore the clotting factors do not react normally with phospholipids and calcium.

Increasing the fibrinolytic activity of blood can be accomplished in several ways, including the intravenous administration of the active proteolytic enzyme plasmin or the infusion of agents that activate the proenzyme plasminogen to plasmin. These agents include urokinase and streptokinase, which produce an immediate increase in fibrinolytic activity, the intensity of which is predictable depending on dosage. The resultant fibrinolytic state can markedly accelerate the rate of dissolution of thrombi or emboli. The digestion of fibrin and other proteins, including fibrinogen, leads to the formation of fibrin degradation products that have anticoagulant activity. This effect contributes to the bleeding complications of thrombolytic therapy.

TREATMENT OF ACTIVE THROMBOEMBOLISM

If patients with established venous thromboembolism do not receive antithrombotic therapy, the thrombotic process may extend, producing obstruction to venous return, or if pulmonary embolization occurs, a fatal outcome may develop. In the vast majority of patients, venous thrombosis in the legs begins in the veins of the calf and will usually remain localized, producing few if any symptoms and no significant long-term consequences. However, in approximately 20% of these patients, the thrombi will extend into the popliteal and low proximal veins, and approximately 40% of these will develop pulmonary embolism, which may lead to a fatal outcome.

In patients with major vein thrombosis, the process of healing often results in residual scarring and loss of venous valve function that produces altered venous return and may lead to the postphlebitic syndrome. Of patients with symptomatic pulmonary embolism, 40% will have recurrence if not treated, of which 20% may be fatal.

Since progression and embolization may develop rapidly and unpredictably, all patients in whom the presence of venous thromboembolism has been confirmed should be treated with anticoagulant therapy (9, 92). There is good evidence that, once treatment is started, the outlook for recovery is favorable, with recurrence, progression or embolization occurring in fewer than 5% of patients. In patients with pulmonary embolism treated with anticoagulants, the recurrence rate is less than 5% with a very low mortality rate. Even those patients with massive emboli have a mortality rate of less than 10%.

Heparin is the drug of choice in primary treatment of venous thromboembolism. Following a course of heparin, the majority of patients require a period of secondary prophylaxis until the risk of recurrence has been eliminated. In some patients, the use of thrombolytic therapy to accelerate the rate of removal of the thrombotic or embolic obstruction may be indicated. This may be achieved by the use of thrombolytic drugs or by surgery. Surgical techniques include thrombectomy and pulmonary embolectomy. In addition, procedures to obstruct vena cava lumen to prevent recurrent embolization may be used and they include caval plication or the use of the Greenfield filter (61).

Anticoagulant Therapy

Heparin

Heparin is the drug of choice in the treatment of acute thromboembolism. Heparin is administered either by continuous intravenous or intermittent intravenous injection or by subcutaneous injection. It is usual to start with an intravenous bolus of 5000 to 7500 units, which will anticoagulate the vast majority of patients. The half-life of heparin is 1 to 2 hours, and in the majority of patients, the bolus will have cleared in 4 hours. if heparin is administered by continuous intravenous fusion, approximately 30,000 units per day will be sufficient to produce an adequate anticoagulant response. If heparin is given by intermittent intravenous injection, approximately 5000 to 10,000 units every 4 to 6 hours are required. Recent evidence shows that heparin may be given by subcutaneous injection in therapeutic doses that will maintain the blood levels at therapeutic concentrations through a 24 hour period.

The response of most patients to heparin falls within a predictable range, however, approximately 15% to 25% of patients will either have an inadequate or excessive response to heparin. Clinical evidence indicates that patients most likely to have recurrent thromboembolism are those who are inadequately anticoagulated, and patients with excessive anticoagulation have an increased incidence of bleeding (11). Therefore, it is desirable to monitor their anticoagulant response by means of one of several clotting tests that are affected by heparin. The choice is usually based on local preference, but it is essential that the test chosen will detect therapeutic levels of heparin and have a reasonably linear response curve. With an appropriately sensitive test, it is possible, immediately upon initiation of heparin therapy, to document that anticoagulation has been achieved. The tests used to monitor heparin therapy are the whole blood clotting time, activated partial thromboplastin time, and more recently, the use of plasma heparin levels. The thrombin clotting time and the prothrombin time are less useful. The precise duration of treatment with heparin is difficult to define, but the objective is to maintain full anticoagulation until active thrombosis has been arrested and the thrombi have been firmly attached to the vessel wall. This requires a minimum of 5 days and may take up to 8 to 10 days to occur. Based on this and on some retrospective data indicating that recurrence is less likely with heparin and compared with warfarin, most authorities recommend the use of heparin for 7 to 10 days followed by a period of secondary prophylaxis with warfarin.

Several complications have been reported with heparin therapy, including hemorrhage, hypersensitivity reactions, and thrombocytopenia. Bleeding is the most important complication and occurs in 5% to 10% of patients. It is particularly likely to occur in patients with an underlying hemostatic defect, patients treated with aspirin, and patients exposed to recent surgery or trauma. There is some evidence that the risk of bleeding increases with the dose of heparin, and in patients at high risk, the use of intermittent intravenous injections is probably associated with a higher risk of bleeding than the continuous infusion of the drug (99, 129). Thrombocytopenia has been reported with varying frequency but probably occurs in less than 2% of patients (15). It is usually seen in the first week of treatment. The mechanism is uncertain and may be immune mediated.

Hypersensitivity is uncommon but may occur and range from cutaneous urticaria to anaphylaxis. The mechanism of hypersensitivity is not understood. Osteoporosis is a rare complication and occurs only after prolonged exposure to heparin (128). This may have some implication regarding its use in spinal cord injury patients.

Bleeding complications of heparin can be prevented by careful attention to the dose. However, if bleeding occurs, heparin should be stopped. If rapid reversal is required, the use of protamine sulfate, which combines with and inactivates heparin, is indicated.

Oral Anticoagulants

After the primary treatment of the thromboembolic episode, usually with 7 to 10 days of heparin, patients require 3 to 6 months of secondary prophylaxis. This may be by the use of oral anticoagulants (21, 25) or by adjusted-dose subcutaneous heparin (74, 76). Oral anticoagulants should begin 5 to 6 days before heparin therapy is discontinued and be maintained for 3 to 6 months. The dose of anticoagulants should maintain prothrombin time in a therapeutic range depending upon the reagent used in the test. For example, there is evidence that, using rabbit brain thromboplastin, the conventional therapeutic range of 24 to 26 seconds results in too high a dose being administered, and the prothrombin time should be maintained between 16 to 18 seconds. The use of human brain thromboplastin, which is more sensitive to changes in coagulation factors, may be safer.

There have been several reports on the use of anticoagulant therapy for the treatment of spinal cord injured patients. The studies involved only small numbers of patients, but in none of the studies was there evidence that the use of anticoagulant therapy in spinal cord injury patients is unsafe (65, 112, 113, 119, 153).

Thrombolytic Therapy

The use of thrombolytic therapy in venous thromboembolism is gaining wide acceptance, but it is contraindicated in the acute phase of spinal cord injury because of the significant risk of hemorrhage (47, 150).

Surgical Therapy

Although the management of venous thromboembolism almost always is medical, a number of surgical procedures are available in patients in whom anticoagulant therapy is contraindicated or has failed. Thrombectomy or pulmonary embolectomy are used only as last resorts. In patients with venous thromboembolism in whom heparin is contraindicated or in whom embolism has occurred despite adequate anticoagulation, caval ligation (126) or insertion of a number of devices to screen the cava may be used. The most recent advance is the use of the Greenfield filter, which may be inserted via the jugular vein (60, 61). The Greenfield filter is a nonthrombogenic structure that lodges in the vena cava below the renal veins and effectively blocks embolization to the lungs from venous thrombi in the legs.

Prevention of Venous Thromboembolism

Two approaches can be taken to prevent venous thromboembolism in high-risk patients: (a) early detection of subclinical venous thrombosis by screening high-risk patients, and (b) the use of primary prophylactic methods. The ideal method of prophylaxis should be safe, effective, and acceptable to patients, nurses, and medical staff. It should be easily administered, inexpensive, and simple to monitor.

Methods of primary prevention of venous thromboembolism that have been evaluated in prospective clinical trials are low-dose heparin, physical methods, platelet function suppressant drugs, dextran, and oral anticoagulants.

Low Dose Heparin

In the late 1960s it was first reported that small doses of heparin, while insufficient to prolong the whole blood clotting time, were effective in reducing the frequency of clinically detectable venous thrombosis. A number of trials using objective methods to diagnose venous thromboembolism have now confirmed the effectiveness of heparin in preventing venous thrombosis among high-risk patients.

There have been over 20 randomized, prospective trials comparing low-dose heparin with placebos (or no treatment) in patients undergoing general abdominothoracic or gynecological surgery. In more than 80% of these trials, heparin reduced the frequency of scan-detected venous leg thrombosis from approximately 30% in the control patients to 7% in the heparin-treated patients (6, 42, 52, 53, 57, 63, 90, 91, 109, 115, 132). In the studies that showed no significant difference between heparin-treated patients and the control group, the frequency of venous thrombosis among the control patients was low or the numbers were too small (1, 38). Patients who had undergone surgery for malignant disease were included in some of the studies, and although the incidence of venous thrombosis was greater in both control and treated patients than in those with nonmalignant conditions, low-dose heparin was again found to be effective in reducing postoperative venous thrombosis.

The reported frequency of clinically significant bleeding in the heparin group has varied. Although in most reports such bleeding was not found, two of the studies noted a clear increase in the percentage of patients who developed postoperative wound hematomas and other postoperative bleeding, but this bleeding was considered to be of minor clinical significance. Major bleeding due to low-dose heparin prophylaxis was very uncommon, and no deaths from bleeding were reported.

Low-dose heparin prophylaxis does not appear to be effective in patients undergoing surgery for hip fractures, and the evidence is suggestive but inconclusive for heparin's effectiveness in patients having elective hip surgery (43, 66, 68, 69, 100, 104, 149). Furthermore, in patients undergoing any orthopedic procedures, the risk of hemorrhage with low-dose heparin prophylaxis is significant. Heparin prophylaxis is also ineffective in open prostatectomy patients.

For general surgical patients, low-dose heparin should be given as 5000 units subcutaneously 2 hours before operation, the same dose 12 hours after surgery, and thereafter two or three times daily until the patient is fully ambulatory.

The efficacy of low-dose heparin prophylaxis is less well-defined in medical patients. There have been four controlled clinical trials in patients with myocardial infarction, and in three of these, heparin did reduce the incidence of scan-detected venous thrombosis of the leg. One study showed the frequency of venous thrombosis following completed strokes to be dramatically reduced with low-dose heparin, but differentiation of thrombotic from hemorrhagic stroke remains imprecise without CAT scanning.

Since most pulmonary emboli originate from venous thrombi in the legs, studies that demonstrate effectiveness of low-dose heparin for prevention of venous thrombosis have supported the hypothesis that low-dose heparin may also prevent pulmonary embolism. Prospective trials of low-dose heparin have confirmed that heparin reduced the incidence of fatal pulmonary embolism (85, 89, 95). Of the trials involving large populations, heparin did not cause clinically significant bleeding.

For medical patients, low-dose heparin should be given as 5000 units subcutaneously every 8 to 12 hours.

Because of the evidence for the efficacy of low-dose heparin prophylaxis in general surgical and medical patients without increased risk of significant hemorrhage, low-dose heparin has been proposed as the method of preventing deep vein thrombosis in spinal cord injured patients; however, there have been no good randomized studies to demonstrate the efficacy and safety of low-dose heparin in these patients. There have been several reports on the use of low-dose heparin in spinal cord injury patients, but these studies have been nonrandomized and involved only small numbers of patients (51, 120, 121, 138, 139, 154). In one study using retrospective controls, there was a highly significant reduction in the frequency of deep vein thrombosis in spinal cord injured patients using objective tests to diagnose deep vein thrombosis. In none of the studies was there a significant increase in bleeding reported. In one randomized controlled trial involving 32 patients with spinal cord injury, the frequency of venous thrombosis was unexpectedly low in both the control and heparinized groups, but in this study, only impedance plethysmography was used, which would be insensitive to calf vein and nonoccluding thrombi. There have been a number of studies that indicate that low-dose heparin may be safe in neurosurgical patients (10, 28, 116).

The majority of the reports indicate that venous thrombosis is most common during the period of flaccidity, and most authors recommend the use of low-dose heparin or other prophylaxis for the first 3 months following injury.

Physical Methods

Because stasis is a major factor in the development of deep vein thrombosis, a number of simple techniques designed to increase blood flow from the legs have been evaluated for the prevention of venous thrombosis in postoperative and other immobile patients. These measures include leg elevation, physiotherapy, elastic stockings, and graduated pressure stockings. More advanced methods for promoting blood flow include electrical calf muscle stimulation and intermittent pneumatic calf compression.

Simple Physical Methods. Studies have reported results of simple physical methods to prevent venous leg thrombosis in general surgical patients. These methods consisted of leg elevation, elastic stockings, a combination of elastic stockings and intensive physiotherapy, and the use of graduated pressure stockings. Results indicated that neither elastic stockings alone nor leg elevation alone reduced the frequency of postoperative venous thrombosis by more than a third.

However, several recent trials demonstrated significant reduction in postoperative venous thrombosis through the use of graduated stockings in a small number of patients. Thus, a combination of simple measures provides some benefit, and the use of graduated pressure stockings, particularly in low-risk patients, may also prove rewarding.

There are no studies on the use of simple physical methods including the use of graduated pressure stockings for the prevention of deep vein thrombosis in spinal cord injury patients. This is a theoretically attractive form of prophylaxis, especially after the period of highest risk is over. Prospective randomized trials are urgently required in this area.

Electrical Calf Muscle Stimulation. Electrical calf muscle stimulation, which prevents venous stasis by contracting the calf muscles, has been evaluated for venous thrombosis prophylaxis in five randomized studies (13, 45, 123). In three studies, it reduced the frequency of leg-scan detected venous thrombosis, and in the other two studies it produced no effect. Electrical calf muscle stimulation has two major disadvantages: (1) it may be used only when patients are anesthetized, and (b) it is unlikely to help patients who remain immobilized for long periods, such as spinal cord injury patients.

Intermittent Pneumatic Calf Compression. Intermittent pneumatic calf compression has been tested extensively for the prevention of postoperative venous thrombosis. A number of devices have been developed utilizing different cycle times and pressures, including a variety of cuffs, boots, and stockings.

Intermittent compression has been shown to empty the deep calf veins of blood and to increase pulsatile blood flow in the femoral veins. Calf compression has also been shown to increase systemic fibrinolytic enzyme activity, which may contribute to venous thrombosis prevention.

A fast compression cycle in 11 of 12 studies has shown a significant reduction in leg-scan detected venous thrombosis among post-operative patients, including patients undergoing knee surgery (75, 140, 148). A slow cycle used in two studies reduced the frequency of venous thrombosis in patients having surgery for nonmalignant disease; however, in one of these studies, it proved relatively ineffective in patients with malignancies (32).

This technique may have special application for patient groups in whom anticoagulant drugs either are contraindicated (e.g. neurosurgical patients) or have been found to be ineffective (e.g. patients undergoing prostatectomy). Intermittent calf compression is, therefore, a promising method of preventing venous leg thrombosis. It is as effective as low-dose heparin and may offer an alternative in selected patient groups. However, there have been no studies designed to demonstrate a reduction in femoral vein thrombosis or pulmonary embolism.

There has been one study on the use of intermittent pneumatic compression devices with and without concomitant antiplatelet therapy with aspirin (300 mg twice daily) and dipyridamole, (75 mg three times per day) which indicated that the use of pneumatic compression alone or pneumatic compression plus platelet suppressant drugs were significantly better than no treatment at all. However, this study can be criticized because the control patients were nonconcurrent and the numbers in the treated group were small (59).

Platelet Suppressant Drugs

Venous thrombosis occurs as a result of fibrin formation and deposition, but the presence of platelet aggregates at sites of some early venous thrombi suggests that platelets do play a role in initiating the process. It is possible, therefore, that drugs to suppress platelet function may help prevent venous thrombosis in some high-risk patients. Of the antiplatelet drugs that have been tested in prospective clinical trials for the prevention of deep vein thrombosis, aspirin is the only one that has been used extensively in practice. However, the aspirin study conclusions have been inconsistent (30, 31, 83, 84, 96, 103, 106, 118, 141, 143, 158, 159).

Early reports on the use of aspirin to prevent postoperative venous thrombosis after general abdominothoracic surgery indicated no benefit, although two studies (one of which made the diagnosis on clinical grounds) demonstrated a trend in favor of aspirin. Several reports on patients undergoing surgery for fractured hip, elective hip replacement, and total knee replacement found aspirin to be beneficial in reducing the frequency of postoperative venous thrombosis; one study of patients undergoing surgery for fractured hip also showed a reduction in the frequency of fatal pulmonary embolism with aspirin.

There is evidence from one of the elective hip studies that the benefit of aspirin for the prevention of venous thrombosis may be confined to male patients. The difference in response between males and females has also been noted in patients with cerebrovascular ischemia receiving aspirin. However, with increasing clinical experience with the use of aspirin as an antithrombotic drug, the sex difference in response may not hold out. Of greater interest is the controversy between the use of low- or high-dose aspirin, an issue which has not yet been resolved.

Oral Anticoagulants

More than 20 studies have attempted to evaluate the effectiveness of oral anticoagulants in preventing venous thrombosis in high-risk (including orthopedic) patients, but only nine protocols had concurrent control patients and objective end points to diagnose venous thromboembolism (105,

107, 114, 130, 131). In each of the controlled studies, oral anticoagulants reduced the frequency of venous thromboembolism, including fatal pulmonary embolism.

Although side effects varied, four studies did report an increase in major bleeding. Thus, oral anticoagulants are effective in preventing venous thromboembolism, but their routine use has not gained general acceptance due to the increased likelihood of bleeding complications. One approach currently being evaluated is the use of low perioperative and early postoperative doses of oral anticoagulants, increasing to more conventional doses when the risk of hemorrhage is over. This method has been shown to reduce the frequency of bleeding without reducing prophylactic efficacy.

There have been no studies on the use of oral anticoagulants for the primary prophylaxis of venous thrombosis in spinal cord injured patients.

Dextran

Dextran is a glucose polymer (originally introduced as a volume expander) with antithrombotic properties. Results of studies evaluating dextran for the prevention of deep vein thrombosis in surgical patients are conflicting, with some reports (especially in patients undergoing hip surgery) indicating significant benefit and others showing no benefit (2, 13, 17, 27, 63, 93).

The major side-effect of dextran is volume overload, which can result in cardiac failure. Also, allergic reactions have been described but are relatively uncommon. Excessive bleeding has been reported in some patients. Since dextran is relatively expensive and must be given by intravenous infusion, it is not an ideal prophylactic agent.

SUMMARY

Table 9.2 summarizes the methods of venous thrombosis prophylaxis and their comparative effectiveness, safety, ease of administration, acceptability and cost. Table 9.3 outlines current application of the various methods to patients in high-risk groups.

Table 9.2.
An Overview of Venous Thromboembolism Prophylaxis

	Effective	Safe	Easy	Acceptable	Inexpensive
Low-dose heparin	+	+	+	+	±
Physical measures in general	−	+	−	−	+
Pneumatic compression	+	+	±	±	±
Aspirin	±	+	+	+	+
Oral anticoagulants	+	−	−	−	+
Dextran	+	±	±	±	−

Table 9.3.
Prevention of Thromboembolism in High-Risk Patients

	Low-dose heparin	Intermittent pneumatic compression	Aspirin	Warfarin	Dextran
Major abdomino-thoracic surgery					
Age under 40	±	±	−	−	−
Age over 40	+	+	±	−	−
Orthopedic surgery*	−	±	+	+	±
Neurosurgery	−	+	−	−	−
Myocardial infarction	+	−	−	−	−
Stroke	−	+	−	−	−

* VT screen with IPG and scan an alternative

REFERENCES

1. Abernethy, E. E., and Hartsuck, J. M. Postoperative pulmonary embolism: A prospective study utilizing low-dose heparin. *Am. J. Surg., 128:*739, 1974.
2. Ahlberg, A., Nylander, G., Robertson, B., Cronberg, S., and Nilsson, I. M. Dextran in prophylaxis of thrombosis in fractures of the hip. *Acta. Chir. Scand. (Suppl.), 387:*83, 1968.
3. Almér, L. O., and Janzon, L. Low vascular fibrinolytic activity in obesity. *Thromb. Res., 6:*171, 1975.
4. Aoko, N., and Narpel, P. C. Inhibitors of the fibrinolytic enzyme system. *Semin. Thromb. Hemost., 10:*24, 1984.
5. Ashford, T. P., and Freiman, D. G. Platelet aggregation at sites of minimal endothelial injury. *Am. J. Pathol., 53:*599, 1968.
6. Ballard, R. M., Bradley-Watson, P. J., Johnstone, F. D., Kenney, A., McCarthy, T. G., Campbell, S., and Weston, J. Low doses of subcutaneous heparin in the prevention of deep vein thrombosis after gynecological surgery. *J. Obstet. Gynecol. Br. Commonw., 80:*469, 1973.
7. Barnes, R. W., Russell, H. E., Wu, K. K., and Hoak, J. C. Accuracy of Doppler ultrasound in clinically suspected venous thrombosis of the calf. *Surg. Gynecol. Obstet., 143:*425, 1976.
8. Barnes, R. W., Wu, K. K., and Hoak, J. G. Fallibility of the clinical diagnosis of venous thrombosis. *J.A.M.A., 234:*605, 1975.
9. Barritt, D. W., and Jordan, S. C. Anticoagulant drugs in the treatment of pulmonary embolism: A controlled clinical trial. *Lancet, 1:*309, 1960.
10. Barnett, H. G., Clifford, J. R., and Llewellyn, R. C. Safety of mini-dose heparin administration for neurosurgical patients. *J. Neurosurg., 47:*27, 1977.
11. Basu, D., Gallus, A., Hirsh, J., and Cade, J. A prospective study of the value of monitoring heparin treatment with the activated partial thromboplastin time. *N. Engl. J. Med., 287:*324, 1972.
12. Baumgartner, H. R., Stemmerman, M. B., and Spaet, T. H. Adhesion of blood platelets to the subendothelial surface: distinct from adhesion to collagen. *Experientia, 27:*283, 1971.
13. Becker, J., and Schampi, B. The incidence of postoperative venous thrombosis of the legs. A comparative study on the prophylactic effect of Dextran 70 and electrical calf-muscle stimulation. *Acta. Chir. Scand., 139:*357, 1973.

14. Bentley, P. G., and Kakkar, V. V. Radionuclide venography for the demonstration of the proximal deep venous system. *Br. J. Surg., 66:*687, 1979.
15. Bell, W. R. Thrombocytopenia occurring during heparin therapy. *N. Engl. J. Med., 295:*276, 1976.
16. Biello, D. R., Mattar, A. G., McKnight, R. C., and Siegel, B. A. Interpretation of ventilation-perfusion studies in patients with suspected pulmonary embolism. *Am. J. Roentol., 133:*1033, 1979.
17. Bonnar, J., and Walsh, J. Prevention of thrombosis after pelvic surgery by British Dextran 70. *Lancet, 1:*614, 1972.
18. Bookstein, J. J. Segmental arteriography in pulmonary embolism. *Radiology, 93:*1007, 1969.
19. Bookstein, J. J., and Silver, T. M. The angiographic differential diagnosis of acute pulmonary embolism. *Radiology, 110:*25, 1974.
20. Brach, B. B., Moser, K. M., Cedar, L., Minteer, M., and Convery, R. Venous thrombosis in acute spinal cord paralysis. *J. Trauma., 17:*289, 1977.
21. Breckenridge, A. Oral anticoagulant drugs: pharmacokinetic aspects. *Semin. Hematol., 15:*19, 1978.
22. Browse, N. L. The ^{125}I-fibrinogen uptake test. *Arch. Surg., 104:*160, 1972.
23. Browse, N. L. Effect of surgery on resting calf blood flow. *Br. Med. J., 1:*1714, 1962.
24. Browse, N. L. and Lea Thomas, M. Source of non-lethal pulmonary emboli. *Lancet, 1:*258, 1978.
25. Brozovic, M. Oral anticoagulants in clinical practice. *Semin. Hematol., 15:*27, 1978.
26. Bynum, L. J., Wilson, J. E., III, Crotty, C. M., Curry, T. S., and Smitson, H. L. Non-invasive diagnosis of deep venous thrombosis by phleborheography. *Ann. Intern. Med., 89:*163, 1978.
27. Carter, A. E., and Eban, R. The prevention of post-operative deep venous thrombosis with Dextran 70. *Br. J. Surg., 60:*681, 1972.
28. Cerrato, D., Ariano, C., and Fiacchino, F. Deep vein thrombosis and low-dose heparin prophylaxis in neurosurgical patients. *J. Neurosurg., 49:*378, 1978.
29. Charkes, N. D., Dugan, M. A., Malmud, L. S., Stern, H., Anderson, H., Kozar, J., and Maguire, R. Labelled leucocytes in thrombi. *Lancet, 2:*600, 1974.
30. Chrisman, O. D., Snook, G. A., and Wilson, T. C. Prevention of venous thromboembolism by administration of hydroxychloroquine. *J. Bone. Joint. Surg., 7A:*918, 1976.
31. Clagett, G. P., Schneider, P., Rosoff, C. B., and Salzman, E. W. The influence of aspirin on postoperative platelet kinetics and venous thrombosis. *Surgery, 77:*61, 1975.
32. Coe, N. P., Collins, R. E. C., Klein, L. A., Bettmann, M. A., Skillman, J. J., Shapiro, R. M., and Salzman, E. W. Prevention of deep vein thrombosis in urological patients: A controlled, randomized trial of low-dose heparin and external pneumatic compression boots. *Surgery, 83:*230, 1978.
33. Collen, D. On the regulation and control of fibrinolysis. *Thromb. Haemost., 43:*77, 1980.
34. Collen, T., Schetz, J., DeCock, F., Holmer, E., and Verstraete, M. Metabolism of antithrombin III (heparin cofactor in man). Effects of venous thrombosis and of heparin metabolism. *Eur. J. Clin. Invest., 7:*27, 1977.
35. Comp, P. C., Jacocks, R. M., and Taylor, F. B., Jr. The dilute whole blood clot lysis assay: a screening method for identifying postoperative patients with a high incidence of deep venous thrombosis. *J. Lab. Clin. Med., 93:*120, 1979.
36. Cook, A. W., and Lyons, H. A. Venous thromboembolic phenomena: their absence in paraplegic or tetraplegic patients. *Am. J. Med. Sci., 218:*155, 1949.
37. Coon, W. W., and Coller, F. A. Some epidemiologic considerations of thromboembolism. *Surg. Gynecol. Obstet., 109:*487, 1959.
38. Covey, T. H., Sherman, L., and Baue, E. Low dose heparin in postoperative patients. *Arch. Surg., 110:*121, 1975.
39. Cranley, J. J., Canos, A. J., and Sull, W. J. The diagnosis of deep venous thrombosis-fallibility of clinical symptoms and signs. *Arch. Surg., 111:*34, 1976.

40. Dalen, J. E., Brooks, H. L., Johnson, L. W., Meister, S. G., Szucs, M. M., and Dexter, L. Pulmonary angiography in acute pulmonary embolism: indications, techniques and results in 367 patients. *Am. Heart. J., 81:*175, 1971.
41. Davie, E. W., and Fukikawa, K. Basic mechanism in blood coagulation. *Annu. Rev. Biochem., 44:*799, 1975.
42. Dechavanne, M., Ville, D., Viala, J. J., Kher, A., Faivre, J., Pousset, M. B., and Dejour, H. Controlled trial of platelet antiaggregating agents and subcutaneous heparin in prevention of postoperative deep vein thrombosis in high-risk patients. *Haemostasis, 4:*94, 1975.
43. Dechavanne, M., Soudin, F., Viala, J. J., Kher, A., Bertrix, L., and DeMourgues, G. Prevention des thromboses veneuses: Succes de l'heparin a fortes doses lors des coxar-throses. *Nouv. Presse Med., 3:*1317, 1974.
44. DeNardo, G. L., Goodwin, D. A., Ravasini, R., and Dietrich, P. A. The ventilatory lung scan in the diagnosis of pulmonary embolism. *N. Engl. J. Med., 282:*1334, 1970.
45. Dejode, L. R., Khurshid, M., and Walther, W. W. The influence of electrical stimulation of the leg during surgical operations on the subsequent development of deep vein thrombosis. *Br. J. Surg., 60:*31, 1973.
46. Drill, V. A., and Calhoun, D. W. Oral contraceptives and thromboembolic disease. *J.A.M.A., 206:*77, 1968.
47. Duckert, F. Thrombolytic Therapy. *Semin. Thromb. Hemost., 10:*87, 1984.
48. Evans, D. S. The early diagnosis of deep vein thrombosis by ultrasound. *Br. J. Surg., 57:*726, 1970.
49. Flanc, C., Kakkar, V. V., and Clarke, M. B. The detection of venous thrombosis of the legs using ^{125}I-fibrinogen. *Br. J. Surg., 55:*742, 1968,
50. Forti, M. E. G., and Gurewich, V. Fibrin degradation products and impedance plethys-mography. Measurements in the diagnosis of acute deep vein thrombosis. *Arch. Intern. Med., 140:*903, 1980.
51. Frisbie, J. H., and Sasahara, A. A. Low dose heparin prophylaxis for deep venous thrombosis in acute spinal cord injury patients: A controlled study. *Paraplegia, 19:*141, 1981.
52. Gallus, A. S., Hirsh, J., O'Brien, S. E., McBridge, J. A., Tuttle, R. J., and Gent, M. Prevention of venous thrombosis with small subcutaneous doses of heparin. *J.A.M.A., 235:*980, 1975.
53. Gallus, A. S., Hirsh, J., Tuttle, R. J., Trebilcock, R., and O'Brien, S. E. Small subcutaneous doses of heparin in prevention of venous thrombosis. *N. Engl. J. Med., 288:*545, 1973.
54. Gibbs, N. M. Venous thrombosis of the lower limb with particular reference to bedrest. *Br. J. Surg., 45:*209, 1957.
55. Gitel, S. N., Stephenson, R. C., and Wessler, S. The activated increased thrombotic tendency induced by estrogen-containing oral contraceptives. *Hemostasis, 7:*10, 1978.
56. Gordon, S. G., Franks, J. J., and Lewis, B. Cancer procoagulant A. The factor X activating procoagulant from malignant tissue. *Thromb. Res., 6:*127, 1975.
57. Gordon-Smith, I. C., le Quesne, L. P., Grundy, D. J., and Newcombe, J. F. Controlled trial of two regimens of subcutaneous heparin in prevention of postoperative deep vein thrombosis. *Lancet, 1:*1133, 1972.
58. Grace, O. S. The fibrinolytic enzyme system in obesity: the effects of venous occlusion and in vitro activation of surface contact. *Clin. Sci., 34:*497, 1968.
59. Green, D., Rossi, E. C., Yao, J. T., Flinn, W. R., and Spies, S. M. Deep vein thrombosis in spinal cord injury: effect of prophylaxis with calf compression, aspirin and dipyrida-mole. *Paraplegia, 20:*108, 1982.
60. Greenfield, L. J. Technical considerations for insertion of vena caval filters. *Surg. Gynecol. Obstet., 148:*422, 1979.
61. Greenfield, L. J., Peyton, R., Crute, S., and Barnes, R. Greenfield vena caval filter experience. *Arch. Surg., 116:*1451, 1981.
62. Griffin, J. H. Clinical studies of Protein C. *Semin. Thromb. Hemost., 10:*162, 1984.

63. Gruber, U. F., Duckert, F., Fridrich, R., Torhorst, J., and Rem, J. Prevention of postoperative thromboembolism by dextran 40, low doses of heparin, or xantinol nicotinate. *Lancet, 1:*207, 1977.

64. Gurewitch, V., Hume, M., and Patrick, M. The laboratory diagnosis of venous thromboembolic disease by measurement of fibrinogen/fibrin degradation products and fibrin monomer. *Chest, 64:*585, 1973.

65. Hachen, H. J. Anticoagulant therapy in patients with spinal cord injury. *Paraplegia, 12:*176, 1974.

66. Hampson, W. G. J., Harris, F. C., Lucas, H. K., Roberts, P. H., McCall, I. W., Jackson, P. C., Powell, N. L., and Staddon, G. E. Failure of low-dose heparin to prevent deep vein thrombosis after hip replacement arthroplasty. *Lancet, 2:*795, 1974.

67. Harpel, P. C., and Rosenberg, R. D. α 2 Macroglobulin and antithrombin-heparin cofactor: modulators of haemostatic and inflammatory reactions. In: *Progress in Hemostasis and Thrombosis, vol 3.* Edited by Spaet, T. H. Grune & Stratton, New York, 1976.

68. Harris, W. H., Salzman, E. W., Athanasoulis, C., Waltman, A. G., Baum, S., and DeSanctis, R. W. Comparison of warfarin, low-molecular-weight dextran, aspirin and subcutaneous heparin prevention of venous thromboembolism following total hip replacement. *J. Bone. Joint. Surg., 49A:*81, 1967.

69. Harris, W. H., Salzman, E. W., and DeSanctis, R. W. The prevention of thromboembolic disease by prophylactic anticoagulants. A controlled study in elective hip surgery. *J. Bone. Joint. Surg., 49A:*81, 1967.

70. Hayt, D. B., Blatt, C. J., and Freeman, L. M. Radionuclide venography; its place as a modality for the investigation of thromboembolic phenomena. *Semin. Nucl. Med., 7:*263, 1977.

71. Henkin, R. E., Yao, J. S. T., Quinn, J. L., and Bergan, J. J. Radionuclide venography (RNV) in lower extremity venous disease. *J. Nucl. Med., 15:*171, 1974.

72. Hirsh, J. Hypercoagulability. *Semin. Hematol., 14:*409, 1977.

73. Hirsh, J., and Hull, R. Comparative value of tests for the diagnosis of venous thrombosis. *World J. Surg., 2:*27, 1978.

74. Hull, R., Delmore, T., Genton, E., Hirsh, J., Gent, M., Sackett, D., McLoughlin, D., and Armstrong, P. Warfarin sodium versus low dose heparin in the long term treatment of venous thrombosis. *N. Engl. J. Med., 301:*855, 1979.

75. Hull, R., Delmore, T. J., Hirsh, J., Gent, M., Armstrong, P., Lofthouse, R., MacMillan, A., Blackstone, L., Reed-Davis, R., and Detwiler, D. C. Effectiveness of intermittent pulsatile elastic stockings for the prevention of calf and thigh vein thrombosis in patients undergoing elective knee surgery. *Thromb. Res., 16:*37, 1979.

76. Hull, R., Delmore, T., Carter, C., Hirsh, J., Genton, E., Gent, M., Turpie, A. G. G., and McLoughlin, D. Adjusted subcutaneous heparin versus warfarin sodium in the long-term treatment of venous thrombosis. *N. Engl. J. Med., 306:*189, 1982.

77. Hull, R., Hirsh, J., Carter, C. J., Jay, R. M., Dodd, P. E., Ockelford, P. A., Coates, G., Gill, G. J., Turpie, A. G. G., Doyle, D. J., Buller, H. R., and Raskob, G. Pulmonary angiography, ventilation lung scanning and venography for clinically suspected pulmonary embolism with abnormal perfusion lung scan. *Ann. Intern. Med., 98:*891, 1983.

78. Hull, R., Hirsh, J., Sackett, D. L., Powers, P., Turpie, A. G. G., and Walker, I. Combined use of leg scanning and impedance plethysmography in suspected venous thrombosis: an alternative to venography. *N. Engl. J. Med., 296:*1497, 1977.

79. Hull, R., Taylor, D. W., Hirsh, J., Sackett, D. L., Powers, P., Turpie, A. G. G., and Walker, I. Impedance plethysmography: the relationship between venous filling and sensitivity and specificity for proximal vein thrombosis. *Circulation, 58:*898, 1978.

80. Hull, R., Hirsh, J., Sackett, D. L., Taylor, D. W., Carter, C., Turpie, A. G. G., and Zielinsky, A. Replacement of venography in suspected venous thrombosis by impedance plethysmography and 125 I-fibrinogen leg scanning. *Ann. Intern. Med., 94:*12, 1981.

81. Hull, R., van Aken, W. G., Hirsh, J., Gallus, A. S., Hoicka, G., Turpie, A. G. G., Walker, I. R., and Gent, M. Impedance plethysmography using the occlusive cuff technique in the diagnosis of venous thrombosis. *Circulation, 53:*697, 1976.
82. Holmes, M. C. G. Deep venous thrombosis of the lower limbs diagnosed by ultrasound. *Med. J. Aust., 1:*427, 1973.
83. Hume, M., Bierbaum, B., Kuriakose, T. X., and Surprenant, J. Prevention of postoperative thrombosis by aspirin. *Am. J. Surg., 133:*420, 1977.
84. Hume, M., Donaldson, W. R., and Suprenant, J. Sex, aspirin and venous thrombosis. *Orthop. Clin. North. Am., 3:*761, 1978.
85. International Multicentre Trial. Prevention of fatal postoperative pulmonary embolism by low doses of heparin. *Lancet, 2:*45, 1975.
86. Jick, H., Slone, D., Westerholm, B., Inman, W. H. W., Vessey, M. P., Shapiro, S., Lewis, G. P., and Worchester, J. Venous thromboembolic disease and ABO blood type. *Lancet, 1:*539, 1969.
87. Johnson, W. C., Patten, D. H., Widrich, W. C., and Nabseth, D. C. Technetium-99ᵐ isotope venography. *Am. J. Surg., 127:*424, 1974.
88. Kakkar, V. V. The diagnosis of deep vein thrombosis using 125 I-fibrinogen test. *Arch. Surg., 104:*152, 1972.
89. Kakkar, V. V. The current status of low-dose heparin in the prophylaxis of thrombophlebitis and pulmonary embolism. *World J. Surg., 2:*3, 1978.
90. Kakkar, V. V., Flanc, C., Howe, C. T., and Clarke, M. B. Natural history of postoperative deep vein thrombosis. *Lancet, 2:*230, 1969.
91. Kakkar, V. V., Spindler, J., Flute, P. T., Corrigan, T., Fossard, D. P., and Crellin, R. Q. Efficacy of low doses of heparin in prevention of deep vein thrombosis after major surgery: A double-blind, randomized trial. *Lancet, 2:*101, 1972.
92. Kanis, J. A. Heparin in the treatment of pulmonary thromboembolism. *Thrombos. Diathes. Haemorrh., 32:*519, 1974.
93. Kline, A., Hughes, L. E., and Campbell, H. Dextran 70 in prophylaxis of thromboembolic disease after surgery: A clinically oriented randomized double-blind trial. *Br. Med. J., 2:*109, 1975.
94. Lahnborg, G., Friman, L., Bergstrom, K., and Lagergren, H. Effect of low-dose heparin on incidence of postoperative pulmonary embolism detected by photoscanning. *Lancet, 1:*329, 1974.
95. Laurent, T. C., Tengblad, A., Thunberg, L., Hook, M., and Lindahl, U. The molecular weight dependence of the anticoagulant activity of heparin. *Biochem. J., 175:*691, 1978.
96. Loew, D., Brucke, P., Simma, W., Vinazzer, H., Dienstl, E., and Boehme, E. Acetylaalicylic acid, low-dose heparin, and a combination of both substances in the prevention of postoperative thromboembolism: A double blind study. *Thromb. Res., 1:*81, 1971.
97. Mackie, M., Bennet, B., Ogston, D., and Douglas A. S. Familial thrombosis: inherited deficiency of antithrombin III. *Br. Med. J., 1:*136, 1978.
98. Mansfield, A. O. Alteration in fibrinolysis associated with surgery and venous thrombosis. *Br. J. Surg., 59:*754, 1972.
99. Mant, M. J., O'Brien, B. D., Thong, K. L., Hammond, G. W., Birtwhistle, R. V., and Grace, M. G. Hemorrhagic complications of heparin therapy. *Lancet, 1:*1133, 1977.
100. Manucci, P. M., Citterio, L. A., and Panajotopoulos, N. Low dose heparin and deep vein thrombosis after total hip replacement. *Thromb. Haemost., 36:*157, 1976.
101. Marciniak, E., and Gockerman, J. P. Heparin-induced decrease in circulating antithrombin III. *Lancet, 2:*581, 1977.
102. McKay, E. J., and Laurell, C. B. The interaction of heparin with plasma proteins: demonstration of different binding sites for antithrombin III complexes and antithrombin III. *J. Lab. Clin. Med., 95:*69, 1980.
103. Medical Research Council. Report of the Steering Committee: Effect of aspirin on

postoperative venous thrombosis. *Lancet, 2:*441, 1972.

104. Morris, G. K., Henry, A. P. J., and Preston, B. J. Prevention of deep vein thrombosis by lowdose heparin in patients undergoing total hip replacement. *Lancet, 2:*797, 1974.

105. Morris, G. K., and Mitchell, J. R. Warfarin sodium in the prevention of deep venous thrombosis and pulmonary embolism in patients with fractured neck of femur. *Lancet, 2:*869, 1976.

106. Morris, G. K., and Mitchell, J. R. A. Preventing venous thromboembolism in elderly patients with hip fractures: Studies of low-dose heparin, dipyridamole, aspirin and flurbiprofen. *Br. Med. J., 1:*535, 1977.

107. Myhre, H. O., and Holen, A. Thromboseprogylakse: Dextran eller warfarin-natrium? *Nord. Med., 82:*1534, 1969.

108. Naso, F. Pulmonary embolism in acute spinal cord injury. *Arch. Phys. Med. Rehabil., 55:*275, 1974.

109. Nicolaides, A. N., Dupont, P.. A., Desais, S., Douglas, J. N., Fourides, G., Lewis, J. D., Hodgworth, H., Luch, K. J., and Jamieson, C. W. Small doses of subcutaneous sodium heparin in preventing deep venous thrombosis after major surgery. *Lancet, 2:*890, 1972.

110. Nicolaides, A. N., Kakkar, V. V., Field, E. S., and Renney, J. T. G. The origin of deep vein thrombosis; a venographic study. *Br. J. Radiol., 44:*653, 1971.

111. Nossel, H. L., Ti, M., Kaplan, K. L., Spanodis, K., Soland, T., and Butler, V. P., Jr. The generation of fibrinopeptide A in clinical samples. *J. Clin. Invest., 58:*1136, 1976.

112. Perkash, A. Experience with the management of deep vein thrombosis in patients with spinal cord injury: Part II: A critical evaluation of the anticoagulant therapy. *Paraplegia, 18:*2, 1980.

113. Perkash, A., Prakash, V., and Perkash, I. Experience with the management of thromboembolism in patients with spinal cord injury: Part I: Incidence, diagnosis and role of some risk factors. *Paraplegia, 16:*322, 1978.

114. Pinto, D. J. Controlled trial of an anticoagulant (warfarin sodium) in the prevention of venous thrombosis following hip surgery. *Br. J. Surg., 57:*349, 1970.

115. Plante, J., Boneu, B., Vaysse, C., Barret, A., Gouzi, M., and Bierme, R. Dipyridamole-aspirin versus low doses of heparin in the prophylaxis of deep venous thrombosis in abdominal surgery. *Thromb. Res., 14:*399, 1979.

116. Powers, S. K., and Edwards, S. B. Prophylaxis of thromboembolism in the neurosurgical patient: A review. *Neurosurgery, 10:*509, 1982.

117. Rabinov, K., and Paulin, S. Roentgen diagnosis of venous thrombosis in the leg. *Arch. Surg., 104:*134, 1972.

118. Renney, J. T. G., O'Sullivan, E. F., and Burke, P. F. Prevention of postoperative deep vein thrombosis with dipyridamole and aspirin. *Br. Med. J., 1:*992, 1976.

119. diRicco, G., Marini, G., Rindi, M., Ravelli, V., Lutzemberger, L., Tusini, G., and Giuntini, C. Pulmonary embolism in neurosurgical patients: diagnosis and treatment. *J. Neurosurg., 60:*972, 1984.

120. Rocha Casas, E., Sanchez, M. P., Arias, C. R., and Masip, J. P. Prophylaxis of venous thrombosis and pulmonary embolism in patients with acute traumatic spinal cord lesions. *Paraplegia, 14:*178, 1976.

121. Rocha Casas, E., Sanchez, M. P., Arias, C. R., and Masip, J. P. Prophylaxis of venous thrombosis and pulmonary embolism in patients with acute traumatic spinal cord lesions. *Paraplegia, 15:*209, 1977.

122. Robin, E. D. Overdiagnosis and overtreatment of pulmonary embolism: The emperer may have no clothes. *Ann. Intern. Med., 87:*775, 1977.

123. Rosenberg, I. L., Evans, M., and Pollock, A. V. Prophylaxis of postoperative leg vein thrombosis by low-dose subcutaneous heparin or preoperative calf muscle stimulation: A controlled clinical trial. *Br. Med. J., 1:*649, 1975.

124. Rosenberg, R. D. Biologic actions of heparin. *Semin. Hematol., 14:*427, 1977.

125. Rosenberg, R. D. Chemistry of the hemostasis mechanism and its relationship to the action of heparin. *Feb. Proc., 36:*10, 1977.

126. Rosenthal, D., Cossman, D., Matsumoto, G., and Callow, A. D. Prophylactic interruption of the inferior vena cava: A retrospective evaluation. *Am. J. Surg., 137:*389, 1979.
127. Rossi, E. C., Green, D., Rosen, J. S., Spies, S. M., and Jao, J. S. Sequential changes in factor VIII and platelets preceding deep vein thrombosis in patients with spinal cord injury. *Br. J. Haematol., 45:*143, 1980.
128. Sackler, J. P., and Liu, L. Heparin-induced osteoporosis. *Br. J. Radiol., 46:*548, 1973.
129. Salzman, E. W., Deykin, D., Shapiro, R. M., and Rosenberg, R. Management of heparin therapy: controlled prospective trial. *N. Engl. J. Med., 292:*1046, 1975.
130. Salzman, E. W., Harris, W. H., and DeSanctis, R. W. Anticoagulation for prevention of thromboembolism following fractures of the hip. *N. Engl. J. Med., 275:*122, 1966.
131. Schondorf, T. H., and Jey, D. Combined administration of low-dose heparin and aspirin as prophylaxis of deep vein thrombosis after hip joint surgery. *Haemostasis, 5:*250, 1976.
132. Scottish Study: A multiunit controlled trial: Heparin versus dextran in the prevention of deep vein thrombosis. *Lancet, 2:*118, 1974.
133. Sevitt, S. The structure and growth of valve-pocket thrombi in femoral veins. *J. Clin. Pathol., 26:*517, 1974.
134. Sevitt, S. Organization of valve pocket thrombi and the anomalies of double thrombi and valve cusp involvement. *Br. J. Surg., 61:*641, 1974.
135. Sevitt, S., and Gallagher, N. Venous thrombosis and pulmonary embolism: A clinicopathological study in injured and burned patients. *Br. J. Surg., 48:*475, 1961.
136. Schull, J. R., and Rose, D. L. Pulmonary embolism in patients with spinal cord injuries. *Arch. Phys. Med. Rehabil. July:*444, 1966.
137. Sigel, E., Ipsen, J., and Felix, W. R. The epidemilogy of lower extremity deep venous thrombosis in surgical patients. *Ann. Surg., 179:*278, 1974.
138. Silver, J. R. The prophylactic use of anticoagulant therapy in the prevention of pulmonary emboli in one hundren consecutive spinal injury patients. *Paraplegia, 12:*188, 1974.
139. Silver, J. R., and Moulton, A. Prophylactic anticoagulant therapy against pulmonary emboli in acute paraplegia. *Br. Med. J., 2:*338, 1970.
140. Skillman, J. J., Collins, R. E., Coe, N. P., Goldstein, B. S., Shapiro, R. M., Zervas, N. T., Bettman, M. A., and Salzman, E. W. Prevention of deep vein thrombosis in neurosurgical patients: A controlled randomized trial of external pneumatic compression boots. *Surgery, 83:*354, 1978.
141. Soreff, J., Johnsson, H., Diener, L, and Goransson, L. Acetylsalicylic acid in a trial to diminish thromboembolic complications after elective hip surgery. *Acta. Orthop. Scand., 46:*246, 1975.
142. Spaet, T. H., and Erickson, R. B. The vascular wall in the pathogenesis of thrombosis. *Thromb. Diath. Haemorrh., 21:*67, 1966.
143. Stamatakis, J. D., Kakkar, V. V., Lawrence, D., Bentley, P. G., Nairn, D., and Ward, V. Failure of aspirin to prevent postoperative deep vein thrombosis in patients undergoing total hip replacement. *Br. Med. J., 1:*1031, 1978.
144. Strandness, D. E., and Sumner, D. S. Ultrasonic velocity detector in the diagnosis of thrombophlebitis. *Arch. Surg., 104:*180, 1974.
146. Stewart, G. J., Ritchie, W. G., and Lynch, P. R. Venous endothelial damage produced by massive sticking and emigration of leukocytes. *Am. J. Path., 74:*507, 1974.
147. Todd, J. W., Frisbie, J. H., Rossier, A. B., Adams, D. F., Als, A. V., Armenia, R. J., Sasahara, A. A., and Tow, D. E. Deep venous thrombosis in acute spinal cord injury: A comparison of 125 I-fibrinogen leg scanning, impedance plethysmography and venography. *Paraplegia, 14:*50, 1976.
148. Turpie, A. G. G., Gallus, G., Beattie, W. S., and Hirsh, J. Prevention of venous thrombosis in patients with intracranial disease by intermittent pneumatic compression of the calf. *Neurology, 27:*435, 1977.
149. Venous Thrombosis Clinical Study Group. Small doses of subcutaneous sodium heparin in the prevention of deep vein thrombosis after elective hip operations. *Br. J. Surg., 62:*348, 1975.

150. Verstraete, M. Biochemical and clinical aspect of thrombolysis: *Semin. Hematol. 15*:35, 1978.
151. Warlow, C., Ogston, D., and Douglas, A. S. Deep venous thrombosis of the legs after strokes. *Br. Med. J., 2:*1178, 1976.
152. Watson, N. Venous thrombosis and pulmonary embolism in spinal cord injury. *Paraplegia, 6:*113, 1968.
153. Watson, N. Anticoagulant therapy in the treatment of venous thrombosis and pulmonary embolism in acute spinal injury. *Paraplegia, 12:*197, 1974.
154. Watson, N. Anticoagulant therapy in the prevention of venous thrombosis and pulmonary embolism in the spinal cord injury. *Paraplegia, 16:*265, 1978.
155. Wessler, S. Thrombosis in the presence of vascular stasis. *Am. J. Med., 33:*648, 1962.
156. Wheeler, H. B., Pearson, D., O'Connell, D., and Mullick, S. C. Impedance phlebography. Technique, interpretation and results. *Arch. Surg., 104:*164, 1972.
157. Wheeler, H. B., O'Donnel, J. A., Anderson, F. A., Penney, B. C., Pevra, R. A., and Benedict, C. Bedside screening for venous thrombosis using occlusive impedance phlebography. *Angiology, 26:*199, 1975.
158. Wood, E. H., Prentice, C. R. M., McGrouther, D. A., Sinclair, J., and McNicol, G. P. Trial of aspirin and RA233 in prevention of postoperative deep vein thrombosis. *Thromb. Diathes. Haemorrh., 30:*18, 1973.
159. Zekert, F. Thrombosen Embolien and Aggregationshemmer in der Chirugie. Schattauer, Stuttgart, 1975.

10

Spasticity in Spinal Cord Injured Patients

ROBERT R. YOUNG
BHAGWAN T. SHAHANI

The term *spasticity* is unsatisfactory, but until research in neuroscience produces much more understanding of motor control, it may be difficult to obtain general agreement about what to call this syndrome. Once we understand the neurophysiology of *normal* motor control, it will be possible, starting from first principles, to describe and characterize various pathophysiological aspects of the complex syndrome known now as spastic paresis.

Spasticity, strictly speaking (38), refers to "a motor disorder characterized by a velocity-dependent increase in tonic stretch reflexes ('muscle tone') with exaggerated tendon jerks, resulting from hyperexcitability of the stretch reflex, as one component of the upper motoneuron syndrome." In everyday parlance however, the term spasticity refers to all aspects of motor dysfunction in patients with lesions of the spinal cord or higher CNS structures. There are at least three separate topics to be considered when one discusses spasticity in a clinical sense.

The first subject to discuss is loss of function. This may range from complete paralysis of voluntary (as opposed to reflex) movement through decreasing degrees of weakness to loss of accurate, coordinated, or discrete movements and an unusual type of fatigability without much loss of peak power. This loss of power and facility is usually most obvious in the human upper extremity. It affects dorsiflexion and extension of fingers more than grip. In legs it also weakens dorsiflexion of the foot and toes out of proportion to plantar flexion. There may also be loss of control of bowels, bladder, and sexual function. There are obviously a number of other causes for such dysfunctions ranging from diseases of peripheral nerves and muscles to disorders of cerebellum and even failure of the patient to try as hard as possible. Symptoms due to loss of function were termed *negative symptoms* by Hughlings Jackson and are presumed to result from disconnection of "descending voluntary motor pathways" from structures within the spinal cord. Such loss of function produces most if not all the disability experienced by a patient with spasticity. These descending pathways include the pyramidal tract, but there are a number of other descending pathways from cerebrum to brainstem and from brainstem to spinal cord (37), so it is unwise to equate spasticity or the upper motor neuron syndrome with the *pyramidal syndrome*. Pure pyramidal lesions, which are extremely rare in man, do produce negative symptoms of this sort but do not give rise to the other aspects of spasticity to be enumerated below.

The second two topics to be considered involve increased reflex function affecting the same muscles that are weak, poorly coordinated, or deficient in voluntary control. Those reflexes that have been the major focus of attention in discussions of spasticity are principally segmental stretch reflexes. Providing a spinal lesion does not damage the segment involved in the reflex arc, stretch reflexes, both phasic (tendon jerk) and tonic (resistance to passive stretch of muscle and perhaps vibratory-induced reflexes), become hyperactive below the level of a lesion in a spastic patient. Such reflexes may become repetitive (clonus); this may disturb patients but increased stretch reflexes produce very little disability. Even increased tonic stretch reflexes, which produce abnormalities of posture such as flexion of the legs (paraplegic dystonia) or extension of the lower extremity and flexion of the upper (hemiplegic dystonia), are very rarely the primary cause of disability. Patients and physicians often feel that the stiff limb might function better voluntarily without increased tonic stretch reflexes, but that rarely proves to be the case (see "tardive hemiplegic dystonia" below.)

The third topic is a second category of reflexes that are abnormal in spasticity and are termed *exteroceptive* (79) rather than proprioceptive. Exteroceptive reflexes include cutaneously induced alterations in posture in addition to those nociceptive or flexor reflexes that are more often the focus of clinical attention (68, 69). These reflexes are particularly hyperactive in patients with lesions of the spinal cord. They sometimes are so labile that what would otherwise be completely innocuous stimuli on the skin of the foot or leg produce what appear to be spontaneous flexor (or even extensor) spasms. In such patients, light rubbing or tickling of the soles of the feet will produce very brisk, involuntary flexor movements, including triple flexion at the hip, knee, and ankle. As one of a subgroup of cutaneous or flexor reflexes, the Babinski response following plantar stimulation has for the past 100 years played a large role in the description of patients with spasticity. Patients with spinal cord lesions may also have reflex hyperactivity of the autonomic nervous system (75), including unexpected rises in blood pressure, emptying of bladder, or fecal incontinence.

Abnormally hyperactive reflexes of all the types listed above were termed "positive symptoms" by Hughlings Jackson. Positive symptoms due to hyperactive cutaneous reflexes may be quite disagreeable or disabling, but these disabilities are not of the same order of magnitude as those caused by negative symptoms. As will be outlined below, various therapeutic modalities can reduce positive symptoms, but there is unfortunately little to be done about negative symptoms.

PATHOPHYSIOLOGY OF SPASTICITY

Our knowledge of the detailed neuronal organization of even the simplest movements is quite deficient and we can only speculate about the complex neuronal arrangements necessary to produce high-level motor control such as the quick, coordinated postural adjustments with extreme accuracy required by world-class musicians or athletes. Therefore, any explanation of the mechanisms responsible for fine motor control or its loss with disease must be patently hypothetical.

Anatomical and Functional Considerations

Kuypers and his colleagues (37) have demonstrated the anatomy of descending pathways regulating behavior of motoneurons, which themselves constitute the final common pathway at the spinal level. Corticospinal fibers from the sensorimotor cortex, after giving off numerous collaterals to structures in the cerebrum and brainstem, descend to the appropriate level within the spinal cord. In addition, there are a number of important subcorticospinal pathways. Kuypers has divided these latter pathways, which descend from brainstem to spinal cord, into a medial and a lateral group. The input to these lateral and medial pathways (that is, their control) comes from various levels of the neuraxis but especially from rostral centers and cerebral cortex. Much of the cerebral cortex outside the sensorimotor and visual or auditory areas has been termed *extrapyramidal* because the striatum (caudate and putamen) receives considerable input from those cortical areas. It is important to remember that the major outflow from those structures making up the extrapyramidal system (the basal ganglia) is to the thalamus and thereby to the cerebral sensorimotor cortex. Lesions of the spinal cord will affect corticospinal and/or the medial and lateral subcorticospinal pathways, thereby disconnecting them from spinal neuronal networks involved with motor performance.

Motor pathways arising in the brainstem and descending to the spinal cord are characterized as medial or lateral depending upon where they terminate within the intermediate zone of the gray matter that one sees in a cross section of the spinal cord. Axons in the medial division of the subcorticospinal system arise from neurons in the medial reticular formation in midbrain, pons, and medulla. They also arise from vestibular nuclei and even from structures that usually have been associated with vision, such as the superior colliculus and the interstitial nucleus of Cajal. Fibers in this medial division descend in the ventral and ventrolateral funiculi to end at all levels of the spinal cord. In the cervical and lumbosacral enlargements, these axons terminate (sometimes bilaterally) in the ventromedial part of Rexed's laminae 7 and 8. At other levels of the cord, the only motoneurons present innervate axial musculature so terminations of these axons must necessarily be concerned, at those levels, with midline structures.

Axons in the lateral subcorticospinal pathways arise from large cells in the red nucleus and from the ventrolateral tegmentum of the pons. These axons cross the midline and descend through the lateral funiculus of the cord to end in the dorsolateral part of the intermediate zone of the spinal gray matter, principally in the cervical and lumbosacral enlargements.

Corticospinal axons arise from cells in the sensorimotor cortex (both the posterior frontal and anterior parietal regions), give off many collaterals, cross the midline at the lower end of the brainstem, and descend in the lateral funiculus of the cord. They end at all levels of the cord and in all areas (both lateral and medial) of the intermediate zone.

Motoneurons and associated interneurons are also organized into medial and lateral groups within the spinal cord. The medial column of motoneurons exists throughout the entire length of the cord and innervates axial muscles. These are paraspinal and trunk muscles that are particularly well-known in the neck and thoracic region but which also exist at the levels where shoulder girdle and pelvic structures increase the anatomical complexity. In the cervical and lumbosacral enlargements, there is also a more lateral column of motoneurons that innervate muscles in the limbs. This lateral column can be subdivided into ventromedial and dorsolateral groups. Those motoneurons that are ventromedial (near the medial cell column) innervate limb girdle and other such proximal muscles. Those motoneurons that lie more dorsolaterally innervate limb muscles and are arranged in such a way that proximal limb muscles are more ventromedial, and the most distal muscles in hands and feet are innervated by motoneurons that lie most dorsally.

In addition to these motoneurons that constitute Rexed's lamina 9, there are many smaller neurons lying in the so-called intermediate zone (laminas 5 through 8) whose axons end upon motoneurons. These interneurons within the motor system are also topographically organized. Those that are in the ventromedial area of the intermediate zone tend to project to ventromedial motoneurons innervating axial and limb girdle muscles. Those interneurons lying dorsolaterally in the intermediate zone project particularly to dorsolateral motoneurons that control muscles of the distal extremities.

From the foregoing, it can be deduced that ventromedial subcorticospinal axons end on interneurons that themselves project to motoneurons of axial and limb girdle muscles. Axons in the lateral subcorticospinal system end upon interneurons that project to motoneurons controlling the distal muscles in the limb. Axons in the corticospinal system end throughout the intermediate zone and overlap the areas innervated by both subcorticospinal pathways. Some axons within the corticospinal system also end directly upon the motoneurons and particularly upon those lying most dorsolaterally innervating distal limb muscles. These particular corticospinal fibers, which are the only supraspinal fibers to end directly upon motoneurons, arise from regions of sensorimotor cortex where foot and hand are highly represented.

Activity within the medial subcorticospinal pathways tends to be concerned with axial and combined body-limb movements such as are important in maintaining an erect posture against gravity and in large total body movements such as walking. On the other hand, activity in the lateral subcorticospinal pathways is particularly concerned with movements of the limbs and especially their distal parts, which are independent of total body movement or more proximal movement within the limb itself. In addition to these types of control, the corticospinal system apparently can regulate both axial and more distal limb movements with a high degree of accuracy, providing very fine motor control with fractionation of individual movements in the distal limbs. Spatial arrangements of proximal limb and axial structures during these complex movements must also be optimized according to the purpose of the movement.

As would be expected from these anatomical observations, Kuypers and his colleagues were able to demonstrate specific and characteristic functional deficits in monkeys where lesions had been made in one of these pathways. For example, lesions of the medial subcorticospinal pathway result in an animal that can manipulate objects in its hand but cannot project its limb into space and has difficulty standing and walking. These animals develop a stooped posture with flexed, adducted dystonia of the limbs. On the other hand, lesions of the lateral subcorticospinal pathway do not affect axial or limb girdle muscles and the animals have normal posture. They can project their limbs out into space and can flex all their fingers together but have great difficulty with dextrous control of their hands and fingers when trying to pick up small bits of food. Similarly, lesions of the corticospinal system produce their maximum deficit by interfering with function of distal limb muscles; in particular, they eliminate the ability of primates to selectively control the function of one finger, for example. It should be remembered, however, that these lateral subcorticospinal and corticospinal lesions that severely reduce voluntary function of the hands and feet do not seem to affect functions of these parts of the limbs when they are used as part of a total body movement such as climbing up a cage. The monkey's fingers flex very nicely to grip the cage in this latter circumstance, even when the animal cannot use them to grasp food.

Although efferent and afferent structures are clearly segregated peripherally, within the central nervous system it becomes increasingly difficult to tell what is "sensory" and what is "motor"—motor performance obviously requires very highly organized and accurate sensory information. In our discussions of descending motor pathways, it is important to include sensory tracts because the final motor performance is continuously adjusted and regulated by means of afferent information as well as efference copy. This latter refers to the fact that collateral branches of descending motor pathways end upon spinal, brainstem, and cerebellar structures that are thereby appraised of motoneuron activity about to take place. This must be integrated with afferent activity coming back from the periphery to produce a maximally well-organized movement. In the absence of knowledge to the contrary, one assumes that lesions of any of these fibers within the cord reduce the quality of the net motor performance by disconnecting higher centers from the spinal motor apparatus. An analogy can be made that likens the production of negative symptoms by spinal lesions to the sorts of negative symptoms that result when lesions of peripheral nerves disconnect spinal motoneurons from their muscle motors. Lesions of peripheral nerves that disconnect motoneurons from their muscles also interfere with afferent information, and this disturbs motor performance even further.

This analogy fails because of the vastly increased complexity of neuronal circuitry within the spinal cord as compared with that in peripheral nerve. Neuroscience has only just begun to recognize the subtle complexity underlying even the simplest voluntary movements. Lesions of the central motor system produce weakness or even complete paralysis by virtue of disconnecting higher centers from spinal structures. They can also produce loss of dexterity out of proportion to loss of peak power, presumably by interfering with corticospinal or lateral subcorticospinal functions with relative preservation of more primitive circuits that can switch motoneurons on to produce good power without particular facility. These lesions also produce a sort of fatigability, causing whatever movements remain to be increasingly less well-performed when attempted seriatim. Hypotheses to explain that sort of pathophysiology are even more difficult to formulate.

Abnormal Control of Single Motor Unit Discharges

Even such apparently simple functions as continuous activation of single motor units are affected by upper motoneuron lesions in very characteristic ways. For example, in the presence of spasticity, patients cannot activate as many motor units in any weak muscle as they should, and many of those that are activated cannot be made to fire rapidly or continuously. It should be stressed, however, that all motor units in any one muscle are not equally affected unless there is a complete spinal transection. Among those motor units that still can be activated voluntarily by the spastic patient some behave more normally than others (82).

In general, however, they function abnormally in an unexpected way. Under normal circumstances during a very accurate isometric contraction, if one compares joint intervals during the prolonged, tonic discharge of a single motoneuron (that is, the interval of time between sequential discharges of that motoneuron), one often finds a weak negative serial correlation (1, 83). If the normal subject is asked to control either the force or motoneuron firing rate so that a motoneuron fires at about 10 Hz, for example, this steady discharge can be maintained for long periods of time with relatively little fluctuation in instantaneous firing frequency. However, there are inevitably small variations in the intervals that occur one after another. Not all such variations occur randomly. Under normal circumstances, the presence of a negative serial correlation means that if an interval is shorter than the mean (100 msec in this case), the very next interval will be, on the average, longer than the mean.

This beat-to-beat automatic control of joint intervals to maintain a specified mean firing rate is absent in patients with spasticity. In these patients, even if the mean discharge frequency is normal, fluctuations from that mean are larger than normal because the negative serial correlation is absent. In this latter case, longer intervals than the mean tend to be followed by longer intervals and shorter intervals by shorter intervals (i.e., a positive serial correlation exists) so that trends develop, and the force or firing frequency produced by the patient fluctuates more than normal.

This quantifiable and subtle abnormality of motoneuron behavior was unsuspected on clinical grounds, but quantitative neurophysiological observations of this sort may permit one to objectify disabilities that are grouped together as the negative symptoms of spasticity. Because these observations also demonstrate that, even in a largely paretic muscle, some motoneurons are much less affected than others, rehabilitative therapies may be devised to take advantage of the presence of these few relatively normal motor units. In any case, the abnormality demonstrable by joint interval histograms is a good example of subtle dysfunctions produced by lesions within the motor system.

See the papers by Mayer and his colleagues for an interesting discussion of alterations in contraction times and fatigability of single motor units in first dorsal interosseous muscles of hemiplegic patients (78) and in triceps surae in paraplegic cats (49).

Exaggerated Segmental Stretch Reflexes

The strict definition of spasticity is concerned entirely with hyperactivity of segmental stretch reflex arcs. See Fig. 10.1 for a schematic diagram of the structures involved. One aspect of this enhancement is the excessively large twitch or phasic contraction of a spastic muscle following a tap either on its tendon or, in the case of extremely hyperactive tendon reflexes, a tap elsewhere in that limb or even on the contralateral limb. This latter behavior is termed *radiation of reflexes* (39). Examples include: (a) contraction of spastic adductors of the thigh following percussion with a reflex hammer on the contralateral limb; (b) a spinal lesion at C5 or C6 that interferes with function of the biceps reflex arc so that contraction of the spastic triceps muscle follows a tap on the biceps tendon; (c) finger flexion following a tap on the distal radius; and (d) during elicitation of a Hoffman's sign, contraction of the flexors of the distal phalanx of the thumb following a quick stretch of the finger flexors. This radiation of reflexes is not entirely due to unusually widespread effects of Ia afferent impulses within the spinal cord, although there is some of that. Spindle primary afferents end predominantly on motoneurons innervating the same muscle in which the spindle lies, but they also end on motoneurons (and interneurons) associated with synergistic muscles. When motoneurons are not hyperexcitable, excitatory postsynaptic potentials (EPSPs) produced by these latter endings are not large enough to activate other motoneurons than those to the spindle's own muscle. When motoneurons *are* hyperexcitable and reflexes *are* hyperactive, however, reflexes may spread into these synergistic muscles. That is not the whole story, however. Lance and de Gail (39) showed there is also peripheral spread of a vibratory wave following a tendon tap. This vibratory wave is most effective in stimulating muscle spindles within the muscle whose tendon was tapped, but as it spreads throughout a limb, even though its amplitude decreases as it gets further from the tendon, it still can activate spindle primary endings. When segmental stretch reflexes are especially brisk, these relatively few endings in other muscles produce enough EPSPs to activate these other muscles just as though they themselves had been tapped upon.

Hyperactive tendon reflexes of a phasic type, such as described above, are hallmarks of spasticity. It must be remembered, however, that immediately following a spinal lesion, in the phase of spinal shock, tendon reflexes in the affected limbs will either be absent or hypoactive. With the passage of time following the spinal lesion (minutes in a frog, an hour or so in cats and dogs, and days or weeks in man), tendon reflexes reappear and become brisker providing the patient is in good general health without excessive stimulation of nociceptive reflex afferents. Flexor and other nociceptive reflexes always predominate over extensor and proprioceptive reflexes even in normal individuals. Following a spinal lesion, pressure sores, cystitis, and other such pathological processes produce tremendous nociceptive afferent input into the isolated spinal cord, although the patient, because of the spinal lesion, often does not feel these inputs. In any case, unless the spinal injured patient is in good general health, a state of modified spinal shock or flexor reflex predominance may persist indefinitely so that tendon reflexes may only reappear and become spastically hyperactive many months after the original injury.

Tonic stretch reflexes, rather than these phasic tendon jerks, are the ones emphasized in the definition of spasticity. Although torque motors and other mechanical stretching devices are available, tonic stretch reflexes are practically always tested at the bedside or in the clinic by the physician who personally moves a limb at a joint thereby stretching a group of muscles.

As a subjective experience, the clinician describes the resistance generated by the stretched muscles in response to passive movement at the appropriate joint. These evaluations of tonic stretch reflex activity are therefore highly subjective and only semiquantitative at best. If a patient fails to relax (rather common with confused or elderly patients where gegenhalten is prominent), if there is severe fibrosis or arthritis that operates mechanically to stiffen a joint, or if various extrapyramidal disorders are present, there is also increased resistance to passive movement, which in the latter case at least, may also be due to increased tonic stretch reflexes. Therefore the strict definition of spasticity includes the term *velocity dependent*—with Parkinsonian rigidity there is little velocity-dependent increase in resistance, there is no *free interval*, and there is no clasp-knife phenomenon, all of which are said to be characteristic of spasticity.

By palpation of a muscle belly or surface EMG recording, it can be ascertained that a classicially spastic muscle about to be stretched passively is completely free of activity at rest. As stretch begins, particularly if the muscle is stretched slowly, there is no increased resistance to passive movement for a fraction of a second and then, depending upon the severity of the spasticity, the examiner notices a gradually increasing resistance as the stretched muscle becomes increasingly activated. If stretch is particularly quick, the brief interval following the onset of stretch before EMG activity is obvious (the free interval) may be very short and hard to recognize clinically. With Parkinsonian rigidity, there is no free interval, and the muscle is usually active, albeit slightly, at rest. The resistance felt when one stretches a rigid muscle is certainly greater as one stretches more rapidly, but this increase with increased velocity of stretch is more dramatic in a spastic muscle. As a spastic muscle is stretched moderately rapidly and its contraction builds up, one may elicit the clasp-knife phenomenon. That is, the resistance suddenly falls off and it becomes much easier to stretch the muscle.

It must be emphasized that these classical definitions of spasticity and rigidity are not particularly helpful clinically. The patients one commonly sees with spasticity, whether it be from cerebral infarction or spinal cord damage, will often have one muscle in a limb that fulfills the criteria listed above for spasticity but another muscle in the same limb may be rigid. The dystonic postures common with spasticity are, in fact, rigidity; there are extremely few lesions within the central nervous system that affect only the pyramidal system. Practically all lesions within the cerebral hemispheres and the spinal cord involve either the cerebral extrapyramidal areas (nonpyramidal cortex and basal ganglia) or subcorticospinal pathways so that it would be surprising if symptoms produced by these lesions were due only to pyramidal dysfunction. Furthermore, when objective evaluations making use of repeatable mechanically induced stretches are studied quantitatively, the clasp-knife phenomenon is extremely uncommon.

Unfortunately, bedside testing in which the motor system of the clinician is evaluating the motor system of the patient is notoriously unreliable. The examiner's stretch reflex mechanisms are brought into action and themselves respond automatically, without the continuous conscious awareness of the examiner. For example, when ankle clonus is generated by an examiner who quickly dorsiflexes the foot of a spastic patient, there is clonic contraction at approximately 6 hertz, not only in the patient's triceps surae but also in the examiner's wrist flexor muscles; activity in these two muscle groups occurs at the same frequency although 180° out of phase. This alternation of activities (of which the examiner is not aware) tends to sustain the rhythmic discharge in the patient's leg. Similar subconscious fluctuations in the examiner's motor behavior probably underlie most bedside demonstrations of other phenomena (such as the clasp-knife effect) thought to differentiate spasticity from rigidity.

Once it was discovered that tendon reflexes and tonic stretch reflexes are driven by afferent input from muscle spindles, it was natural to image that hyperactive reflexes might be due to excessive input from unusually sensitive spindles. Evidence from the effect of peripheral neuropathies, dorsal rhizotomies, local cooling of muscle (which decreases spindle sensitivity), and temporary blockade of peripheral nerves clearly demonstrated that stretch reflexes of all types, both normally active and hyperactive, were reduced or eliminated by conditions that interfere with stretch reflex afferent activity. Such observations, however, do *not* give particular insight into the mechanism of hyperactive stretch reflexes. The fact that reflexes can be diminished by the production of lesions (temporary or permanent) in the stretch reflex arc (cordotomies, cordectomies, rhizotomies, neurectomies, etc.) and spasticity can be reduced by these lesions, local cooling of muscle and so on does not prove that spasticity is due to hyperactivity within the afferent limbs of the reflex arc. With the development of microneurography, a method for recording spindle afferent activity with microelectrodes inserted into peripheral nerves of unanesthetized human beings (73), the concept of increased spindle sensitivity due to increased gamma motoneuron efferent activity failed to receive confirmation. That is to say, no one has yet demonstrated increased primary spindle afferent activity in response to a quantified tap or stretch of muscle in patients with spasticity as compared to normal subjects (13).

It therefore appears that, in spastic patients, normal input from spindles produces excess motoneuron discharge because of an enhanced central excitatory state at the level of the motoneuron pool; hyperactive stretch reflexes in spastic patients are due to excessively sensitive spinal motor circuits rather than to excessively sensitive peripheral sensory endings.

Another reason many had assumed that spastic hyperreflexia was due to increased spindle sensitivity was the supposed similarity between spasticity and decerebrate rigidity in the cat where, among other abnormalities, increased activity of static gamma motoneurons has been demonstrated. However, on closer inspection, decerebrate rigidity has proven to be a poor model of spasticity. First, decerebrate rigidity is maximal immediately after the brainstem transection, lessens progressively, and disappears after a day or so whereas human spasticity only develops after a delay of days and increases slowly. Second, lesions responsible for spasticity may affect, among other structures, only corticospinal and subcorticospinal pathways, whereas decerebrate rigidity is produced by transection of the entire brainstem. Third, there are no direct, monosynaptic endings of corticospinal fibers onto spinal motoneurons in cats as there are in man. Fourth, Hultborn, Pierrot-Deseilligny, and their colleagues (13) have demonstrated different pathological physiology in these two situations. They have also pioneered the development of animal models more similar to human spasticity (30).

About 25 years ago the concept of presynaptic inhibition was developed. In brief, this describes the observation that inhibitory mechanisms do not always operate postsynaptically by adding inhibitory postsynaptic potentials (IPSPs) to the next neuron to hyperpolarize it. It is possible, by means of impulses in axons ending on primary afferent terminals (axoaxonic synapses), to reduce the efficacy of impulses in these presynaptic terminals—to reduce the extent to which they depolarize the neuron on which they synapse. This alteration can occur very selectively on certain primary afferent terminals before they get to their first synapse. Calcium influx into axon terminals is necessary if an impulse is to release the neurotransmitter stored there. Presynaptic receptors may be effective by controlling the magnitude of calcium current moving into the terminals. Receptors that, when activated, decrease the inward calcium current would produce presynaptic inhibition. It appears that much information coming into the spinal cord through dorsal root afferent fibers is "turned down" before it gets to the first postsynaptic cell upon which those fibers end.

In any case, once this mechanism had been described, Delwaide (16) and others suggested that spasticity may be the result of insufficient presynaptic inhibitory activity. In that way, normal impulses coming into the cord from muscle spindles (impulses which would normally have been turned down by presynaptic inhibition) are now maximally effective in depolarizing motoneurons so that a larger reflex output develops. Among the evidence that supports this hypothesis is the fact that tonic vibratory inhibition of tendon reflexes or H reflexes is decreased in spastic patients. Normally, when a vibrator is applied to the Achilles (or other) tendon, the amplitude of the ankle jerk or H reflex in that muscle is considerably reduced compared to the same reflexes without vibration (24). A second subsidiary hypothesis states that vibratory stimulation of muscle spindles (which have been demonstrated to be very sensitive to stimuli of this sort) produces a barrage of activity entering the cord, and that activity tends to increase presynaptic inhibition in these same fibers so that the motoneuron pools discharge less than they normally would following any stretch reflex afferent input. Because this vibratory-induced suppression of tendon or H reflexes is reduced or absent in patients with spasticity, Delwaide's hypothesis is that presynaptic inhibition may be less in such patients and therefore tendon reflexes greater. As will be seen later in discussions of diazepam as an antispastic drug, these clinical neurophysiological concepts have some very practical implications.

What other changes within the central motor system might be responsible for spastic hyperreflexia? Since lesions rostral to the segment under study produce spasticity, it is reasonable to assume that such lesions result in abnormalities of descending control of the segmental spinal motor apparatus. For example, excessive hyperactivity at the segmental level could be due to excessive descending excitation and/or deficient descending inhibitory activity. Even with a complete spinal transection, where spinal hyperexcitability has been assumed to be due to deficient descending inhibition, transection of descending excitatory or inhibitory activity that normally ends on upper spinal interneurons may either facilitate or disinhibit descending excitatory propriospinal activity ending at the lower segmental level. In addition, there may be primary or secondary alterations in the segmental neuronal circuitry consequent to rostral lesions as a result of degeneration of descending tracts, including their terminals on segmental neurons.

Well-known local circuits might be involved in spasticity (13, 14, 30). Spindle afferent activity automatically excites motoneurons of the muscle being stretched and, by activation of an interneuron, reciprocally inhibits antagonist motoneurons. With voluntary contraction, descending pathways simultaneously activate those alpha and gamma motoneurons going to the contracting muscles. At the same time, these descending influences activate inhibitory neurons that lie in the pathway going from spindle primary endings in the contracting muscles to the antagonist motoneuron pools. Coactivation of these and the related inhibitory neurons during voluntary contraction is also important to minimize stretch reflexes from muscles that are passively lengthened during voluntary contraction of the agonist muscle groups. Deficient descending activation of this latter inhibitory system could tend to produce cocontraction of antagonist muscle groups, generalized stiffening of the limb, and slowing of rapid alternating movements with inability to produce isolated contraction of individual muscles— difficulties that are present in spastic patients.

When radiation of reflexes was discussed above, mention was made of direct connections of spindle afferents that end on motoneurons of synergistic muscles. It has been established that spindle primary afferents, in addition to these monosynaptic connections, also produce polysynaptic excitation of motoneurons, innervating their own muscles and synergistic muscles. Loss of inhibitory control over these interneurons would produce hyperactive and radiated reflexes.

Ib afferents from Golgi tendon organs (which are particularly sensitive to active muscle contraction) produce di- and trisynaptic inhibition of motoneurons of their own muscle and synergistic muscles. These Ib afferents are active during all normal movements and provide a regulatory mechanism whereby the CNS can continuously sample and regulate muscle force. Decreased activity (that is, lack of descending facilitation) of these inhibitory interneurons due to rostral lesions would interfere with this negative feedback force-regulating system and produce stretch reflex hyperactivity.

Although it was originally assumed that the clasp-knife phenomenon was due to increasing Ib inhibition, that has always been a largely unsubstantiated hypothesis. It should be remembered that there are many other muscle afferent fibers than those coming from spindle primary endings or Golgi tendon organs. Houk and colleagues (63) suggested that impulses in small myelinated group III or group IV fibers produced by intramuscular activity are responsible for inhibition underlying the clasp-knife phenomenon.

Spinal motoneurons have axon collaterals that activate Renshaw cells; their discharges inhibit alpha and gamma motoneurons in the same motoneuron pool. These Renshaw cells are also under facilitatory supraspinal control and if their negative feedback activity were decreased by supraspinal lesions, increased stretch reflex activity would be the result.

As further evidence for the inadequacy of decerebrate rigidity as a model for human spasticity, note the following. In the decerebrate preparation, polysynaptic Ia excitatory pathways are very active and presynaptic inhibition is not suppressed, so Delwaide's hypothesis certainly does not apply to decerebrate rigidity. On the other hand, Ib inhibition is quite reduced in decerebrate cats. Decreased activity of Renshaw cells has not been reported in decerebrate animals.

Two approaches have been taken to work out the pathophysiology of spasticity. In the first, spinal transections have been produced in cats. Second, increasingly complex and well-controlled studies are being undertaken in human beings. More thorough and invasive physiological investigations can clearly be carried out in spastic cats. Although complete transection in cats produces a clinical picture of spasticity similar in many respects to that seen in the human, the amount of care and attention required to keep such spinal cats alive and healthy is so great that few studies of these animals have been undertaken. On the other hand, following a hemisection of the cord, cats require little special attention, and relatively large numbers of them can be studied for long periods of time. Unfortunately, clinical inspection of motor performance in the hind legs of a hemispinalized cat shows little spasticity. Fortunately, careful physiological recordings do demonstrate reflex abnormalities on the side of the cord below the transection (14).

Direct stimulation of alpha motoneurons by passage of current through a microelectrode inside the cell has not shown changes in excitability of motoneurons in chronic spinal cats when compared with normal ones. There is some evidence, however, that the spastic motoneurons may be smaller than normal ones, perhaps in response to partial denervation of their dendritic trees. If they are shrunken, excitatory presynaptic endings that remain intact would be expected to be more effective.

In these spinal cats, as in the human studies mentioned above, investigators have not demonstrated increased activity in static gamma motoneurons although decreased activity has been demonstrated in the acute phase of spinal shock after a spinal transection. Transmission in polysynaptic excitatory Ia pathways is increased in chronic spinal cats but decreased presynaptic inhibition of Ia terminals has not been clearly demonstrated. Renshaw cell activity seems to be increased in the chronic phase after a spinal lesion, which should tend to decrease the activity of tonic stretch reflexes. In summary, Hultborn and his colleagues are not yet able to demonstrate precisely which spinal mechanisms are responsible for the hyperactive stretch reflexes in cats with chronic spinal lesions. In particular there is no evidence for hyperexcitability intrinsic to the alpha motoneuron itself nor for excessive fusimotor (gamma motoneuron) or spindle activity. Hyperactive stretch reflexes in these cats at least must therefore be due to abnormalities in local interneuronal circuitry.

Neurophysiological investigations of humans with various types of spasticity are necessarily more indirect and therefore more difficult to interpret than similar studies of laboratory animals. Studies using H reflexes attempt to evaluate the excitability of alpha motoneuron pools but the results of such experiments are modified in addition by presynaptic events in the Ia terminals. H reflex studies are also difficult to interpret because subtle and often poorly controlled variability in posture (sitting versus standing versus lying), joint angles, neck and head orientation, exteroceptive and interoceptive influences, such as discomfort due to the recording procedure or to a full bladder, and background level of voluntary activation all contribute to fluctuations in motoneuron excitability. These have little or nothing to do with added alterations resulting from CNS lesions. H reflex excitability curves in which two identical stimuli are delivered to the tibial nerve at varying intervals from one to many hundred msec have been used in an attempt to test motoneuron excitability cycles; the hope has been that typical or specific abnormalities in these cycles would be found in spasticity, Parkinson's disease, etc. Unfortunately, very long-lasting and significant changes in excitability of peripheral axons follow the first stimulus so that even though the second stimulus is electrically identical to the first, the number of axons stimulated by it is apt to be significantly less during the first hundred msec after the initial stimulus (61). Naturally this second, less effective stimulus produces a smaller H reflex but that has little to do with fluctuations of excitability within the motoneuron pool. Conclusions drawn from H reflex studies must be examined very critically.

A few investigations have been fully aware of these difficulties and have taken great pains in their experiments to control most of them, but it is unfortunately still not possible to draw firm conclusions from most H reflex studies in patients with spasticity. For example, studies that suggest muscle spindle sensitivity to static stretch is increased in spasticity await confirmation by more direct methods, microneurography for example. New and better clinical neurophysiological investigative techniques are being developed that may eventually allow us to quantitate such phenomena as polysynaptic Ia excitation, presynaptic inhibition, Renshaw cell inhibition, and reciprocal inhibition—some or all of which may be abnormal in spasticity.

Using H reflexes, one can test pathways mediating reciprocal Ia inhibition in spastic man. Yanagisawa and colleagues (77) reported a high level of reciprocal inhibition from triceps surae to anterior tibial motoneurons in hemiplegic patients. They then blocked nerves to triceps surae, following which the patients could produce stronger voluntary dorsiflexions of the foot. On the other hand, in patients with spasticity due to spinal lesions, reciprocal inhibition from anterior tibial motoneurons onto ankle extensors seemed to be unusually strong.

Paired H reflexes have also been used to test Renshaw inhibition. In hemiplegic patients, Renshaw cells, contrary to expectations, appear to function normally or to have increased activity. Supraspinal control of Renshaw cell activity seems to be abnormal, however and, because this sort of appropriately regulated negative feedback is particularly important during ongoing tonic motoneuron activity (as opposed to phasic activation with a tendon jerk), abnormalities in it might account for spastic difficulty in fractionation of movements if not for increased stretch reflexes (31, 60).

Our investigative methods, either clinical or electrophysiological, tend to focus attention on stretch reflex activity while the patient is at rest. Although such activities (e.g., tendon reflexes) are of interest to physicians, they clearly have little functional or pathophysiological significance. It is when a patient begins to move that difficulties are noted. By extrapolation from their exaggeration at rest, it has been suggested that stretch reflexes may somehow interfere with voluntary movement. Dietz (19, 20), Knutsson (33–35), and McLellan (50) have studied stretch reflexes during voluntary movement, a situation in which their activity (and effects upon it by medications or other therapies) may be of considerable significance. As a summary of the initial reports from these studies, it may be said that stretch reflexes are often increased even further during the course of a movement but most of the disability experienced by the patient still appears to be the result of negative symptoms.

Kinesiological EMG studies from multiple muscles in the lower extremities reveal characteristic abnormalities of timing and pattern of muscle discharge during natural voluntary movements in patients with spasticity due to spinal cord lesions such as multiple sclerosis. Conrad and his colleagues (59) reported recordings of this type from patients pedaling a stationary bicycle. This sort of motor performance was chosen because it produces a reproducible sequence of voluntary leg movements similar to activity during a step cycle, but EMGs during pedaling are more easily recorded since the patient does not move across the floor. Comparing activity of spastic patients with normal controls, they showed that the time during each cycle when rectus femoris is derecruited came abnormally late in about half the patients. That is, during any one cycle of pedaling, quadriceps continue to be active much longer than normal, overlapping activity in the antagonist hamstring group. In a separate study of multiple sclerosis patients without evidence of an upper motoneuron lesion, they found that one-third of them also had this same abnormality. These studies of a relatively complex natural movement can therefore reveal abnormalities at a time when stretch reflexes, plantar responses, and motor performance, as judged clinically, appear normal. Other elegant automated studies of mechanical (as well as electromyographic) aspects of gait have been reported by Conrad and associates (11) and Crenna and Frigo (12). These techniques constitute a powerful method for analysis of gait abnormalities that, in spastic patients, are often associated with poorly timed (abnormally long) contractions of muscles leading to cocontraction of antagonists.

Hultborn's experiments with chronic spinal hemisection in the cat also provide important evidence for permanent changes of the spinal segmental level in response to lesions rostral in the neuraxis (30). For example, he transected the left half of the spinal cord at T12 and, days or weeks later, carried out experimental evaluation of stretch and cutaneous reflexes on both sides at the S1 level. In addition, on the day of the final experiment, he produced a complete transection of the spinal cord at L1, one segment caudal to the initial hemisection. Even after the lower cord was disconnected from the site of the old lesion, ventral root reflex responses to peripheral nerve stimulation (monosynaptic and polysynaptic reflexes produced by muscle and cutaneous afferent stimulation) were considerably increased on the left side. Although these reflexes were larger on the side downstream from the original lesion (an abnormality revealed by this experiment to be due to some permanent change caudal to the old lesion), various tests of inhibition at the segmental level showed it either to be equal on the two sides or slightly greater on the side of the hemisection. This reflex hyperactivity cannot therefore be explained simply as local loss of inhibition. Furthermore, these experiments demonstrate permanent alterations produced at a spinal segmental level far removed from the more rostral lesion.

Because spindle primary afferent fibers are known to make monosynaptic connections with motoneurons innervating their own muscles, it was generally assumed that not only phasic stretch reflexes but also tonic stretch reflexes are mediated entirely by monosynaptic Ia EPSPs on spinal motoneurons. Hultborn and colleagues (14) have recently demonstrated the existence of polysynaptic excitatory pathways from spindle primary afferents onto alpha motoneurons. These circuits appear to require tonic facilitation by serotonergic pathways that descend from the rostral part of the magnocellular raphe nucleus in the brainstem. This polysynaptic circuit with its Ia activation permits greater integration of afferent activity from different muscles with activity in afferents coming from skin, joints and so on. It also permits prolonged excitation of motoneurons as a result of intermittently changing activity from muscle spindles. Tonic stretch reflexes, especially in cats with long-standing spinal lesions, appear to be mediated primarily through this polysynaptic Ia network rather than by monosynaptic activity.

Are Longer Latency Stretch Reflexes Involved?

The simple answer to the question posed above is, "they must be," but it has not yet been possible to define an experimental paradigm that gives a more clear-cut answer. The concept of long loop stretch reflexes arose from two separate groups of observations. It has long been known that when Ia and other stretch-activated afferents enter the spinal cord they end not only on segmental motoneurons and interneurons but also turn rostrally and project to a number of higher centers including the cerebellum. Phillips, working with laboratory primates, recorded stretch-induced afferent activity that, with very short latency, activates corticospinal neurons in the sensorimotor region of cerebral cortex (59). One of Phillips' suggestions was that this paucisynaptic circuit (Ia input activating upper motoneurons that then project directly down onto lower motoneurons) could be considered a transcortical stretch reflex of relatively inflexible, semiautomatic type (58).

Later several groups studied EMG responses in voluntarily contracting human (and laboratory animal) muscles that were suddenly stretched (42, 47, 48). A single, apparently smooth brisk ramp stretch of an already contracting muscle produces EMG activity that appears to compensate for the stretch with relatively short latency. This stretch-induced EMG activity is segmented into two or three bursts, roughly 20 to 25 msec apart in the human arm. The earliest burst that comes with spinal stretch reflex latency is generally agreed to be due to activity of these relatively simple spinal segmental mechanisms. A second or second and third EMG burst follows the first with a latency that depends upon the size of the animal, distance of the stretched muscle from the spinal cord, and perhaps the distance of the spinal segmental level from the cerebrum in that animal. The initial assumption was that a single burst of stretch-induced muscle afferent input activated the motoneuron pool via a local stretch reflex arc but also passed rostrally, perhaps through motor cortex, in a longer loop to return to activate the same spinal motoneuron pool once or twice more.

It was then suggested that lesions anywhere in this longer loop pathway, even in motor cortex, would produce characteristic disturbances in the later EMG bursts. Patients with complete transections could, of course, have no transcortical loops intact, but it is very difficult to test them because they also cannot provide background contraction of muscles below the lesion. However, increases in the first EMG burst (usually referred to as M1) and decreases in the second or third bursts (M2 and M3) were recorded in patients with discrete lesions of the cerebral motor system (41). This was taken to be confirmation of the long loop theory, but that is certainly not a necessary conclusion. For example, lesions of the suprasegmental motor system will produce changes of a long lasting spastic nature at the spinal segmental level as is described above. In the presence of these segmental changes, the spinal motor system will respond differently to Ia input even without the necessity for that input to go all the way up to cerebral cortex and back down. As another example, after cerebral cortical lesions, the plantar reflex changes so a Babinski sign develops and abdominal reflexes disappear, but no one suspects that the afferent limbs of these reflexes extend up through sensorimotor cortex.

Furthermore, Hagbarth and Young (26, 27) demonstrated, by recording human spindle Ia activity using microneurography, that even an apparently smooth brisk ramp stretch produces 40 to 50 Hz oscillations within the stretched muscles. These oscillations, particularly in the presence of alpha-gamma coactivation, produce several bursts of spindle afferent activity 20 or 25 msec apart during or following each single stretch. When these segmented afferent bursts enter the cord, the bursts of EMG activity that follow at the same latency after each of them appear to be a repetitive spinal stretch reflex. There probably are contributions to the later EMG bursts by long loop mechanisms (49), but it is not possible to recognize any such contributions simply by recording EMG activity. Chronic changes in muscle stiffness, produced by spasticity for example, will alter muscle afferent responses produced by stretch. Furthermore, in the presence of enhanced spinal stretch reflex mechanisms, a larger percentage of any motoneuron pool will be activated by the first burst of Ia activity leaving more motoneurons in a refractory or hypoexitable state so that the subsequent M2 or M3 would naturally be smaller. None of this can be used as support for the hypothesis that recording these long latency stretch reflexes gives direct anatomical information about supraspinal motor pathways.

In summary, both afferent and efferent pathways rostral to the spinal segmental level are clearly disturbed in patients with spasticity, but one cannot demonstrate unequivocally how much of the abnormal motor control in patients with spasticity is due to any one of these mechanisms.

Hyperactive Exteroceptive Reflexes in Spinal Spasticity

Many nonproprioceptive reflexes are also abnormal in patients with spasticity, particularly exteroceptive reflexes that are organized around afferent input from skin and subcutaneous tissue (Fig. 10.1). Nociceptive reflexes, which require painful or damaging stimuli, are only one subgroup of exteroceptive reflexes. As an example of the difference among these latter reflexes, cutaneous abdominal reflexes are usually decreased or absent in the presence of spasticity whereas cutaneously induced nociceptive flexor reflexes are typically hyperactive. Spinal reflexes in the autonomic system, the output of which regulates sweating, blood pressure, and bowel and bladder function, are also abnormally hyperactive, particularly in patients with spinal cord lesions. In such patients, autonomic reflex behavior takes the form of a gross, nonselective "mass response." The old concept that normally some sort of generalized "autonomic tone" exists throughout the

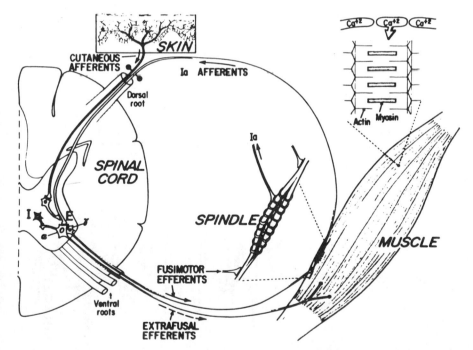

Figure 10.1. Structures involved in the segmental stretch reflex arc (see the text for details). E is an excitatory presynaptic ending, I an inhibitory interneuron, α an alpha motoneuron and γ a gamma motoneuron. Note that for muscle to contract, calcium must be released from sarcoplasmic reticulum (Ca+2) into the sarcoplasm where ATP, actin, and myosin are present. Cutaneous afferents are also illustrated. (From Young, R. R., and Delwaide, P. J. Drug therapy-spasticity. *New Engl. J. Med.*, 304:28–33, 96–99, 1981.)

body has been disproved. Wallin and his colleagues (76) have demonstrated the existence of very elegantly specialized autonomic reflex responses that are regionally organized, highly selective, and functionally discrete. However, in the presence of spinal lesions, this discriminative behavior disappears and is replaced by a crude, generalized reflex found throughout the body caudal to the spinal lesions (75). This is therefore the counterpart of spasticity within the autonomic system.

As Hagbarth and Finer (25) demonstrated, normal cutaneous reflex behavior is also highly organized to produce automatic movements that remove the stimulated body part from a noxious stimulus. In simplest and crudest form, a pinprick or brief noxious electrical stimulus to a finger or toe will produce a relatively short latency flexor reflex of the arm or leg, accompanied by appropriate alterations in posture in the other leg or body parts to compensate for changes produced by the short latency flexor reflex activity. In patients with spinal lesions, the threshold for production of abnormally massive flexor (or, depending upon the exact site of stimulus, extensor) nociceptive reflexes is very much lower (Fig. 10.2). Previously innocuous stimuli such as a puff of air on the foot will product massive triple flexion at hip, knee, and ankle as well as dorsiflexion of toes in a patient with spinal lesions whereas there would be no response in a normal

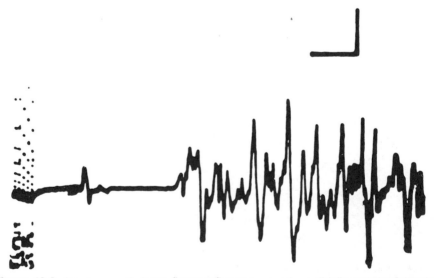

Figure 10.2. An abnormally large flexor reflex recorded from tibialis anterior following a train of electrical stimuli to the tibial nerve in a patient with a partial lesion of the spinal cord. Note the small short-latency "first component" and the massive "second component". Calibration is 50 msec and 200 uV. (From Shahani, B. T., and Young, R. R. The flexor reflex in spasticity. In: *Spasticity: Disordered Motor Control.* Edited by Feldman, R. G., Young, R. R., and Koella, W. P. Yearbook Medical Publishers, Chicago, 1980, pp. 287–295.)

subject. Most spontaneous flexor spasms (Fig. 10.3) are probably hyperactive reflex responses to unidentified trivial stimuli. Furthermore, local sign, an important aspect of cutaneous reflexes, is also lost in spasticity. In other words, the elegantly integrated contractions and relaxations of various muscle groups, which serve to preserve body posture but remove the part of the body being stimulated from the stimulus, are absent. Under normal circumstances a pinprick on the ball of the great toe will produce dorsiflexion of that toe, an entirely appropriate response. A pinprick elsewhere on the sole of the foot will produce plantar flexion of the toes in order to reduce tension on the skin of the sole of the foot and thereby remove it from the pin. If the stimulus to the sole of the foot is massive enough, there may be triple flexion at ankle, knee, and hip as well as plantar flexion of the toes. A stimulus to the dorsum of the foot will produce plantar flexion to remove the foot from the noxious stimulus. All these appropriate behaviors disappear in patients with spasticity. In them, a stimulus anywhere in the lower leg will produce triple flexion and dorsiflexion of the toe—a Babinski response. This may or may not remove the noxious stimulus from the foot, depending on where the stimulus is. Natural reflexogenic stimuli may produce responses only in flexor muscles (Fig. 10.4) or, when reciprocal inhibition is deficient, in both extensors and flexors (Fig. 10.5).

Obviously, a Babinski response is abnormal because scratching of the lateral side of the foot produces great toe dorsiflexion, which does not serve a useful function. It should also be noted that EMG studies of plantar cutaneous nociceptive reflexes have shown that what happens is not simply contraction of plantar flexing muscles under normal circumstances and dorsiflexing muscles in spasticity. Even in normal subjects, there is cocontraction of muscles that plantar flex and dorsiflex the great toe whenever the sole is stimulated, but the plantar flexing muscles are stronger so that

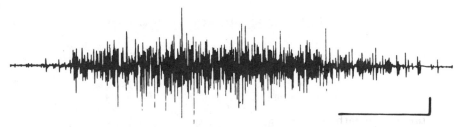

Figure 10.3. A spontaneous flexor spasm recorded from tibialis anterior in a patient with a spinal cord lesion. Note the recruitment pattern here is very much like a normal voluntary recruitment pattern; the smaller unit which was recruited first was also the last to be de-recruited. Like other "spontaneous" flexor spasms, this could be a reflex response to a small unrecognized cutaneous stimulus. Calibration is 1 sec and 200 uV. (From Shahani, B. T., and Young, R. R. The flexor reflex in spasticity. In: *Spasticity: Disordered Motor Control.* Edited by Feldman, R. G., Young, R. R., and Koella, W. P. Yearbook Medical Publishers, Chicago, 1980, pp. 287–295.)

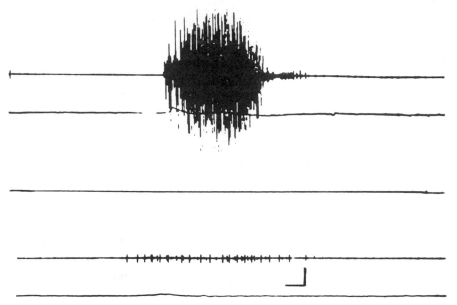

Figure 10.4. Two spontaneous flexor spasms recorded only from tibialis anterior (the upper tracing in each pair) in a patient with a thoracic cord lesion. No activity is recorded from triceps surae (the lower tracing in each pair.) Some spasms (the upper one) produce a full recruitment pattern whereas others (the lower one) are the discharge of only a few motor units. Calibration is 250 msec and 200 uV. (From Shahani, B. T., and Young, R. R. The flexor reflex in spasticity. In: *Spasticity: Disordered Motor Control.* Edited by Feldman, R. G., Young, R. R., and Koella, W. P. Yearbook Medical Publishers, Chicago, 1980, pp. 287–295.)

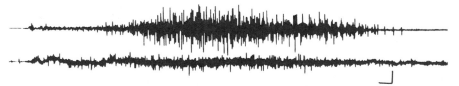

Figure 10.5. A spontaneous flexor spasm recorded in both tibialis anterior (upper tracing) and triceps surae in a patient with a high cervical cord lesion. Note more or less simultaneous activity in both these antagonistic muscle groups. Calibration is 200 msec and 200 uV. (From Shahani, B. T., and Young, R. R. The flexor reflex in spasticity. In: *Spasticity: Disordered Motor Control.* Edited by Feldman, R. G., Young, R. R., and Koella, W. P. Yearbook Medical Publishers, Chicago, 1980, pp. 287–295.)

movement takes place. Similar cocontraction is seen in patients with spasticity, but cutaneously induced flexor activity is then predominant. There exists, therefore, a continuum between clear dorsiflexion and clear plantar flexion rather than a binary situation where the toe either goes up or down.

Abnormal hyperactivity of exteroceptive reflexes is clearly a fundamental part of the upper motoneuron syndrome even though the strict definition of spasticity does not mention such reflexes (38). Polysynaptic spinal flexor reflex circuits are more complex than the stretch reflex circuits mentioned above and far less is known about them.

PHARMACOLOGICAL MANAGEMENT

General Principles

Drug therapy for spasticity necessarily has a narrow range of realistic goals. Most of the functional deficit in patients with spasticity is due to negative symptoms such as loss of facility, for which there is no effective therapy. Therapies do exist for several of the positive symptoms, but even if it were possible to eliminate the positive symptom required for a diagnosis of spasticity (exaggerated stretch reflexes), the patient would probably not notice any change in handicap. Our most effective therapies diminish flexor spasms and are useful for patients with lesions affecting the spinal cord even though they do not alter enhanced stretch reflexes and therefore do not affect spasticity in the strict sense of that word. For a recent review of drug therapy for spasticity, see Young and Delwaide (80).

Spasticity is not one circumscribed disorder of motor performance. Both the functional deficits and positive symptoms vary from patient to patient depending upon the site and extent of the CNS lesion. Patients with lesions in the spinal cord experience flexor spasms as well as adducted and flexed legs—a very different picture from the extended legs of patients with cerebral lesions producing hemiplegic dystonia. Even if one looks at a group of spinal cord injury patients with spasticity, there is not a uniform, homogeneous clinical picture. Any really effective therapy, whether pharmacological or otherwise, must be tailored to the patient's specific disabilities. It is unlikely, therefore, that there will be one single therapy for spasticity—even under the best of circumstances in the future, there will probably be a number of therapies for different types of spasticity.

As neurobiology provides us with more details of the CNS circuits involved in motor control, including the neurotransmitters involved, it should be possible to produce more specific pharmacological agents that will enhance or block excitatory and inhibitory activity in those circuits. By that time, clinical neurophysiology should have provided methods for identifying and quantifying the elemental functional subdivisions of the motor system that are defective in any one particular patient. This information will enable the therapist to identify the particular therapeutic modalities necessary for that individual patient and will also provide objective monitoring of improvement, thereby elevating the science of Neurological Rehabilitation to a quantitative level. As William Thompson Lord Kelvin said, "When you can measure what you are speaking about, and express it in numbers, you know something about it, but when you cannot measure it, when you cannot express it in numbers, your knowledge is of a meager and unsatisfactory kind; it may be the beginning of knowledge, but you have scarcely in your thoughts advanced to the stage of science." Once Neurological Rehabilitation has reached that stage, appropriate pharmacologic and other manipulations should lead to a rational therapy for movement disorders.

Meanwhile, the drugs available must be used to treat this chronic disability, which will presumably require therapy for the remainder of a patient's life. The long-term safety and efficacy of these drugs are poorly understood. Nevertheless, long-term treatment is justifiable providing the medication produces clear-cut reduction in patient discomfort or disability, or improvement in function. It is necessary to objectify that beneficial effect, because without it, unless a medication has practically no side effects or expense, there is no justification for its long-term employment. Documentation of drug-related improvement in terms of quantitative variables defined by clinical neurophysiology laboratories is a significant problem. The paucity of such techniques has resulted in a severe limitation in medical science's ability to be certain about the efficacy of pharmacologic or physical therapies. Once the physiologic building blocks of the motor system have been discovered and the "game plan" by which they are employed to produce normal motility is clear, it should be possible to measure the function of each of these elemental building blocks objectively and probe the value (or lack of it) of each mode of treatment. Meanwhile, even simple measurements such as counting the number of flexor spasms per day are preferable to the subjective impressions obtained by those people observing the patient, including physicians, paramedical personnel, family members, and the patient himself.

Baclofen for Flexor Spasms

Baclofen is the most effective therapy for patients whose spasticity results from spinal cord lesions, and it also has the least side effects (21). It produces considerable, often dramatic reduction in number and severity of flexor spasms or similar cutaneously induced extensor spasms. It also reduces tonically increased flexor tone in the legs of these patients. It is effective in the isolated spinal cord below a complete transection, which proves that most of its action takes place at the spinal level even in patients without complete transection.

Although baclofen is known to be a powerful neuronal depressant with actions over a wide area of the nervous system, its precise mechanisms of action are not yet clear. Because it is a parachlorophenyl derivative of gamma-aminobutyric acid (GABA), it is usually assumed to operate at GABA synapses, but even that is not entirely clear. Baclofen's action is not antagonized by at least one specific antagonist (bicuculline), which is effective in blocking GABA's action at certain synapses, as in its role as presynaptic inhibitory transmitter. There are other GABA-mediated presynaptic actions including decreased release of excitatory transmitter, an activity usually ascribed to baclofen's action (Fig. 10.6). This may include reduction in the release of substance P, which is a neurotransmitter active at the central ends of afferent nerves coming from skin and elsewhere, in which impulses tend to produce flexor and other nociceptive reflex activity.

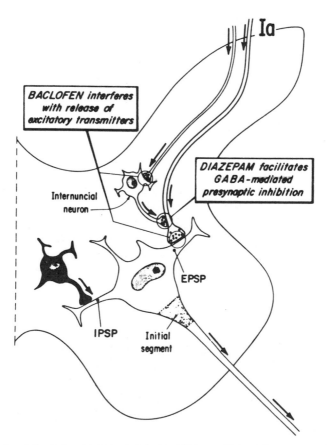

Figure 10.6. An enlargement of the left half of Figure 10.1 to illustrate putative sites of action of baclofen and diazepam. GABA is gamma aminobutyric acid, a neurotransmitter supposed to mediate presynaptic inhibition. EPSP represents excitatory postsynaptic potentials on the motoneuron and IPSP, inhibitory postsynaptic potentials produced by inhibitory interneurons. If EPSP's exceed IPSP's on dendrites and the cell body so the initial segment of the axon is depolarized by about 10 mV, an impulse arises there and is conducted out to the muscle fibers in that motor unit (see the text for details.) (From Young, R. R., and Delwaide, P. J. Drug therapy-spasticity. *New England J. Med.*, 304:28–33, 96–99, 1981.)

Whatever its mechanism of action, baclofen is quite effective in reducing both the frequency and severity of *flexor spasms*—a term used to include even extensor spasms when these are produced spontaneously or by various cutaneous stimuli. Baclofen also reduces tonic flexor muscle dystonia in the lower extremities in spinal cord injured patients. It is not particularly effective in patients with cerebral lesions, and the incidence of side effects is much higher in these patients than in those whose lesions are limited entirely or predominantly to the spinal cord.

Flexor spasms are often painful and may awaken patients frequently at night. They are also unpleasant in the daytime and can produce unexpected falls in ambulatory patients. Patients are therefore grateful for reduction in the number of flexor spasms and for decreased severity of those that remain. Baclofen may also reduce spasms affecting pelvic floor muscles and thereby improve bowel and bladder control, but these effects are less dramatic than those listed above. Personal hygiene and nursing care in nonambulatory patients can be improved when baclofen relaxes the tightly flexed and adducted legs. By reducing the number of stimulus-induced flexor spasms, baclofen may also permit the use of orthotic devices and facilitate transfers. Despite this reduction of flexor activity, baclofen does not improve the stiff spastic gait in patients with spinal lesions, nor does it increase manual dexterity in the hands of such patients.

Baclofen is probably more effective than diazepam in patients with spinal lesions. It certainly produces less sedation. Therapy usually begins with half a 10 mg tablet twice a day and can be increased by half a tablet every 3 days until the patient either is considerably improved or is taking two tablets four times a day. If it is necessary to discontinue baclofen, it should not be abruptly withdrawn because that often produces a temporary rebound increase in the number and severity of spasms.

Baclofen has remarkably few significant side effects. Large doses given acutely, particularly in patients whose lesions also effect the cerebrum, can produce sedation, somnolence, and ataxia. When employed as suggested above, the most frequent side effect of baclofen is temporary drowsiness, which usually disappears within a few days even though the medication is continued. Because of the sedation and because any such side effects of alcohol or other CNS-active drugs would be additive, patients should be cautioned with regard to driving or operating dangerous machinery. Baclofen may occasionally be counterproductive in patients who have learned to use the stiffness of their limbs to assist in activities of daily living. Fortunately it is extremely rare that baclofen results in a poorer motor performance.

In some patients with spinal lesions, episodic spasms of pain are more troublesome than any accompanying movements of the legs, and in such patients, baclofen may also be quite useful.

In summary, baclofen is clearly the most effective agent for treatment of patients with spasticity caused by lesions of the spinal cord. Its effect is to reduce flexor spasms and it has little effect on stretch reflexes.

Dantrolene to Weaken Muscles

Dantrolene reduces the amount of calcium released from sarcoplasmic reticulum following each muscle action potential. Because this movement of calcium from the reservoir cisternae into the sarcoplasm is necessary for activation of myosin-ATPase, which results in movement of actin and myosin filaments past one another to produce tension, dantrolene interferes with excitation-contraction coupling and weakens muscles. It does not affect conduction of the muscle action potential and therefore has no effect on the EMG. Any given level of dantrolene has more effect on type II muscle fibers than on type I fibers.

Dantrolene has little effect on cardiac or smooth muscle, so levels of dantrolene can be elevated gradually (providing side-effects such as diarrhea or hepatitis don't supervene) until skeletal muscles have been weakened to a suitable extent considering the patient's general situation. It must be admitted that dantrolene's antispastic (myorelaxant) effect is due to its ability to produce mild to moderate generalized muscle weakness, and there are relatively few spinal cord injured patients who are improved overall by weakening their muscles. It may be useful in those nonambulatory patients whose nursing care is compromised by severe muscle contractions, especially if such patients will not be further handicapped by loss of voluntary power. In our experience, it is remarkably rare to find a patient whose function is improved by dantrolene.

Patients can begin taking one 25 mg dantrolene tablet each day and the dosage can be increased by one tablet twice a week. Benefits will not be recognized for 5 or 10 days after any given therapeutic level has been reached so increase in medication should not be made too frequently. Maximum dantrolene doses are about 100 mg four times a day. As the doses increase, generalized weakness or diarrhea will eventually result. Some patients are made drowsy or lightheaded by dantrolene, which suggests it may also have CNS effects. If no clear cut benefit is obtained within 6 weeks, dantrolene therapy should be discontinued because of the risk of hepatic toxicity. This risk is increased in patients who have been given intermittent short courses of high dose dantrolene therapy or in patients who receive more than 300 mg per day for longer than 2 months. The risk of dantrolene-induced hepatic toxicity is greatest in women, in patients older than 35 years, and in patients receiving estrogens. Liver function tests should be carried out before dantrolene is given and periodically during therapy.

Diazepam

Diazepam appears to enhance presynaptic inhibition by facilitating or potentiating the postsynaptic effect of GABA. Benzodiazepines such as diazepam have no direct GABA-mimetic effect but they increase the efficiency of GABA-ergic transmission when such synapses are already activated. Diazepam binds to a receptor near the GABA receptor and increases the affinity of these latter receptors for GABA (Fig. 10.6). This renders them more efficient at increasing chloride and possibly decreasing calcium conductance.

Diazepam's effect is a particularly interesting one. Direct GABA agonists would stimulate all GABA receptors indiscriminately whereas diazepam only increases the efficiency of those GABA receptors that are already being stimulated in the normal course of physiological events. In other words, diazepam operates in the fine-tuning of these synapses by turning up their gains. It therefore produces an effect similar to that of GABA wherever its effect has been tested. Naturally occurring agonists for these diazepam receptors have been identified; diazepam appears to mimic the action of these naturally occurring transmitters in the same way that opiates mimic the action of endogenous opioids.

Diazepam is useful alone or together with other agents in the treatment of patients with spasticity due to lesions of the spinal cord. Painful spasms are often reduced but there is no evidence that diazepam is better than baclofen in that role.

Delwaide has pioneered in physiological studies of patients with spasticity (17, 18). Within a group of clinically indistinguishable patients, diazepam will enhance vibratory inhibition of tendon reflexes in some and baclofen will normalize H reflex recovery curves in others. These effects allow one to predict which patients are more likely to benefit from diazepam therapy or from the use of baclofen.

Diazepam therapy can begin with one 2 mg tablet twice a day and this dose can be increased slowly by one tablet every few days until unwanted side effects develop or the patient reaches a level of two 10 mg tablets three or four times a day. Diazepam's major side effect is drowsiness, but if the doses are increased very slowly, certain patients can take remarkably large amounts of diazepam with few untoward reactions. Diazepam should also be used cautiously in patients who take alcohol or other CNS-active medications. Patients should be cautioned against driving or using dangerous equipment. Abrupt withdrawal of diazepam may produce seizures. Diazepam may also increase depression. Large acute doses of diazepam may produce coma and respiratory depression.

Newer Agents

Propranolol can be used orally to suppress ankle clonus, a symptom that is occasionally annoying but rarely of functional significance. When given intravenously, the alpha-adrenergic blocking agent thymoxamine can also depress clonus but is not effective orally (46). Phenoxybenzamine has not proven to be effective in the therapy of spasticity. Autonomic effects on spasticity have once again become fruitful areas for research.

Tizanidine has been used in Europe for the treatment of spasticity in patients with spinal cord lesions but is not yet available for routine use in North America. Tizanidine, an imidazoline derivative, reduces tonic stretch reflexes and enhances presynaptic inhibition in animals. In patients, it enhances vibratory inhibition of H reflexes (Delwaide's definition of a presynaptic inhibitory enhancer) and reduces abnormal cocontraction of antagonist muscle groups. Its effects on spasticity are similar to those of diazepam but tizanidine has many less side effects (22, 40, 72). Baclofen is probably more effective than tizanidine in reducing flexor spasms in patients with spinal cord disease but both agents are useful together; they appear to operate by different mechanisms and together produce useful therapeutic responses with fewer side effects.

A clinically useful GABA agonist should be helpful in the therapy of spasticity but such a medication is not available at this time. In Europe, studies of THIP (tetrahydroisoxazolopyridin) suggest it is a relatively specific and potent GABA agonist in animals. Preliminary studies in patients with spinal lesions showed reduction in stretch reflex activity and increases in vibratory suppression of H reflexes (57). It may also increase the flexor reflex threshold, but more studies are necessary before its clinical utility can be demonstrated.

A new use for an old pharmacological agent has recently been described by Struppler and his colleagues (71). They found that epidural opioids (fentanyl and morphine) repeatedly suppressed flexor reflexes (including flexor spasms) and adduction spasm in the legs of a patient with spasticity of spinal origin (due to multiple sclerosis). These opioids did not affect ankle clonus or the patient's ability to produce voluntary dorsiflexion of the foot. Perhaps clinically useful techniques can be developed to deliver opioids to the spinal cords of patients such as this; high concentrations near the cord probably affect enkephalinergic interneurons but the amount of opioids in the general circulation is so low that systemic effects including addiction may not be a problem.

NEUROSURGICAL MANAGEMENT

One has tended to think of neurosurgical therapies for spasticity as being destructive of peripheral or central nervous system tissue, principally in an effort to interrupt pathways necessary for operation of stretch and exteroceptive reflexes. In this way, certain of the more objectionable positive symptoms in spastic patients can be reduced or eliminated but there is little chance for improvement in function. Sometimes, what little function was present is also reduced by these destructive lesions.

Two more recent neurosurgical developments tend to contradict the stereotype listed in the first sentence above. The first of these was the development of stereotactic ablation of small targets within deep nuclei such as the thalamus. Although these procedures are also destructive of nervous tissue, they do not, when properly placed, produce negative symptoms themselves; that is, one cannot recognize the loss of any function despite the fact that these lesions interrupt the outflow from cerebellum or basal ganglia into thalamus and thalamocortical circuits. In fact, in the ideal patient, such lesions permit an improvement in function by eliminating tardive posthemiparetic dystonia as discussed later.

Even more recently, neurosurgeons have been employing dorsal column stimulation, a relatively noninvasive and nondestructive technique that may improve function in patients with spinal cord lesions.

Eventually neurosurgical techniques may be developed that will assist in the regeneration of axons within the spinal cord and thereby restore certain functions that otherwise would have continued to be lost. For a discussion of experimental aspects of neuronal replacement and reconstruction of damaged CNS circuits, see the review by Bjorklund and Stenevi (6).

Neurectomies and Rhizotomies

Because stretch reflexes and nociceptive reflexes cannot be elicited in the absence of afferent input, dorsal rhizotomies eliminate these reflexes. Unfortunately, large areas of the body are simultaneously rendered anesthetic and usually develop pressure sores or unrecognized traumatic lesions. Also, with the loss of all proprioceptive input, movements become extremely ataxic, poorly coordinated, and nearly useless, at least from many patients' standpoints. Attempts have therefore been made to reduce some but not all afferent input into the cord by producing partial rhizotomies. Dilute solutions of alcohol or phenol injected into mixed nerves within muscles or placed around dorsal roots certainly do produce lesions of the most superficial and smaller afferent fibers. It was originally hoped that such chemical lesions would preferentially damage small diameter fibers such as gamma efferents that innervate muscle spindles and pain and temperature afferents coming into the cord. The selective action of phenol or alcohol, at least in terms of actions upon axons of varying diameters, proves to be disappointing. Such lesions tend to destroy more superficial axons of all diameters within nerves or roots, which nevertheless may sometimes be useful.

Thermal effects on smaller diameter axons have been possible in animal laboratories for many years, but producing a differential block of small fibers in the clinical situation is difficult. Attempts were made at one time to bathe the roots in iced artificial spinal fluid; there were reports of improvement in patients with spasticity but that technique no longer seems popular. Focused high energy ultrasound produces a discrete thermal (heat) lesion primarily affecting smaller diameter nerve fibers (81), but the application of this technique to multiple nerves or roots has never been feasible. There are more recent reports of thermal probes placed within roots to heat fibers and destroy the smaller ones. These thermal rhizotomies may produce dramatic relief of spasticity in patients (30a), but more research and more widespread application of this technique is necessary before it can be evaluated objectively.

The original rationale for the use of chemical or thermal agents to destroy small rather than large diameter axons was the assumption that spasticity was due to increased fusimotor tone. That no longer seems likely, although disruption of fusimotor activity in spastic patients will obviously reduce stretch reflexes, which usually is of little benefit. More often, lesions in nerves or roots that were thought to be specific for axons of smaller diameters prove, upon close postmortem inspection, to have affected fibers of all diameters. Any relief of spasticity produced by such nonspecific lesions must reflect the role of the mass action of large numbers of afferents in setting the level of intensity of spasticity. It may be that, in the presence of increased central excitability due to lesions causing spasticity, some motor circuits are activated, in part at least, by various nonspecific afferent inputs.

As another example of this possibility, selective neurectomies are sometimes remarkably effective. For example, in patients with little motility of the legs and difficulties in personal hygiene because of tightly adducted thighs, obturator neurectomies on one or both sides will certainly paralyze adductor muscles and make nursing care easier. When such operations are done, one often finds that spasticity in quadriceps or hamstring muscles (or even in muscles below the knee) is also considerably reduced even though these muscular groups have no immediate relationship to the obturator nerve. The explanation for such nonspecific relief of spasticity has been that decreased input from adductor muscles also cuts down on the general level of spinal excitability in motoneuron pools distinct from those supplying muscles innervated by the obturator nerve.

Production of Spinal Lesions

If pain is a particular problem in spinal cord injured patients with spasticity, a median cordotomy that transects those fibers crossing the midline near the central canal can disconnect the second neuron in the pain circuit from its higher centers, producing a clinical picture similar to that seen with syringomyelia. This cordotomy, which would be placed in the lumbar and lower thoracic region in patients with particular difficulty in the legs, would not disconnect stretch reflex and other local circuits and therefore would do little to reduce spasticity.

In patients with absolutely no function of legs, bowels, or bladder, and with disagreeable spasms or dystonic legs, surgeons have resorted to localized cordectomy. In these procedures, the spinal cord is removed over a number of segments in the appropriate region. This produces complete anesthesia, flaccidity of limbs, and paralysis of bowel and bladder function. Even in patients with a more rostral complete cord transection who are unaware of the loss of sensation produced by this procedure, the absence of automatic regulation of bowel and bladder activity and the absence of locally mediated flexor reflexes in response to painful stimuli may be a retrograde step. After all, these functions, even in an isolated cord, tend to be useful. With the advent or newer therapies, cordectomy is now rarely necessary.

Dorsal Column Stimulation

Approximately 20 years ago, Melzack and Wall (51) developed the *gate theory* of analgesia. According to this theory, afferent activity in smaller diameter, slower conducting axons (which mediate the sensations of pain) can be presynaptically inhibited or otherwise reduced after they enter the spinal cord but before they reach their first synapse. This suppression of painful afferent activity can be produced by impulses in larger diameter, more rapidly conducting afferent fibers. In order to effect this therapy, electrodes are placed around or near peripheral nerves and chronic stimulation of large diameter fibers is carried out. Transcutaneous electrical nerve stimulation (TENS) is also used. For a recent review of endogenous pain control systems, see the article by Basbaum and Fields (3).

For technical reasons, it proved easier to place stimulating electrodes over the dorsal columns of the spinal cord so that chronic stimulation could be used for reduction of pain. It was then discovered that spinal cord stimulation for pain also had beneficial effects on motor abnormalities in those same patients. Dorsal column stimulation is now used routinely in several centers in North America for the therapy of specific motor disorders including spasticity in patients with spinal cord lesions. The electrodes are usually placed percutaneously into the epidural space in the cervical area. A short chain of electrodes is placed because maximum improvement depends upon finding exactly the correct location for the electrodes and discovering the intensity and frequency of stimuli necessary to optimize improvement. The location of electrodes and stimulus parameters vary to a certain extent from one patient to the next and must be adjusted empirically in any given patient. Stimulation in this region will obviously produce no effects in the lower extremities of patients who have complete spinal transections in the lower cervical or thoracic regions. In patients with partial transections and in patients with multiple sclerosis, dorsal column stimulation may be quite useful. Waltz reports (personal communication) marked or moderate improvement (see below) in 60% to 70% of more than 75 patients with multiple sclerosis. No patient was worsened by stimulation. Complications include infection in less than 1% and electrode or stimulator failure that may occur in 10% to 15% requiring a further operative procedure.

Improvements in such patients include decreased spasticity, abolition of ankle clonus, reduction in the number of painful spasms, and increased range of motion. Bladder control may also be improved and, in ambulatory patients, stability of gait may be increased and ataxia decreased.

Chronic epidural spinal cord stimulation is apparently capable of improving a wide variety of motor disabilities including spasticity. Mechanisms underlying this effect are probably of a relatively nonspecific nature but are basically unclear; benefits may result either from direct electrical influences on central nervous tissue or from the release of neurotransmitters or neuromodulators produced by this stimulation.

Stereotactic Thalamotomy

An appropriately placed tiny lesion within ventrolateral or ventral intermediate thalamic nuclei can certainly reduce dystonia in patients with spasticity secondary to cerebral lesions, but it would not be useful for patients with complete or nearly complete spinal lesions. Furthermore, even in patients with cerebral spasticity, relief of dystonia is practically never accompanied by improvement because negative symptoms such as lack of dexterity persist. However, there are rare patients with cerebral lesions who do benefit from relief of this dystonia. In these infrequent patients, hemiplegic dystonia developed 6 to 18 months after a stroke (which usually involves thalamus or upper brainstem), and their motor systems were seen to be functioning at an extremely high level following recovery from the stroke and before development of dystonia. Such patients should profit from stereotactic neurosurgery to relieve this tardive posthemiparetic dystonia. As far as we know, the existence of such patients with spasticity due to spinal cord lesions has not been demonstrated.

ROLE OF PHYSICAL MODALITIES

With improved nursing care and rehabilitation techniques (for example, prevention of decubitus ulcers and bladder infection), every patient with spinal cord injury recovers from spinal shock and develops spasticity within a few days to a few months after the injury. Management emphasis has shifted from surgical treatment of severe spasticity to preventive and conservative management that has made destructive surgery unnecessary for most patients.

The goal of conservative management is to prevent complications of spasticity so the patient can function at the highest level of performance in activities of daily living (ADL). Since clinical manifestations of spinal cord lesions also include negative symptoms, such as weakness, a certain amount of spasticity may be useful. For example, reflex activation of quadriceps (by cutaneous stimulation of upper thigh) may help the patient stand up. Excessive spasticity on the other hand creates a number of problems that interfere with all levels of the rehabilitation process. Examples of excessive spasticity are spontaneous flexor and extensor spasms, heel cord shortening, extension or flexion contractures of the hip and knee, and adductor spasms. Methods to prevent these complications, which interfere with ambulation, wheelchair independence, and ADL, include: (a) Elimination of intrinsic and extrinsic factors resulting in increased afferent input to the spinal cord; (b) Proper positioning; and (c) Passive range of motion.

Elimination of Factors Evoking a Reflex Response

A variety of extrinsic and intrinsic stimuli can produce flexor reflexes in patients with spinal cord injury. Distension of any internal organ including bladder, colon, and rectum can result in severe flexor spasms. The smaller the capacity of the bladder, the smaller the amount of urine required to activate the flexor reflex pathways. Intermittent catheterization of the bladder is preferred to indwelling catheterization, which results in a small contracted bladder. Evacuation of a distended rectum often results in dramatic reduction in the degree of spinal spasticity. Intercurrent infections, especially of the urinary tract, result in increased flexor spasms. Decubitus ulcers should be prevented because they, along with plantar warts, burns, and infected ingrown toe nails, can be a cause of abnormal sensory input resulting in increasing reflex activity. Toxemia secondary to infected bed sores may produce severe spontaneous spasms. Sometimes infection may produce increased reflex activity long before an increase in body temperature. Other factors that may increase spasticity are lesions affecting sexual organs (phimosis or paraphimosis), infections of the vagina, or infected retained birth control devices. Hemorrhoids, anal fistulae, and fractures or dislocations of bones (often unrecognized) also produce increased flexor spasms. In addition to factors described above, changes in patients' environments, such as extremes of temperature, may result in excessive spasticity. Finally, emotional stress can cause severe increases in spasticity. This type of excess spasticity lends itself to successful therapy by human contact, diversion into work and sports, and judicious treatment with appropriate drugs (54).

Proper Positioning

Proper positioning of limbs below the level of the neurological lesion is essential and should be done early to avoid contractures. In the supine position there is a tendency for the hip and knee joints to acquire a flexed posture. In prone and upright positions the extensor synergy is predominant. The position of the ankle joint should be such that the foot is kept in the midline and at a right angle to the leg. Splints should not be used because they and the bandages with which they are held tend to produce pressure sores. The knee and hip joints should be kept in full extension when the patient is lying on his back and at 20° flexion when the patient is lying on his side. Both legs must be kept in about 10° abduction. A pillow should never be kept under the knee because it tends to produce flexion, not only at the knee but also at the hip. A pillow between the knees is, however, useful because it prevents pressure sores on the medial aspect of the knee. Guttmann (23) used the "earliest possible standing position" in parallel bars for paraplegic patients as a means of overcoming exaggerated action of the flexors of hips and knees. In patients with high thoracic and cervical lesions, extensor synergy of the trunk and lower limbs is greatly increased by putting the patient in a prone position for several hours a day.

Passive Range of Motion (ROM)

Passive ROM at all joints below the level of the lesion is useful for prevention of increased spasticity and contractures. Passive movements must be carried out gently through the full ROM of each joint several times a day for the first few weeks. Thereafter, ROM must be performed at least once a day. The relaxing effect of passive movements in spastic muscles is increased by placing the patient in a warm bath. It must be emphasized that, during the period of flaccidity, passive ROM must be carried out carefully by a trained physical therapist because excessive movements may be a factor contributing to the disabling complication of paraarticular ossification seen in paraplegic patients (62). It has been found that alternating passive movement of paralyzed spastic lower limbs, as produced by cycling action in a pedal exerciser controlled by the patient's arms, has a remarkable relaxing action that lasts for several hours in spastic limbs.

Electrical Stimulation Techniques

Continuous tetanizing of muscle groups with low voltage currents (43, 74) to relieve spasticity has not been used widely (23). In one paraplegic patient, a peroneal nerve stimulator was implanted on both sides. Using a cycle exercise module attached to the stimulator, each leg was stimulated for longer and longer periods, eventually 6 to 8 hours daily (15). There was significant increase in the bulk, not only of the anterior compartment muscles but also of the calf and thigh muscles, within 6 to 12 months. There was marked reduction in spasticity and improved ability to ambulate with crutches. Further studies to evaluate the usefulness of this technique must be carried out because it provides a method for electrical exercise, reduction of spasticity, and promotion of circulation in lower extremities as well as an opportunity to study and promote reflex movements (15).

In recent years, functional electrical stimulation (FES) has been used not only to strengthen weak paraparetic muscles (and reduce their spasticity) but also for simple FES-assisted standing and restoration of a biped gait in patients with complete transection of the spinal cord. Using four to six channels of FES, two of three paraplegic patients with complete transections of the spinal cord were able to walk in parallel bars, the third patient could perform independent unassisted walking over short distances with the aid of a roller walker (36).

Ultrasound

An objective method has been developed to determine the effect of ultrasonic energy on spasticity (44). Preliminary studies suggest that with lower ultrasonic doses (0.76 watts/cm2) applied over appropriate spastic muscles, there is a significant increase in spasticity whereas with higher doses (1.9 watts/cm2) there is significant decrease in spasticity lasting for 10 to 15 miutes (70). Further studies are needed in order to evaluate the usefulness of this technique.

Local Cryotherapy

Local cold therapy for the treatment of spastic patients has received wide acceptance for the management of abnormal muscle tone. Hartviksen (29) applied granular ice packs to spastic muscles for 20 minutes and found reduction of spasticity both during the application and for many hours after removal of the ice. Deep tendon reflexes were diminished and muscle tone was depressed. Reflexes returned to normal within one-half to 1 hour after the packs were removed, but muscle tone remained suppressed for a number of hours after return of the reflexes. Other investigators have used local applications of cracked ice in wet towels for 10 minutes and believe that reduction of spasticity permits the patient to: (a) perform self-care exercise programs in a more active and functional manner; (b) assist with forceful stretching; (c) perform active exercises of antagonistic muscle groups; and (d) improve his gait (45). Since intramuscular temperatures remain normal even when the ice pack is in place for approximately 30 minutes, reduction in reflex activity is probably related to blocking of cutaneous afferents (29, 55). Miglietta (56) found that clonus frequency dropped or it disappeared for 4 hours after spastic extremities were immersed in water at 65°F for 15 minutes.

Biofeedback

With modern technology, it is possible to monitor different physiological parameters, including blood pressure, skin temperature, EEG, and electromyographic (EMG) activity, which provide an individual with immediate and continuing audiovisual demonstration of changes in bodily function. EMG audiovisual feedback techniques (EMGAVF) have been widely used to improve motor performance in normal subjects and in patients with a variety of neurological disorders (4, 7, 65–67). The rationale for using EMGAVF is that while receiving instantaneous information from their muscles, individuals can be trained to improve motor performance in a relatively short time with the hope that eventually such control can be achieved without continued use of instrumentation. In patients who develop spasticity due to partial lesions of the spinal cord, EMGAVF is used (7) to: (a) improve strength in weak muscles; (b) relax overactive spastic muscles; and (c) improve coordination of movement.

ORTHOPEDIC MANAGEMENT

Orthopaedic surgeons have operated on peripheral structures (muscle transplantations, tenotomies, myotomies, partial or complete resection of peripheral nerves, and osteotomies) for the treatment of spasticity for many years. Both orthopaedic and neurosurgical procedures, however, are less likely to be necessary if the patient receives early preventive treatment in a spinal cord injury center. Surgical procedures on peripheral structures must be given preference over destructive operations on the spinal cord, especially in patients with incomplete lesions who have satisfactory bladder and sexual function (23). The choice of surgical procedure depends upon the type and degree of spasticity and which specific muscle groups are affected. In some patients who have had severe spasticity and contractures for a long time, it may be necessary to use two or more procedures to achieve the desired results. It has been found (as noted above) that, in addition to correcting contractures and reducing spasticity locally, surgery can at times have general beneficial effects, reducing spasticity beyond the local site. In order for every surgical procedure to be successful it must be followed by carefully planned conservative treatment. Some of the common orthopaedic procedures used in patients with spasticity due to spinal cord injury are described below.

Relief of Spasticity by Chemical Interruption of the Reflex Arc

In a few patients who have severe debilitating illness or who have severe contactures and decubitus ulcers, intensive medical and nursing programs may not be sufficient to reduce their spasticity. In these cases it may be necessary to perform selective motor point or peripheral nerve blocks (2, 28, 32). Before injecting a neurolytic agent, such as alcohol or phenol, it is necessary to evaluate the usefulness of selective blocks by observing the effects of injecting local anesthetic (e.g., procaine) into the appropriate region. If local anesthesia produces useful, albeit temporary, relief of spasticity, longer lasting neurolytic agents such as 3%, 5%, or 10% phenol in water or absolute alcohol may be injected. Following the use of these agents, beneficial effects can last for months. Blocking of cutaneous nerves leading from areas with decubitus ulcers may also be of considerable value. For example, blocking the sural nerve at midcalf and blocking the lateral femoral cutaneous nerve in the thigh near the anterior superior iliac spine produce marked reduction of tone and flexor deformities in the lower limbs. Phenol or alcohol block of the obturator nerve can produce significant reduction in adductor spasms facilitating bowel and bladder training. If one particular muscle is in spasm, local injection of phenol into its motor point may be useful.

Tenotomies

Tenotomies are indicated when patients develop contractures of leg muscles due to improper preventive management, especially faulty positioning, during the stage of spinal shock. In long-standing cases, both flexor and extensor tendons of the toes may need open division (54). When plantar flexion synergy is combined with inversion of the foot, it is important to combine tenotomy of the tibialis posterior muscle at the ankle with plantar flexor tenotomy. Knee flexion contractures may require open tenotomies of medial and lateral flexors of the knee joint. This procedure is sometimes combined with a capsulotomy and division of heads of the gastrocnemius muscle in order to obtain full extension at the knee joint. Occasionally medial and lateral knee ligaments and their bursae have to be dissected free in order to relieve the contracture. Adductor tenotomy should never be performed because results are only partially successful. Moreover, incisions for adductor tenotomy are so situated that sweating favors infection that may delay the healing process.

Lengthening of Tendons

Achilles tendon lengthening is one of the most useful and widely performed surgical procedures for treatment of spasticity. It is a safe surgical procedure that produces long-term benefits. In patients with spinal spasticity, lengthening of the Achilles tendon is indicated if its shortened state acts as a trigger point for generalized spasticity or results in a localized spastic pes equinus deformity. Operation on one side may produce beneficial effects beyond the local site, with relief of spasticity at the contralateral ankle joint and the knee and hip joints bilaterally. In patients in whom both ankles are equally affected, lengthening operations can be performed on both sides under the same anesthetic. At least 6 weeks or 2 months must elapse before one can recognize long-term beneficial effects of surgery and determine postsurgical treatment. After the surgical procedure there may be an increase in the degree of spasticity for a few days, followed by permanent correction of the localized deformity at the ankle and reduction in generalized spasticity. Postoperative care with splints requires careful daily attention in order to prevent pressure sores. When the patient is allowed to stand up and walk, he is taught to put full weight on the entire plantar surface of the foot.

When an equinus deformity of the foot is combined with fixed supination and pronation deformities, it is necessary to perform appropriate tenotomies in addition to heel cord lengthening. Elongation of the biceps femoris tendon, with resection of the inner hamstrings, is occasionally performed in some patients in whom flexion contractures at the knee act as trigger points for severe flexor spasms.

Myotomy

One of the most disabling and incapacitating features of heightened flexor reflex synergy is violent hip flexor spasms. This results in hip flexion contractures if this synergy is not treated from the beginning. For patients with established flexion contractures of the hip, myotomies are preferred to tenotomies, which produce only partial and temporary effects. Some degree of hip flexion can be preserved if the long head of the biceps is retained. Beneficial effects of iliopsoas myotomy last for a number of years (54, 52, 53). Whenever bilateral myotomies are performed for hip flexion contractures, these can be combined with obturator neurectomies if the patient suffers from both hip flexion and adductor spasms or contractures.

Neurectomy

Obturator neurectomy, like lengthening of Achilles tendons, is one of the most commonly used surgical procedures for the treatment of spinal spasticity. Some patients develop severe adductor spasms, sometimes with crossing of legs, that do not respond to conservative therapy. In these patients, obturatory neurectomy has resulted in relief not only of adductor spasm but also of generalized spasticity. A subinguinal approach (10) should not be used because it is only partially effective and the incision lies in a sweaty areas with accompanying risks of infection (54). The intrapelvic, extraperitoneal abdominal approach of Selig (64) is the most reliable method for resection of the obturator nerve. This method gives a good exposure of the nerve, even when it is enclosed in adhesions. Postoperatively the leg should be placed in only slight abduction because wide abduction may result in abduction contracture due to unopposed action of the gluteus medius muscle. In patients who have both severe adductor spasm and hip flexion contractures, obturator neurectomy and iliopsoas myotomy can be performed through the same incision.

Other neurectomies (sciatic, femoral, external popliteal) have been performed but are not as widely accepted for the treatment of spasticity as is obturator neurectomy.

Tendon Transplantations

Tendon transplantations have occasionally been used for the treatment of pes equinus varus and severe equinovalgus. Part or all of the tendon of the tibialis anterior muscle or peroneal muscles are transferred to the extensor digitorum depending upon the type of deformity. With improved conservative management, these procedures are rarely used.

REFERENCES

1. Andreassen, S., and Rosenfalck, A. Regulation of the firing pattern of single motor units. *J. Neurol. Neurosurg. Psychiatry,* 43:897–906, 1980.
2. Avad, E. A. Phenol block for control of hip flexor and adductor spasticity. *Arch. Phys. Med.,* 53:554–557, 1972.
3. Basbaum, A. I., and Fields, H. L. Endogenous pain control systems. *Annu. Rev. Neurosci.,* 7:309–338, 1984.
4. Basmajian, J. V., Kukulka, C. G., Narayan, M. G., and Takebe, K. Biofeedback treatment of foot-drop after stroke compared with standard rehabilitation techniques: effects on voluntary control and strength. *Arch. Phys. Med. Rehabil.,* 56:231–236, 1975.
5. Benecke, R., Conrad, B., Meinck, H. M., and Hoehne, J. Electromyographic analysis of bicycling on an ergometer for evaluation of spasticity of lower limbs in man. In: *Motor*

Control Mechanisms in Health and Disease. Edited by Desmedt, J. E. Raven Press, New York, 1983, pp. 1035–1046.

6. Bjorklund, A., and Stenevi, U. Intracerebral neural implants. *Annu. Rev. Neurosci.*, 7:279–308, 1984.

7. Brudney, J., Korein, J., Grynbaum, B., Friedmann, L., Weinstein, S., Sachs-Frankel, G., and Belandres, P. EMG feedback therapy: review of treatment of 114 patients. *Arch. Phys. Med. Rehabil.*, 57:55–61, 1976.

8. Burke, D. Critical examination of the case for or against fusimotor involvement in disorders of muscle tone. In: *Motor Control Mechanisms in Health and Disease.* Edited by Desmedt, J. E. Raven Press, New York, 1983, pp. 133–150.

9. Cheney, P. D., and Fetz, E. E. Corticomotoneuronal cells contribute to long-latency stretch reflexes in the rhesus monkey. *J. Physiol.*, 349:249–272, 1984.

10. Comarr, A. E. Peripheral oeprations for relief of spasticity and/or contracture in patients with spinal cord injuries, a preliminary report. In: *Proceedings 9th Annual Spinal Cord Injury Conference.* United States Veterans Administration, Long Beach, California, 1960, pp. 91–103.

11. Conrad, B., Benecke, R., and Meinck, H. M. Gait disturbances in paraspastic patients. In: *Clinical Neurophysiology in Spasticity.* Edited by Delwaide, P. J., and Young, R. R. Elsevier, Amsterdam, 1985, pp. 155–174.

12. Crenna, P., and Frigo, C. Monitoring gait by a vector diagram technique in spastic patients. In: *Clinical Neurophysiology in Spasticity.* Edited by Delwaide, P. J., and Young, R. R. Elsevier, Amsterdam, 1985, pp. 109–124.

13. Crone, C., and Hultborn, H. Spinal pathophysiology of spasticity. In: *Actual Problems in Multiple Sclerosis Research.* Edited by Pedersen, E., Clausen, J., and Oades, L. FADL's Forlag, Copenhagen, 1983, pp. 87–95.

14. Crone, C., Hultborn, H., Malmsten, J., and Mazieres, L. Tonic stretch reflexes and their dependence on polysynaptic excitation from muscle spindle Ia afferents. In: *Actual Problems In Multiple Sclerosis Research.* Edited by Pedersen, E., Clausen, J., and Oades, L. FADL's Forlag, Copenhagen, 1983, pp. 99–102.

15. Davis, R. D. Spasticity following spinal cord injury. In: *Clinical Orthopaedics and Related Research.* Edited by Urist, M. Lippincott, Philadelphia, 1975, pp. 66–75.

16. Delwaide, P. J. Human monosynaptic reflexes and presynaptic inhibition. In *New Developments in Electromyography and Clinical Neurophysiology*, vol. 3. Edited by Desmedt, J. E. Karger, Basel, 1973, pp. 508–522.

17. Delwaide, P. J. Electrophysiological testing of spastic patients: its potential usefulness and limitations. In: *Clinical Neurophysiology in Spasticity.* Edited by Delwaide, P. J., and Young, R. R. Elsevier, Amsterdam, 1985, pp. 185–204.

18. Delwaide, P. J., Martinelli, P., and Crenna, P. Clinical neurophysiological measurement of spinal reflex activity. In: *Spasticity: Disordered Motor Control.* Edited by Feldman, R. G., Young, R. R., and Koella, W. P. Yearbook Medical Publishers, Chicago, 1980.

19. Dietz, V., and Berger, W. Normal and impaired regulation of muscle stiffness in gait: a new hypothesis about muscle hypertonia. *Exp. Neurol.*, 79:680–687, 1983.

20. Dietz, V., Quintern, J., and Berger, W. Electrophysiological studies of gait in spasticity and rigidity. Evidence that altered mechanical properties of muscle contribute to hypertonia. *Brain*, 104:431–449, 1981.

21. Duncan, G. W., Shahani, B. T., and Young, R. R. An evaluation of baclofen treatment for certain symptoms in patients with spinal cord lesions. *Neurology*, 26:441–446, 1976.

22. Gonsette, R. E., and Demonty, L. Clinical experience with a new antispastic agent (tizanidine) in 152 multiple sclerosis patients. In: *Actual Problems in Multiple Sclerosis Research.* Edited by Pederson, E., Clausen, J., and Oades, L. FADL's Forlag, Copenhagen, 1983, pp. 123–127.

23. Gutmann, L. *Spinal Cord Injuries. Comprehensive Management and Research.* Blackwell, Oxford, 1976, pp. 543–557.

24. Hagbarth, K. E., and Eklund, G. Motor effects of vibratory muscle stimuli in man. In:

Muscular Afferents and Motor Control. Edited by Granit, R. Wiley, New York, 1966, pp. 177–186.

25. Hagbarth, K. E., and Finer, B. The plasticity of human withdrawal reflexes to noxious skin stimuli in lower limbs. *Prog. Brain Res., 1:*65–78, 1963.

26. Hagbarth, K. E., Hagglund, J. V., Wallin, E. U., and Young, R. R. Grouped spindle and electromyographic responses to abrupt wrist extensor movement in man. *J. Physiol., 312:*81–96, 1981.

27. Hagbarth, K. E., Young, R. R., Hagglund, J. V., and Wallin, E. U. Segmentation of human spindle and EMG responses to sudden muscle stretch. *Neurosci. Lett., 19:*213–217, 1980.

28. Halpren, D., and Meelhuysen, F. E. Phenol motor point block in management of muscular hypertonia. *Arch. Phys. Med., 47:*659, 1966.

29. Hartviksen, K. Ice therapy in spasticity. *Acta. Neurol. Scand. (Suppl. 3), 8:*79, 1962.

30. Hultborn, H., and Malmsten, J. Changes in segmental reflex transmission following chronic spinal hemisection in the cat and the rat. In: *Actual Problems in Multiple Sclerosis Research.* Edited by Pedersen, E., Clausen, J., and Oades, L. FADL's Forlag, Copenhagen, 1983, pp. 96–98.

30a. Kasdon, D. L., and Lathi, E. S. A prospective study of radiofrequency rhizotomy in the treatment of posttraumatic spasticity. *Neurosurgery, 15:*526–529, 1984.

31. Katz, R., and Pierrot-Deseilligny, E. Recurrent inhibition of alpha-motoneurons in patients with upper motor neuron lesions. *Brain, 105:*103–124, 1982.

32. Khalili, A. A., Harmel, M. H., Forster, S., and Benton, J. G. Management of spasticity by selective peripheral nerve block with dilute phenol solutions in clinical rehabilitation. *Arch. Phys. Med., 45:*513, 1964.

33. Knutsson, E. Studies of gait control in patients with spastic paresis. In: *Clinical Neurophysiology in Spasticity.* Edited by Delwaide, P. J., and Young, R. R. Elsevier, Amsterdam, 1985, pp. 175–184.

34. Knuttsson, E., and Martensson, A. Dynamic motor capacity in spastic paresis and its relation to prime mover dysfunction, spastic restraint and antagonist co-activation. *Scand. J. Rehabil. Med., 12:*93–106, 1980.

35. Knuttson, E., and Richards, C. Different types of disturbed motor control in gait of hemiparetic patients. *Brain, 102:*405–430, 1979.

36. Kralj, A., Bajd, T., Turk, J., and Benko, H. Gait restoration in paraplegic patients: A feasibility demonstration using multichannel surface electrode FES. *J. Rehabil. R. D., 20:*3–20, 1983.

37. Kuypers, H. G. J. M. Anatomy of the decending pathways. In: *Handbook of Physiology, Section 1: The Nervous System, Vol. II Motor Control.* Edited by Brooks, V. B. American Physiological Society, Bethesda, Maryland, 1981, pp. 597–666.

38. Lance, J. W. Symposium synopsis. In: *Spasticity: Disordered Motor Control.* Edited by Feldman, R. G., Young, R. R., and Koella, W. P. Yearbook Medical Publishers, Chicago, 1980, pp. 485–494.

39. Lance, J. W,, and deGail, P. Spread of phasic muscle reflexes in normal and spastic subjects. *J. Neurol. Neurosurg. Psychiatry, 28:*328–334, 1965.

40. Lataste, X., and Coward, D. Selective mode of action of tizanidine. In: *Actual Problems in Multiple Sclerosis Research.* Edited by Pedersen, E., Clausen, J., and Oades, L. FADL's Forlag, Copenhagen, 1983, pp. 121–122.

41. Lee, R. G, Rohs, G. L., and White, D. G. Long latency EMG responses to load perturbations in hemiplegic patients. *Can. J. Neurol. Sci., 6:*384, 1979.

42. Lee, R. G., and Tatton, W. G. Motor responses to sudden limb displacements in primates with specific CNS lesions and in human patients with motor system disorders. *Can. J. Neurol. Sci., 2:*285–293, 1974.

43. Lee, W. J., McGovern, J. P., and Duvall, E. N. Continuous tetanizing (low voltage) currents for relief of spasm. A clinical study of twenty-seven spinal cord injury patients. *Arch. Phys. Med., 31:*366–771, 1950.

44. Lehmann, J. F. Ultrasound therapy. In: *Therapeutic Heat and Cold.* Edited by Licht, S.

Waverly Press, Baltimore, 1965, pp. 321–386.

45. Licht, S. Local cryotherapy. In: *Therapeutic Heat and Cold.* Edited by Licht, S. Waverly Press, Baltimore, 1965, pp. 538–563.

46. Mai, J. Depression of spasticity by alpha-adrenergic blockade. *Acta Neurol. Scand., 57:*65–76, 1978.

47. Marsden, C. D., Merton, P.A., and Morton, H. B. Is the human stretch reflex cortical rather than spinal? *Lancet, 1:*759–761, 1973.

48. Marsden, C. D., Merton, P. A., and Morton, H. B. Stretch and servo action in a variety of human muscles. *J. Physiol., 259:*531–560, 1976.

49. Mayer, R. F., Burke, R. E., Toop, J., Walmsley, B., and Hodgson, J. A. The effect of spinal cord transection on motor units in cat medial gastrocnemius muscles. *Muscle Nerve, 7:*23–31, 1984.

50. McLellan, D. L. Co-contraction and stretch reflexes in spasticity during treatment with baclofen. *J. Neurol. Neurosurg. Psychiatry, 40:*30–38, 1977.

51. Melzack, R., and Wall, P. D. Pain mechanisms: A new theory. *Science, 150:*971–979, 1965.

52. Michaelis, L. S. Myotomy of iliopsoas and obliquus externus abdominis for severe spastic flexion contracture at the hip. *Paraplegia, 2:*287–294, 1964.

53. Michaelis, L. S. Neurological terminology, prognosis and classification of para- and tetraplegia. In: *Proceedings 17th Annual Spinal Cord Injury Conference.* Veterans Administration, Washington, D.C., 1969, U.S. Government Printing Office.

54. Michaelis, L. S. Spasticity in spinal cord injuries. In: *Handbook of Clinical Neurology, Injuries of the Spine and Cord, Vol. 26, Part II.* Edited by Vinken, P. J., and Bruyn, G. W. Elsevier, New York, 1976, pp. 477–487, 1976.

55. Miglietta, O. E. Evaluation of cold in spasticity. *Am. J. Phys. Med., 41:*148, 1962.

56. Miglietta, O. E. Electromyographic characteristics of clonus and influence of cold. *Arch. Phys. Med., 45:*508, 1964.

57. Mondrup, K., and Pedersen, E. The acute effect of THIP in human spasticity—A pilot study. In: *Actual Problems in Multiple Sclerosis Research.* Edited by Pederson, E., Clausen, J., and Oades, L. FADL's Forlag, Copenhagen, 1983, pp. 132–134.

58. Phillips, C. G. Motor apparatus of the baboon's hand. *Proc. Roy. Soc. [B.], 173:*141–174, 1969.

59. Phillips, C. G., Powell, T. P. S., and Wiesendanger, M. Projection from low-threshold muscle afferents of hand and forearm to area 3a of baboon's cortex. *J. Physiol., 217:*419–446, 1971.

60. Pierrot-Deseilligny, E., and Mazieres, L. Spinal mechanisms underlying spasticity. In: *Clinical Neurophysiology in Spasticity.* Edited by Delwaide, P. J., and Young, R. R. Elsevier, Amsterdam, 1985, pp. 63–76.

61. Potts, F. A., and Young, R. R. Long-term post-stimulus reduction in axon excitability when tested with submaximal electrical stimulus in vivo or vitro. *Soc. Neurosci. Abstr., 78:*188, 1981.

62. Rossier, A. B, Bussat, P. H., Infante, F., Zender, R., Courvoisier, B., Mutheim, G., Donath, A., Vasey, H., Taillard, W., Lagier, R., Gabbiani, G., Baud, C. A., Pauezat, J. A., Very, J. M., and Hachen, H. J. Current facts on para-osteo-arthropathy (POA). *Parapelgia, 11:*36–78, 1973.

63. Rymer, W. Z., Houk, J. C., and Crago, P. E. Mechanisms of the clasp-knife reflex studied in an animal model. *Exp. Brain Res., 37:*93–113, 1979.

64. Selig, R. C. Die intrapelvine extraperitoneale Resektion des Nervus obturatorius und anatomische Studien uber die Topographie dieses Nerven. *Arch. f. Klin. Chir. (Berl.), 103:*994–1011, 1914.

65. Shahani, B. T. Control of voluntary activity in man and physiological principles of biofeedback. In: *Electromyography in CNS Disorders: Central EMG.* Edited by Shahani, B. T. Butterworth, Boston, 1984, pp. 161–175.

66. Shahani, B. T., Connors, L., and Mohr, J. P. Electromyographic audiovisual training effect in the motor performance in patients with lesions of the central nervous system. *Arch. Phys. Med. Rehabil.*, 58:519, 1977.

67. Shahani, B. T., Newfeld, S., and Peteet, J. Effects of training with EMG audiovisual feedback (EMG AVF) on proximal musculature in patients with lesions of the central nervous system (CNS). In: *Programme of the Annual Scientific Meeting of the American Academy of Physical Medicine and Rehabilitation.* Honolulu, 1979.

68. Shahani, B. T., and Young, R. R. Human flexor reflexes. *J. Neurol. Neurosurg. Psychiatry*, 34:616–627, 1971.

69. Shahani, B. T., and Young, R. R. The flexor reflex in spasticity. In: *Spasticity: Disordered Motor Control.* Edited by Feldman, R. G., Young, R. R., and Koella, W. P. Yearbook Medical Publishers, Chicago, 1980, pp. 287–295.

70. Stillwell, D. M., and Gersten, J. W. Effect of ultrasound on spasticity. *American Institute of Ultrasound in Medicine, Proceedings of 4th Annual Conference on Ultrasonic Therapy.* Detroit, 1955, pp. 124–131.

71. Struppler, A., Ochs, G., Burgmayer, B., and Pfeiffer, H. G. The therapeutic use of epidural opioids in flexor reflex spasm. *Electroencephalogr. Clin. Neurophysiol.*, 56:S178, 1983.

72. Toerring, J., Hansen, P. H., Klemar, B., and Pedersen, E. Effect of tizanidine on proprioceptive and flexor reflexes in spastic patients. In: *Actual Problems in Multiple Sclerosis Research.* Edited by Pederson, E., Clausen, J., and Oades, L. FADL's Forlag, Copenhagen, 1983, pp. 128–129.

73. Vallbo, A. B., Hagbarth, K. E., Torebjork, H. E., and Wallin, B. G. Somatosensory, proprioceptive and sympathetic activity in human peripheral nerves. *Physiol. Rev.*, 59:919–957, 1979.

74. Vogel, M., Weinstein, L., and Abramson, A. S. Use of tetanizing current for spasticity. *Phys. Ther. Rev.*, 35:435–437, 1955.

75. Wallin, B. G., and Stjernberg, A. Sympathetic activity in man after spinal cord injury. *Brain*, 107:183–198, 1984.

76. Wallin, G. Intraneural recording and autonomic function in man. In: *Autonomic Failure.* Edited by Bannister, R. Oxford University Press, Oxford, 1983, pp. 36–51.

77. Yanagisawa, N., Tanaka, R., and Ito, Z. Reciprocal Ia inhibition in spastic hemiplegia in man. *Brain*, 99:555–574, 1976.

78. Young, J. L., and Mayer, R. F. Physiological alterations of motor units in hemiplegia. *J. Neurol. Sci.*, 54:401–412, 1982.

79. Young, R. R. The clinical significance of exteroceptive reflexes. In: *New Developments in Electromyography and Clinical Neurophysiology.* Edited by Desmedt, J. E. Karger, Basel, 1973, pp. 697–712.

80. Young, R. R., and Delwaide, P. J. Drug therapy-spasticity. *New Engl. J. Med.*, 304:28–33, 96–99, 1981.

81. Young, R. R., and Henneman, E. Functional effects of focused ultrasound on mammalian nerves. *Science*, 134:1521–1522, 1961.

82. Young, R. R., and Shahani, B. T. A clinical neurophysiological analysis of single motor unit discharge patterns in spasticity. In: *Spasticity: Disordered Motor Control.* Edited by Feldman, R. G., Young, R. R., and Koella, W. P. Yearbook Medical Publishers, Chicago, 1980, pp. 219–231.

83. Young, R. R., and Wierzbicka, M. M. Behavior of single motor units in normal subjects and in patients with spastic paresis. In: *Clinical Neurophysiology in Spasticity.* Edited by Delwaide, P. J., and Young, R. R. Elsevier, Amsterdam, 1985, pp. 27–40.

11

Heterotopic Ossification After Spinal Cord Injury

SAMUEL L. STOVER

The term *heterotopic ossification* is used to describe the formation of bone in abnormal anatomic locations, usually soft tissues. This extraskeletal bone has been described in almost every organ system of the body and appears to have many inciting causes (3).

Because of the diversity of medical diagnoses with which ossification in soft tissues occurs, attempts at classification are numerous and often exclusive. A simple classification of such ossification is probably the best: (a) progressive, and (b) nonprogressive self-limiting. The only truly progressive form is known as myositis ossificans progressiva, which is a congenital form first appearing in early childhood and frequently progressing to severe immobility by adulthood. The nonprogressive self-limiting forms of heterotopic ossification usually occur secondary to another diagnosis and have associated pathological changes that seem to initiate the formation of bone (3). In a few instances, however, the bone formation is spontaneous and occurs in otherwise healthy individuals (40, 47).

Nonprogressive heterotopic ossification occurs most commonly following severe neurological injury and is especially common following spinal cord injury. This soft tissue bone formation in spinal cord injury patients has been referred to by many names: ectopic ossification, ectopic bone, ectopic calcification, paraarticular calcification, periarticular ossification, dystrophic ossification, neurogenic ossifying fibromyopathy, myositis ossificans, myositis ossificans circumscripta, and paraosteoarthropathy (POA), the term that is used frequently in the European literature. Although it has been referred to as calcification, it is actually distinguishable from soft tissue calcification by the fact that there is true osteoblastic activity with bone formation rather than simply a deposition of amorphous calcium phosphate into the tissues.

Dejerine, a French neurologist, is generally credited with the first descriptive account of heterotopic ossification in spinal cord injury patients in

1918 (9). Soft tissue ossification had been recognized in certain other medical conditions centuries earlier, although Dejerine and his coauthors proposed that metaplasia of connective tissue secondary to hemorrhage and edema may be the cause of this soft tissue bone formation. In 1926 Leriche and Policard (34) suggested that mature connective tissue may be transformed into primitive cells as a result of trauma or infection, and this damaged tissue eventually ossifies. In a radiological report in 1941 Brailsford (6) reported that traumatic stripping of the periosteum at the site of muscular attachments may cause heterotopic ossification in patients with disease or injury of the central nervous system. In 1945 Soule (50) proposed that unrecognized trauma to soft tissues led to hemorrhage in the tissues with subsequent ossification. Hardy and Dickson studied this problem and in 1963 reported the occurrence of soft tissue ossification in three groups of patients with paraplegia: (a) no known associated factors except the possibility of fractures; (b) in association with skin and joint sepsis; and (c) in areas of pressure ulcers (22). They did not think there was any relationship between trauma and eventual ossification.

The etiology of heterotopic ossification remains unknown. Similarly, there is no uniform agreement about its pathogenesis. Diathesis or metaplasia of bone marrow-derived cells or local mesenchymal and endothelial cells in the intramuscular connective tisue are most commonly accepted (41). Primitive or embryonic mesenchymal cells, which are known to be present in connective tissue, appear to be stimulated by some as yet unknown factor. Two recently identified proteins may eventually give some insight into this bone formation. The first is bone morphogenetic protein (BMP), which has a primary function of inducing bone cell differentiation. When implanted into muscle tissue, BMP induces perivascular connective tissue and other unspecialized cells to become bone-forming cells (35). The second protein is called human skeletal growth factor (hSGF), which regulates the total number of bone cells produced (10). The actual inducing agent of these cellular changes that lead to osteogenesis remains unknown. Some investigators feel these unknown inducing agents are influenced by genetic factors, and studies of human leukocyte antigens (HLA) have suggested positive correlations with HLA-B 18 (37) and HLA-B 27 (33). Others, however, do not find any significant differences of HLA when patients with heterotopic ossification are compared to healthy, matched controls (59). Since heterotopic ossification is common in conditions with neurological impairments, neurological and bioelectric factors have also been implicated.

The reported incidence of heterotopic ossification following spinal cord injury ranges from 16% to 53% (58). For unknown reasons, there appear to be geographical differences in the incidence; even within a geographic area there may be cyclic changes, where the incidence may be greater some years than others. In many spinal cord injury patients the extent of heterotopic ossification is minimal and is only an incidental x-ray finding. However, in 18% to 37% of those patients who develop heterotopic ossification, the extent of ossification is of such a magnitude that limitation of joint mobility occurs, resulting in joint ankylosis in the more severe cases (32, 60, 61).

Heterotopic ossification always develops below the neurological level of spinal cord injury. While most common about the hips, it also occurs fairly frequently about the knees (5, 32, 51, 60) (Fig. 11.1). Heterotopic lesions occur less frequently about the shoulders, elbows, paravertebral area, along the length of the femurs, and very rarely in the hands and feet. If not present about the hips, it is only rarely observed at other joints or locations. Several specific anatomic locations are especially predisposed to the development of heterotopic ossification. These include the adductor, flexor and abductor areas of the hips, and along the medial collateral ligaments of the knees. It is found less frequently in patients with incomplete neurological injuries than in patients with complete lesions (32). It occurs equally on the right and left sides. There is little difference in the incidence in men or women. It is very rare in children with spinal cord injury. Persons with associated long bone fractures do not appear to have any higher incidence of heterotopic ossification.

The onset of heterotopic ossification is most frequently observed between

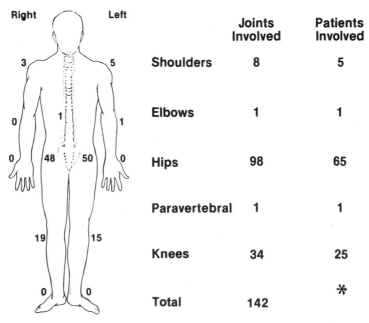

	Joints Involved	Patients Involved
Shoulders	8	5
Elbows	1	1
Hips	98	65
Paravertebral	1	1
Knees	34	25
		*
Total	142	

Figure 11.1. Location and incidence of heterotopic ossification found in 77 patients by prospective x-ray survey of 250 spinal cord injury patients. The total number of patients is more than 77 because some patients have multiple joint involvement.

1 and 4 months after injury. It has been reported to be evident on x-ray as early as 19 days following trauma (22). With newer diagnostic techniques such as the three phase radioisotope bone scan, it is suggested that the actual onset may even occur earlier (19). Heterotopic ossification rarely occurs more than 1 year after injury unless there are other, unusual inciting factors that are described later.

In some patients who develop minimal heterotopic ossification, there are no clinical signs or symptoms. The condition is discovered by x-ray, and it has no further clinical significance. Patients who develop more extensive heterotopic lesions may clinically present with all the signs and symptoms of a localized inflammatory reaction of the involved area. In these patients, the area may have soft tissue swelling, heat, and erythema; a systemic febrile reaction may also be present. Heterotopic ossification must be suspected in any patient with fever of undetermined origin (FUO), even if other clinical signs are not yet evident. Low grade fever in the more extensive cases may persist for a couple of weeks. When an acute heterotopic lesion develops about the hips or knees, it is often difficult to clinically distinguish from thrombophlebitis. Hydroarthrosis of the knee may also be present if heterotopic ossification is forming at either the hip and/or the knee, but this occurs with thrombophlebitis also. When acute heterotopic ossification develops about the hips, the swelling is often greater in the proximal extremity compared to the distal extremity. After a day or two, the swelling becomes firmer and more indurated in the local area where bone is forming in comparison to the swelling typically associated with thrombophlebitis. Several days later, a rather firm mass may be felt in the subcutaneous tissues, which gradually becomes more demarcated from the surrounding tissues. Within a week, the mass has a bony consistency and there is usually a progressive loss of range of motion of the affected joints.

Radiographic evidence of heterotopic ossification is often absent for 1 to 2 weeks after clinical signs appear (5, 19, 56). Radioisotope bone scans, however, may be diagnostic as soon as clinical signs are evident (43) (Fig. 11.2), or may even precede clinical signs by as long as 6 weeks (19, 55). The three-phase bone scan can be useful in early detection of heterotopic ossification. An increase of radioisotope uptake during the first minute after injection is known as phase I, or the blood-flow study phase. In heterotopic ossification studies, it is known also as the early vascular proliferative or precursor phase. Phase II is observed 2 minutes after injection and is known as the blood pool or osteoid phase, and phase III is observed 2 hours after injection and recognized as the active bone or bone-seeking radioisotope phase. Repeating the three-phase bone scans at 2 week intervals shows a progression of these phases as heterotopic ossification develops (19). When using Gallium-67 scans to search for a cause of fever of undetermined origin in the absence of clinical signs, positive results are sometimes reported as heterotopic ossification develops (55). Angiography may also demonstrate

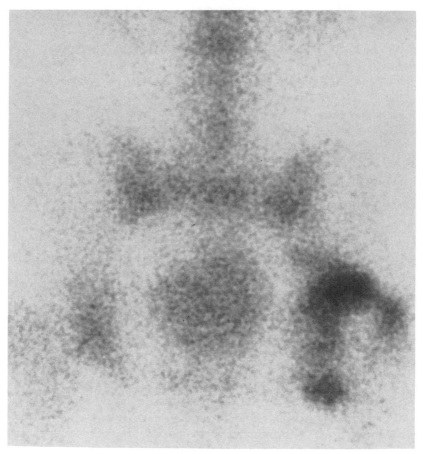

Figure 11.2. Radioisotope bone scan shows increased uptake in left hip area.

hypervascularity, increased arterial diameter, and early venous return (45). Serial alkaline phosphatase determinations may be helpful (39), but neither a normal nor an abnormal level of alkaline phosphatase is diagnostic (45). Elevated levels are suggestive of active bone formation, but, it must be remembered that associated healing fractures may also cause an elevation of the serum alkaline phosphatase. The level of alkaline phosphatase does not necessarily reflect the severity or extent of the heterotopic ossification lesion being formed. Serum calcium levels are usually normal following spinal cord injury.

When an inflammatory reaction is noted, the differential diagnosis must include thrombophlebitis, cellulitis, periostitis, sepsis of the joint, hematoma, localized trauma, and fracture. Although venograms, plethysmography, and I-125 labeled fibrinogen scans may be helpful in differentiating thrombophlebitis from heterotopic ossification, it is now recognized that as many as 78% (20) of all spinal cord injury patients with complete neurological lesions develop some degree of thrombophlebitis; therefore, the presence of thrombophlebitis does not rule out the possibility of coexistent heterotopic ossification. The bone scan then becomes the most important test for an accurate differential diagnosis. Biopsies are rarely needed for differential diagnosis following spinal cord injury. It has even been suggested that the performance of biopsies before lesions are mature may lead to stimulation and formation of increased bone (3). Because of the variation of cellular activity within the bony mass, biopsy samples must be of sufficient size to make an accurate diagnosis. When heterotopic ossification has a very late onset and an inciting cause is not apparent, a biopsy may be much more important to rule out bone malignancy, which is another diagnosis that must be included in the differential diagnosis of patients who do not have spinal cord injury and develop soft tissue ossification.

About 7 to 10 days after the appearance of clinical signs, x-rays begin to show a flocculent, patchy appearance as an increased amount of amorphous calcium phosphate is deposited. The acute inflammatory reaction appears to predispose the involved tissues to imminent calcification followed by ossification, which then proceeds more slowly, giving the appearance of coalescence and enlargement on x-ray. During the next 2 to 3 months, bone boundaries become more distinct, and with further time, immature bone is replaced by more mature-appearing bone on x-ray (Fig. 11.3).

The increase of ossification tends to give the appearance of gradual

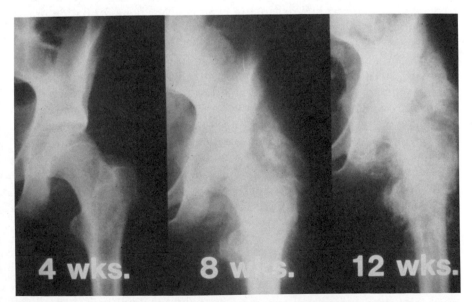

Figure 11.3. X-ray signs of heterotopic ossification development, with minimal evidence just medial to the head of the femur 4 weeks postinjury, progressing with increased size, more distinct bone boundaries, and more mature appearing bone by 12 weeks postinjury.

progression of the pathological process. It is believed, however, that the inflammatory process is a rather sudden event with ossification of the inflammatory mass taking place as a gradual process. The bone matures most rapidly along the outer aspects of the bony mass, with multiple foci of osteogenesis being formed throughout the heterotopic bone (22, 45).

Anatomically, the heterotopic lesion is extraarticular, but it may be firmly attached to the joint capsule or aponeurosis. At times, the heterotopic mass is attached to the cortex of adjacent bone with or without disruption of that cortex. The bone mass lies outside the tendons and muscles, which are usually well preserved; however, atrophic muscle fibers occasionally become incorporated into the heterotopic bone mass (45).

Microscopically, the immature inflammatory mass consists of a highly cellular, pleomorphic stroma, including fibroblasts, ground substance, and collagen fibers (1). Hypervascularity is abundant where centers of ossification develop. Except for lymphocytes, there is relatively little inflammatory infiltration (45). Eventually, hyperchromatic osteoblasts become irregularly placed in the crude osteoid. The newly formed bone consists of woven trabeculae that are undergoing osteoclastic erosion. An undifferentiated inner zone is surrounded by an outer layer of well-differentiated bone, suggesting a neoplastic-like appearance. Immature edematous fibroblastic connective tissue without inflammatory infiltration sometimes surrounds the heterotopic mass. At the periphery, atrophic muscle fibers are sometimes found undergoing lysis (22, 45). Amorphous calcium phosphate is replaced gradually by enlarging hydroxyapatite crystals. New bone formation arises multicentrically in the immature fibrous tissue with areas of mature bone intermixed with areas of immature bone. Approximately 6 months after onset, the heterotopic lesion begins to evolve into bona fide bone, complete with trabeculae, marrow, and lamellar arrangements around abundant vascular channels. The glycosaminoglycan content is similar to normal compact bone (49). Adipose tissue, however, is increased in the bone marrow spaces, and hematopoesis is virtually absent. This bone has been described as corticospongiosal bone of lamellar structure, with occasional haversian systems. The structural features are similar to all nontumoral new bone formation, such as fracture callus, which distinguish it from normal bone (45). During the first 18 months after the appearance of the heterotopic lesion, there is a progressive increase in the amount of mineralization. The degree of mineralization approaches that of mature, adult bone 24 to 36 months after its first appearance.

Once the heterotopic ossification mass is fairly well-delineated by x-ray examination several months after the onset, further increases in the size of the bony mass or evidence of onset at other sites of the body are rare. However, certain precipitating factors occasionally do induce increased bone growth or new foci of heterotopic ossification many months or even years after a spinal cord injury in persons with or without previous heterotopic ossification. Factors that have been observed to induce the late onset of heterotopic ossification include: severe systemic type of illness, hepatic trauma with hepatic failure, surgery in the immediate area of new bone formation or even at a distant location, and infection. A septic hip joint will often induce new heterotopic ossification in the infected hip area. A trochanteric bursitis of one hip has been associated with induced heterotopic ossification formation along the femur of the opposite leg. Pressure ulcers that extend to the bone may induce additional bone formation, which has an irregular appearance of bone destruction and new bony spur-like formation. Although it is sometimes treated as chronic osteomyelitis, this diagnosis seems doubtful since pressure ulcers heal over these bony irregularities without prolonged antibiotic treatment. Rotational skin flap surgery is also often successful over these areas with or without excision of the involved bone. Occasionally, surgery to close pressure ulcers will induce additional heterotopic bone formation. This seems to be especially true when proximal resections of the femur are done along with rotational skin flaps for trochanteric ulcers.

Once heterotopic bone has formed and its outlines are fairly well delineated, the bony mass rarely regresses spontaneously. It has been observed to decrease in size very occasionally, particularly, in areas where muscles override the mass and either active or passive muscle movement causing friction or pressure on the bone leads to secondary remodeling or partial resorption of the bony mass.

Prevention and treatment of heterotopic ossification have been subject to a wide variety of opinions. Without an adequate understanding of the etiology and pathogenesis, approaches to the treatment of developing or mature heterotopic ossification have been limited. There is still debate about the effect and value of exercise and physical therapy on the development of heterotopic ossification (28, 32, 51). If one considers myositis ossificans traumatica as a model, bleeding and hematoma formation in the predisposed areas of the musculoskeletal system at the time of injury or subsequent to the spinal cord injury have been considered as inducing factors of heterotopic ossification. For this same reason, some have postulated that early physical therapy exercise programs may be a source of trauma (24, 48) and bleeding into the soft tissue leading to the development of heterotopic ossification. The combination of immobilization and forcible mobilization is reported to cause heterotopic ossification in the quadriceps muscle of rabbits (36). There is little additional evidence, however, to support the idea that trauma or exercise programs play a part in the development of heterotopic ossification following spinal cord injury. There is growing evidence that rest leads to decreasing joint range of motion without diminishing the extent of heterotopic ossification (51).

If ossification is taking place, the continuation of aggressive range of motion exercise can also lead to the development of a pseudarthrosis, whereas a small bridge of bone can lead to ankylosis in the absence of continued exercises (51). Successive forceful manipulation to fragment the ossification followed by repeated manipulation and an aggressive range of motion exercise program has even been advocated to improve the range of motion and possibly eliminate the need for surgery (60). In patients with incomplete spinal cord injuries who have preservation of sensation below the level of injury, maintaining joint range of motion with a passive exercise program may be difficult because of pain that frequently accompanies the development of heterotopic ossification. Depending on the extent of sensory preservation, severe pain may, therefore, be caused by an aggressive exercise program, making it impossible to continue that program.

Antiinflammatory agents have been used without success. Calcitonin has also been ineffective (4, 38). Diathermy and ultrasound have not demonstrated any beneficial effects (14, 31, 60). Although not proven in patients with spinal cord injury, radiation following hip arthroplasty has been stated to be effective to some extent in preventing postoperative recurrence of heterotopic ossification. A total of 2000 Rads has been used in ten divided doses over 12 days (8).

Recognition of the early clinical signs and symptoms of heterotopic ossification has led to more appropriate management. Improved diagnostic techniques discussed previously are permitting earlier and more accurate diagnosis. This is especially important in making the differential diagnosis between thrombophlebitis and heterotopic ossification since treatments are completely different. Thrombophlebitis is generally treated with anticoagulation and rest of the involved extremity. When early heterotopic ossification is recognized, anticoagulation is contraindicated and aggressive joint range of motion exercises should be continued.

Etidronate disodium (Didronel) was the first therapeutic agent proven to be effective in actually preventing heterotopic ossification formation when given prophylactically (11, 12, 52). Etidronate disodium is one of the diphosphonates [disodium-1-hydroxyethane diphosphonate (EHDP)]. This simple inorganic compound possesses properties similar to the naturally occurring inorganic pyrophosphates, which are hypothesized to be regulators of biological calcification (15). The diphosphonates, however, have the advantage of being absorbed intact from the gut, are not metabolized, and are excreted into the urine in unchanged form. Etidronate disodium has a high affinity for the calcium ion of hydroxyapatite (15, 27) and localizes primarily on bone (17), particularly bone that is metabolically active (18). Etidronate disodium appears to act by chemisorption onto the hydroxyapatite crystal surface, and although this mechanism is not clearly understood, inhibition of crystalline growth of hydroxyapatite seems to be an integral part of the process (46). It may also be deposited in soft tissues where calcium ion accumulates (7). Etidronate disodium inhibits in vitro dissolution and growth of hydroxyapatite crystals (15); it also prevents experimentally induced soft tissue calcification in vivo (13, 16), and the resorption and accretion of bone are reduced (30). Evidence for direct effects of disodium etidronate on bone cells is controversial, but some pathological changes have been noted in bone cells subjected to this compound (42). Collagen synthesis does not appear to be affected by etidronate disodium (21). However, in a bone-induction model the matrix that forms in the presence of etidronate disodium is atypical (42).

In 1976 a preliminary report was first published showing the effectiveness of etidronate disodium in the prevention of heterotopic ossification following spinal cord injury (52). Starting 20 to 121 days after injury, male patients were treated for 8 to 12 weeks with etidronate disodium in a double-blind, placebo-controlled study. Effectiveness was assessed by the amount of heterotopic ossification formed during the 8 to 12-week treatment period as determined by routine x-rays using a 0 to 4 numerical grading scale. The 4.0 grade was defined as the maximum amount of heterotopic ossification expected around the hips or knees, and which invariably caused ankylosis. The amount of heterotopic ossification in the etidronate disodium-treated patients was significantly less ($p < 0.05$) compared with the placebo-treated patients up to the time treatment was discontinued. Therefore it has been shown that heterotopic ossification formation can be successfully prevented during etidronate disodium treatment. Follow-up in a subset of patients showed that some degree of ossification may still occur after the drug is discontinued. The final amount of heterotopic ossification that developed in the etidronate disodium-treated group was considerably less than that in the placebo-treated group, and functional limitations were usually prevented. The final incidence of heterotopic ossification, however, was about the same in both the etidronate disodium and placebo-treated patients.

The fact that the final incidence remains about the same in both groups after 8 to 12 weeks of treatment with etidronate disodium suggests the drug does not prevent the inflammatory process that predisposes the soft tissues to ossification. Plasmans and associates (42) described this as inhibition of ossification without inhibition of osteoinduction. During treatment with etidronate disodium, ossification of this inflammatory mass is prevented. The predisposition for ossification appears to decrease with time, suggesting that there is a maturation process of this inflammatory mass. The ultimate effectiveness of etidronate disodium therefore appears to be dependent upon the time of initiation of treatment and the length of treatment. Further studies are under way to determine if longer periods of treatment are more beneficial. Present recommendations are to use etidronate disodium prophylactically in spinal cord injury patients beginning at about the third week after injury. The recommended dosage is 20 mg/kg/day for 2 weeks, decreasing to 10 mg/kg/day for 10 weeks. The drug is given in a single dose 1 hour before breakfast with a glass of fruit juice. Should gastrointestinal side effects occur, the dose can be divided and given one hour before meals twice daily. If there have not been any clinical signs or symptoms of heterotopic bone formation during the time of prophylactic treatment, the 12-week treatment regimen is probably adequate to prevent any significant heterotopic ossification. Since etidronate disodium does not prevent the inflammatory reaction, it is possible that all the clinical signs and symptoms of acute heterotopic ossification can still occur during the treatment period. If this occurs, and heterotopic bone is suspected or is proven by bone scan or x-ray, treatment with etidronate disodium should probably be continued for at least 6 months and possibly even as long as a year. Further studies are necessary to determine the optimal length of treatment and dosage.

The safety of etidronate disodium has been assessed in studies of patients with spinal cord injury (52), total hip replacement (11, 12), and Paget's disease (29). Gastrointestinal disturbances such as nausea, occasional vomiting, and diarrhea have been documented in both etidronate disodium and placebo-treated groups, with only a slightly higher incidence totaling 10% to 20% in the etidronate disodium-treated group (52). No other more serious or permanent gastrointestinal side effects have been observed. Dividing the dosage, giving half before breakfast and half before lunch, usually eliminates these side effects. A rise in the serum phosphorus is a well-documented finding during etidronate disodium therapy and has no known clinical side effects (46). It is completely reversible when the drug is discontinued. In fact, compliance in taking the medication can often be monitored by this parameter. Osteomalacia is a recognized side effect when etidronate disodium is given at higher doses for prolonged periods of time; however, no adverse side effects on skeletal bone metabolism have been observed in spinal cord injury patients despite the fact that they are developing rather severe disuse osteoporosis. There is no observed increase in the number of fractures during treatment and long bone fractures continue to heal during treatment. In a review of fracture experience during treatment of Paget's disease with etidronate disodium, it was concluded that the risk of fractures at lower doses may actually be decreased, but, with higher doses for extended periods of time, there may be a slightly increased fracture risk (26). Animal studies have shown that fracture healing is interfered with only at much higher doses of etidronate disodium than those recommended for treatment of spinal cord injury patients (44).

In a very small number of patients who continue to have progression of ossification during etidronate disodium treatment, the major concern must be drug compliance. If drug compliance is satisfactory, the next question that must be answered is whether or not the patient is absorbing the drug adequately from the gastrointestinal tract. This can be determined to some extent by the serum phosphorus that is usually elevated during treatment. Finally, there are probably occasional persons who must be considered as drug failures at the recommended doses since the ossification process continues to progress even when treatment, which is considered to be adequate, is administered.

In those patients who develop heterotopic ossification to the extent that limitation of joint motion leads to functional impairment, surgical intervention is the only remaining method of treatment. Surgery is considered only in patients who have functional impairment or who develop abnormal skin pressure areas because of limited joint motion. When mobility is either decreased or there is complete ankylosis unilaterally or bilaterally, abnormal pressure distribution in the sitting or lying positions can predispose to pressure ulceration of the overlying skin (23).

Attempts at surgical resection, however, have been followed by many reported complications (2, 22, 25). These complications include hemorrhage, severe postoperative infections that may eventually necessitate amputation, and postoperative recurrence of heterotopic ossification. It is commonly accepted that postoperative recurrence of the heterotopic bone is somewhat dependent on its maturity (25, 45, 56). Therefore the accurate assessment of maturity has created considerable interest.

The x-ray appearance of heterotopic ossification, although helpful, is inadequate to confirm maturity. Areas of immature bone may be obscured by masses of more mature bone (56, 61). The alkaline phosphatase is of little help in evaluating maturity since it often is transiently elevated and then returns to normal levels quite some time before actual bone maturity takes place. Bone biopsies may be helpful but are not completely accurate since the heterotopic ossification mass has intermixed areas of mature and immature bone and the results of biopsies depend on the exact site of the biopsy. A bone scan is presently the most reliable parameter to determine the maturity of heterotopic ossification. Decreasing radioisotope-uptake ratios determined by serial bone scans suggest maturity of the bony mass. And yet this single criterion does not appear to be sufficient. A continuing decrease of the radionuclide-uptake ratio should be followed by a steady state and demonstrated by serial scanning over several months (56). Qualitative scans are inadequate. At the present time absolute values of uptake on isolated images are not available to accurately determine maturity. Therefore, in an attempt to be most accurate, quantitative scan data is required at precisely the same anatomic location on the serial scans. Quantification, however, is also somewhat difficult with the present scan equipment, and proper positioning of the patient is very important on serial scanning. It is also recognized that a very active site of bone turnover within the heterotopic bone mass demonstrated on the scan may shift from one region to another during the course of maturation (56). This suggests that there is some mechanism after onset, in addition to time, that is responsible for alteration of bone turnover within the heterotopic mass.

Determination of maturity of heterotopic ossification therefore continues to be elusive. Some areas of heterotopic ossification continue to have increased radioisotope uptake for many years (53, 57). In areas where ankylosis is incomplete and a pseudarthrosis is present, constant motion appears to prolong radioisotope uptake indefinitely.

Excessive blood loss and postoperative hemorrhage have also complicated surgical resection. The heterotopic bone mass is quite vascular, and therefore meticulous hemostasis is quite important during surgery. Suction drainage should be used postoperatively as long as necessary, usually 48 to 72 hours, but the length of time depends more importantly on the amount of drainage than on a specified period of time. Postoperative hematoma without adequate drainage may predispose to infection.

Postoperative infection has probably been the leading cause of morbidity associated with surgery, and to the greatest extent possible, all potential sources of infection must be eliminated before surgery is begun. For this reason, surgery should not be performed in patients with open skin lesions such as pressure ulcers or other suspected skin infections. Transient bacteremia from such lesions can seed the hematoma following surgery and lead to severe infection at the operative site. Open skin lesions should be allowed to heal conservatively or surgical closure should be performed with adequate time for healing before considering resection of heterotopic ossification.

Another source of infection may possibly come from the urinary tract. A urine culture and sensitivity should be obtained prior to surgery, with appropriate antibiotic treatment initiated preoperatively so that a sterile urine can be demonstrated. Antibiotic therapy is continued postoperatively for 2 to 3 weeks and can either be the antibiotic used to clear the urinary tract or another broad-spectrum antibiotic.

Patient evaluation and planning for surgery must be done in advance of anticipated surgery. Etidronate disodium should be started 2 weeks preoperatively at a dosage of 20 mg/kg/day (53). To avoid complications and have a successful outcome of surgery, close attention must be given to details as previously described and outlined in Figure 11.4.

    I. Eliminate sources of infection
      A. Avoid infected skin lesions
      B. Secure sterile urine
        1. Perform urine culture and sensitivity
        2. Initiate appropriate antibiotic treatment
      C. Use broad-spectrum antibiotic postoperatively
   II. Use wedge resection
  III. Careful hemostasis
  IV. Use suction drainage postoperatively
   V. Careful progressive range-of-motion exercises postoperatively

Figure 11.4. Outline of special considerations when performing surgical resection of heterotopic ossification.

The goal of surgery is to restore functional joint motion. It is not necessary or even wise to excise the entire heterotopic bone mass, especially about the hip joint. A wedge resection is performed with the size of the wedge determined by the amount of bone removed, which is necessary to obtain 90° of hip flexion or adequate functional joint motion about other joints. Such a resection leads to a rather large dead space. Exactly what happens in this dead space is poorly understood. One way to reduce the dead space is to remove and trim down the edges of the bone from which the wedge was removed, allowing a more gentle saucerization of the dead space. Following resection of heterotopic ossification about the hip, Wharton (61) recommended that the postoperative management include keeping the hip and knee flexed to 90° to decrease the dead space. This requires support in a well-padded sling. Sacral pressure ulcers can be a hazard with this type of positioning.

The time to start range of motion exercises depends on other postoperative conditions rather than on a strict time protocol. As soon as the flow of hematoma into the hemavac stops, the drainage tube can be removed. Very gentle passive range of motion exercises are started 2 or 3 days later. Limited active exercises are also permitted if the patient has voluntary movement. Once the exercise program has been started, one must not try to achieve the maximum motion obtained at surgery immediately, but rather should attempt to achieve this motion postoperatively by gradual progression. In patients who have had heterotopic ossification removed about the hips, reclined sitting is begun several days after the range of motion exercises are started, usually occurring 1 to 2 weeks postoperatively with gradual progression to full sitting. It must be remembered that most of these patients have rather marked disuse osteoporosis, and the degree of osteoporosis may even be greater in patients who have had prolonged bony ankylosis as a result of the heterotopic ossification. This factor must be considered during the postoperative mobilization program to avoid fractures from therapy that might be too aggressive.

Etidronate disodium is continued postoperatively at a dosage of 10 mg/kg/day for at least 12 months (54). When etidronate disodium is used to prevent heterotopic ossification following total hip arthroplasty, it is recognized that 10 mg/kg/day is usually inadequate, and continuation of 20 mg/kg/day postoperatively is recommended (12). The lower dose has been adequate in most spinal cord injury patients, but patients should be followed closely with routine x-rays after surgery, and if there are signs of early recurrence in the postoperative site, the higher dose should be reinstituted. If there is no evidence of recurrence by routine x-rays during the first 3 weeks postoperatively, it is unlikely that recurrence will take place later during drug treatment (53). The optimal length of treatment still remains to be determined. It appears as though the surgical procedure again sets off an inflammatory reaction similar to that seen when heterotopic ossification first forms. This inflammatory mass must again undergo maturation with time and eventually has less predisposition to ossification. Because there is some evidence that recurrence is less when the bone is more mature at time of surgery, there have been many questions about the timing of surgery. The effectiveness of etidronate disodium in prevention of the recurrence of ossification does not seem to completely depend on the state of maturation; therefore, if etidronate disodium is used, surgical excision can be performed as early as 6 months after onset. Prior to that time, the bone may not have very clear demarcation and the hypervascularity of the immature bony mass may make surgical resection and control of bleeding difficult. Decisions about the correct time for surgery will often depend on the experience of the surgeon until more data is available to support decision making.

When surgical resection has been successful and recurrence is either absent or minimal and functional joint motion has been maintained, it is still important to continue passive joint range of motion exercises indefinitely after surgery to maintain the joint motion. Soft tissues in the areas of surgical resection of heterotopic ossification sometimes have a tendency to form contractures to a greater degree than uninvolved joints. Late contractures can still develop.

REFERENCES

1. Ackerman, L. V. Extra-osseous localized non-neoplastic bone and cartilage formation (so-called myositis ossificans). *J. Bone Joint Surg., 40A:*279–298, 1958.
2. Armstrong-Ressy, C. T., Weiss, A. A., and Ebel, A. Results of surgical treatment of extra-osseous ossification in paraplegia. *N. Y. State J. Med., 59:*2548–2553, 1959.
3. Bayley, S. J. Resident Review #14—Funnybones: A review of the problem of heterotopic bone formation. *Orthop. Review, 8:*113–120, 1979.
4. Bethel, R. G. H., and Doran, D. M. L. Calcitonin for myositis ossificans. *Rheumatol. Rehabil., 18:*188–189, 1979.
5. Blane, C. E., and Perkash, I. True heterotopic bone in the paralyzed patient. *Skeletal Radiol., 7:*21–25, 1981.
6. Brailsford, L. F. Changes in bones, joints and soft tissues associated with disease and injury of the central nervous system. *Br. J. Radiol., 166:*320–328, 1941.
7. Buja, L. M., Tofe, A. J., Pakey, R. W., Francis, M. D., Lewis, S. E., Kulkarni, P. V., Bonte, F. J., and Wilerson, J. T. Effect of EHDP on calcium accumulation and technitium-99m pyrophosphate uptake in experimental myocardial infarction. *Circulation, 64:*1012–1017, 1981.
8. Coventry, M. B., and Scanlon, P. W. The use of radiation to discourage ectopic bone. *J. Bone Joint Surg., 63A:*201–208, 1981.
9. Dejerine, Mme., and Ceillier, A. Para-osteo-arthropathies des paraplegiques par lesion medullaire (etude clinique et radiographique). *Ann. Med. Interne, 5:*497–535, 1918.
10. Farley, J. R., and Baylink, D. J. Purification of a skeletal growth factor from human bone. *Biochemistry, 21:*3502–3507, 1982.
11. Finerman, G. A. M., Krengel, W. F., Lowell, J. D., Murray, W. R., Volz, R. G., Bowerman, J. W., and Gold, R. H. Role of diphosphonate (EHDP) in the prevention of heterotopic ossification after total hip arthroplasty: a preliminary report. In: *The Hip, Proceedings of the Fifth Open Scientific Meeting of the Hip Society.* C.V. Mosby Co., St. Louis, Mo. 1977, pp. 222–234.

12. Finerman, G. A. M., and Stover, S. L. Heterotopic ossification following hip replacement or spinal cord injury. Two clinical studies with EHDP. *Metabol. Bone Dis. Relat. Res., 4 & 5:*337–342, 1981.
13. Fleisch, H. A., Russell, R. G. G., Bisaz, S., Mulhaubauer, R. C., and Williams, D. A. The inhibitory effect of phosphonates on the formation of calcium phosphate crystals *in vitro* and on aortic and kidney calcification *in vivo. Eur. J. Clin. Invest., 1:*12–18, 1970.
14. Fleming, W. C. Preliminary observations on the use of ultrasonics in treatment of soft tissue calcification in paraplegia. *Proc. Annual Clin. Spinal Cord Injury Conf., 6:*18–19, 1957.
15. Francis, M. D., Russell, R. G., and Fleisch, H. Diphosphonates inhibit formation of calcium phosphate crystals *in vitro* and pathological calcification *in vivo. Science, 165:*1264–1266, 1969.
16. Francis, M. D., Flora, L., and King, W. R. The effects of disodium ethane-1-hydroxy-1, 1-diphosphonate on adjuvant induced arthritis in rats. *Calcif. Tissue Res., 9:*109–121, 1972.
17. Francis, M. D., Slough, C. L., and Tofe, A. J. Factors affecting uptake and retention of technitium-99m-diphosphonate and 99m-pertechnetate in osseous, connective and soft tissues. *Calcif. Tiss. Res., 20:*303–311, 1976.
18. Francis, M. D., Slough, C. L., Black, H. E., Tofe, A. J., and Cloyd, G. G. Diphosphonate treatment of a primary osteosarcoma in a dog: a case report. *Vet. Radiol., 21:*168–176, 1980.
19. Freed, J. H., Hahn, H., Menter, R., and Dillon, T. The use of the three-phase bone scan in the early diagnosis of heterotopic ossification (HO) and in the evaluation of Didronel therapy. *Paraplegia, 20:*208–216, 1982.
20. Green, D., Rossi, E. C., Yao, J. S. T., Flinn, W. R., and Spies, S. M. Deep vein thrombosis in spinal cord injury: Effect of prophylaxis with calf compression, aspirin, and dipyridamole. *Paraplegia, 20:*227–234, 1982.
21. Guenther, H. L., Guenther, H. E., and Fleisch, H. The effects of 1-hydroxyethane-1, 1-diphosphonate and dichloromethandiphosphonate on collagen synthesis by rabbit articular chondrocytes and rat bone cells. *Biochemistry, 196:*293–301, 1981.
22. Hardy, A. G., and Dickson, J. W. Pathological ossification in traumatic paraplegia. *J. Bone Joint Surg., 45B:*76–87, 1963.
23. Hassard, G. H. Heterotopic bone formation about the hip and unilateral decubitus ulcers in spinal cord injury. *Arch. Phys. Med. Rehabil., 56:*355–358, 1975.
24. Hossack, D. W., and King, A. Neurogenic heterotopic ossification. *Med. J. Aust., 1:*326–328, 1967.
25. Hsu, J. D., Sakimura, I., and Stauffer, E. S. Heterotopic ossification around the hip joint in spinal cord injured patients. *Clinic. Orthop., 112:*165–269, 1975.
26. Johnston, C. C., Altman, R. D., Canfield, R. E., Finerman, G. A. M., Taulbee, J. D., and Ebert, M. L. Review of fracture experience during treatment of Paget's Disease of bone with etidronate disodium. *Clinic. Orthop., 172:*186–194, 1983.
27. Jung, A., Bisaz, S., and Fleisch, H. The binding of pyrophosphate and two diphosphonates by hydroxyapatite crystals. *Calcif. Tiss. Res., 11:*269–280, 1973.
28. Kewalramani, L. S., and Ortho, M. S. Ectopic ossification. *Amer. J. Phys. Med., (3)56:*99–120, 1977.
29. Khairi, M. R. A., Johnston, C. C., Jr., Altman, R. D., Wellman, H. N., Serafini, A. N., and Sankey, R. R. Treatment of Paget disease of bone (osteitis deformans). Results of a one-year study with disodium etidronate. *J.A.M.A., 230:*562–567, 1974.
30. King, W. R., Francis, M. D., and Michael, W. R. Effect of disodium ethane-1-hydroxy-1, 1-diphosphonate on bone formation. *Clin. Orthop., 78:*251–270, 1971.
31. Knapp, M. E. After care of fractures. In: *Handbook of Physical Medicine and Rehabilitation.* Edited by Krusen, F. H., Kottke, F. J. and Ellwood, P. M. W.B. Saunders, Philadelphia, 1971, pp. 579–585.

32. Knudsen, L., Lundberg, D., and Ericsson, G. Myositis ossificans circumscripta in para-/ tetraplegics. *Scand. J. Rheumatol., 11:*27–31, 1982.

33. Larson, J. M., Michalski, J. P., Collacott, E. A., Eltorai, D., McCombs, C. C., and Madorsky, J. B. Increased prevalence of HLA-B 27 in patients with ectopic ossification following traumatic spinal cord injury. *Rheumatol. Rehabil., 20:*193–197, 1981.

34. Leriche, R., and Policard, A. Les problemes de la physiologie normale et pathologique de l'os. Masson, Paris, 1926.

35. Maugh, T. H., II. Human skeletal growth factor isolated. *Science, 217:*819, 1982.

36. Michelsson, J. E., Granroth, G., and Andersson, L. C. Myositis ossificans following forcible manipulation of the leg. *J. Bone Joint Surg., 62A:*811–815, 1980.

37. Minaire, P., Betuel, H., Girard, R., and Pilonchery, G. Neurologic injuries, paraosteoarthropathies, and human leukocyte antigens. *Arch. Phys. Med. Rehabil., 61:*214–215, 1980.

38. Naftchi, N. E., Viau, A. T., Sell, G. H., and Lowman, E. W. Spinal cord injury: Effects of thyrocalcitonin on periarticular bone formation in three subjects. *Arch. Phys. Med. Rehabil., 60:*280–283, 1979.

39. Nicholas, J. J. Ectopic bone formation in patients with spinal cord injury. *Arch. Phys. Med. Rehabil., 54:*354–359, 1973.

40. Ogilvie-Harris, D. J., Hons, Ch. B., and Fornasier, V. L. Pseudomalignant myositis ossificans: Heterotopic new-bone formation without a history of trauma. *J. Bone Joint Surg., 62A:*1274–1283, 1980.

41. Ostrowski, K., and Wlodarski, K. Induction of heterotopic bone formation. In: *Biochemistry and Physiology of Bone, Vol. III.* Edited by Comar, C. L., and Bronner, J. Academic Press, New York, 1971, pp. 229–336.

42. Plasmans, C. M. T., Jap, P. H. K., Kuijpers, W., and Slooff, T. J. J. H. Influence of a diphosphonate on the cellular aspect of young bone tissue. *Calcif. Tiss. Int., 32:*247–256, 1980.

43. Prakash, V. Radionuclide assessment of heterotopic ossification in spinal cord injury patients. *J. Am. Paraplegia Soc., 6:*10–12, 1983.

44. Procter and Gamble Co. Unpublished data.

45. Rossier, A. B., Bussat, P. H., Infante, F., Zender, R., Courvoisier, B., Muheim, G., Donath, A., Vasey, H., Taillard, W., Lagier, R., Gabbiani, G., Baud, C. A., Pouezat, J. A., Very, J. M., and Hachen, H. J. Current facts on para-osteo-arthropathy (POA). *Paraplegia, 11:*36–78, 1973.

46. Russell, R. G. G., and Smith, R. Diphosphonates; experimental and clinical aspects. *J. Bone Joint Surg., 55B:*66–68, 1973.

47. Samuelson, K. M., and Coleman, S. S. Nontraumatic myositis ossificans in healthy individuals. *J.A.M.A., 235:*1132–1133, 1976.

48. Silver, J. R. Heterotopic ossification, clinical study of its possible relationship to trauma. *Paraplegia, 7:*220–230, 1969.

49. Solheim, K. Microradiography and the glycosaminoglycans in myositis ossificans. *J. Oslo City Hosp., 18:*51–55, 1968.

50. Soule, A. B. Neurogenic ossifying fibromyopathies: A preliminary report. *J. Neurosurg., 2:*485–497, 1945.

51. Stover, S. L., Hataway, C. J., and Zeiger, H. E. Heterotopic ossification in spinal cord-injured patients. *Arch. Phys. Med. Rehabil., 56:*199–204, 1975.

52. Stover, S. L., Hahn, H. R., and Miller, J. M. Disodium etidronate in the prevention of heterotopic ossification following spinal cord injury (preliminary report). *Paraplegia, 14:*146–156, 1976.

53. Stover, S. L., Niemann, K. M. W., and Miller, J. M. Disodium etidronate in the prevention of postoperative recurrence of heterotopic ossification in spinal cord injury patients. *J. Bone Joint Surg., 58A:*683–688, 1976.

54. Stover, S. L., and Niemann, K. M. W. Unpublished data.

55. Suzuki, Y., Hisada, K., and Masanori, T. Demonstration of myositis ossificans by 99 mTc pyrophosphate bone scanning. *Radiology, 111:*663–664, 1974.
56. Tanaka, T., Rossier, A. B., Hussey, R. W., Ahnberg, D. S., and Treves, S. Quantitative assessment of para-osteo-arthropathy and its maturation on serial radionuclide bone images. *Radiology, 123:*217–221, 1977.
57. Tibone, J., Sakimura, I., Nickel, V. L., and Hsu, J. D. Heterotopic ossification around the hip in spinal cord injured patients. A long-term follow-up study. *J. Bone Joint Surg., 60A:*769–775, 1978.
58. Venier, L. H., and Ditunno, J. F., Jr. Heterotopic ossification in paraplegic patient. *Arch. Phys. Med. Rehabil., 54:*475–479, 1971.
59. Weiss, S., Grosswasser, Z., Ohri, A., Mizrachi, Y., Orgad, S., Efter, T., and Gazit, E. Histocompatibility (HLA) antigens in heterotopic ossification associated with neurological injury. *J. Rheumatol., 6:*88–91, 1979.
60. Wharton, G. W., and Morgan, T. H. Ankylosis in paralyzed patient. *J. Bone Joint Surg., 52A:*105–112, 1970.
61. Wharton, G. W. Heterotopic ossification. *Clinic. Orthop., 112:*142–149, 1975.

12

The Psychosocial Adjustment to Spinal Cord Injury

ROBERTA B. TRIESCHMANN

Spinal cord injury is a low-incidence, high-cost disability that imposes tremendous changes on a person's lifestyle. The majority of persons who face these changes are young, male, and action oriented. Young, Bowen, Burns, and McCutchen (36) report that males account for 82% of the spinal injuries in the United States. A majority of these injuries (62.5%) occur to those aged 15 to 29. Within this age group, the causes of spinal cord injuries are vehicular/pedestrian accidents (52%), penetrating wounds (14%), sports–diving (13%), sports–other (6%), falls (11%), falling or flying objects (4%), and other (2%). The incidence of paraplegia is 47% and quadriplegia 53%. Paraplegia and quadriplegia occur equally from most of these accidents except for four categories. Penetrating wounds (72%) and accidents associated with falls or flying objects (72% and 28%) are more likely to result in paraplegia. However, sports injuries are more likely to result in quadriplegia to a dramatic degree. A full 98% of sports-diving injuries result in quadriplegia as do 80% of the sports-other injuries. Although women account for a small percentage of the spinal injuries, it is interesting to note that their etiologies are somewhat different than their male counterparts: vehicular/pedestrian (60%), penetrating wound (14%), and falls (16%). These statistics have been gathered from 1973 to 1981 at the Model Regional Spinal Injury Treatment Systems in the United States and thus may be slightly biased in favor of the incidence of quadriplegia since the more difficult and complicated injuries were more likely to be referred to specialized treatment centers. However, the general distribution of the data should be fairly representative of the population seen in most major hospitals and rehabilitation centers (37).

Thus, the population is young and predominantly male, and the injuries occur through vigorous activities in a large number of cases, with misjudgment or poor judgment being a factor in the injuries of quite a few. It should be noted, however, that there are no data to suggest a tendency toward psychological self-destructiveness in this group. Rather, the base rate of injudicious motor behavior during the teenage years and the early twenties in males is high and a subset of these individuals acquire a spinal cord injury. This should not be confused with self-selection. Considering the advances in medical science, this group can be expected to live almost a normal life span, but the quality of that life will be influenced by a variety of psychological, social, and environmental variables (31).

Persons who acquire spinal cord injuries are often in the midst of mapping out careers or courses of action that will characterize their adult lives, but they suddenly find themselves paralyzed, with no sensation in their limbs and no control over bladder and bowel. Life as they had known it will be interrupted by months of hospitalization and an often lengthy period during which new techniques must be mastered as a necessity for survival and independent function. The changes in lifestyle will be significant. The spinal injured person must learn how to deal with a world designed for and dominated by able-bodied persons who are not very accepting of those with disabilities. They must learn to face people who now communicate that they are different from whom they used to be and perhaps "less" than they used to be. They must learn new types of recreation and leisure activities, and, in many cases, new vocation. However, after an educational or vocational training program, they must learn to face potential employers who do not want to hire them, not because of lack of qualifications for the job but because of the disability. They must learn that many of their previous friends drift away, and thus they must seek opportunities to meet new people and to make new friends. Yet strangers tend to avoid any interaction with them; consequently, new techniques must be learned to put others at ease and to make them forget the presence of the wheelchair. They must learn a sense of humor in order to cope with the daily frustrations and hard work that living with a disability entails. And they must learn to maintain some sense of dignity and self-worth when faced with a social welfare system that penalizes their efforts to become independent and self-sufficient. This, then, constitutes the impact of a disability on a person's life, and there are many factors that influence the ultimate adjustment the person will make. In this chapter, we will consider some of the psychosocial variables that influence adjustment, but it would be a mistake for health care professionals to assume that these are the only issues that influence the outcome of rehabilitation efforts (31, 33).

THE REHABILITATION PROCESS

Rehabilitation is the process of learning to live with one's disability in one's own environment. This learning experience is a dynamic process that starts at the moment of injury and continues for the remainder of the person's life. There is no definable end point that can be labeled as "rehabilitated" or "adjusted" because, as with all people in all areas of life, disabled persons are continually learning to adapt to their environment in hopefully more functional and satisfying ways. It may take as long as 2 years for the new ADL and mobility techniques to become an automatic part of daily life, and this does not consider the changes in social, recreational, and vocational behaviors that the person must incorporate into his or her repertoire of functional activities. Thus it is most important for health care professionals to understand the principles of learning and the multiplicity of factors that are involved in the process of adjusting to a disability. In the first several weeks after the onset of spinal cord injury, survival of the patient is the concern of hospital personnel, and the person becomes the passive recipient of treatment designed to fix his or her body: skeletal traction or surgery, treatment of associated injuries, management of bladder and bowel, prevention of skin problems, etc. When medical stability has been achieved and the person is no longer sick but now physically disabled, a rehabilitation program will be outlined to teach the person how to manage the activites of daily living and the mobility techniques necessary to negotiate the world. At this point the person can no longer be the passive recipient of treatments but must become an active participant in the process of learning to live with the spinal injury.

Unfortunately, the operational policies and procedures of hospitals and rehablitation centers have been designed to dispense units of organic treatment. The person is a patient, and the staff delivers treatments, usually according to a schedule and sequence designed by the staff and for the convenience of the staff. This is not an optimal environment in which to teach new behaviors to persons who are not sick and who essentially are students. Therefore, two models of rehabilitation must be examined so that we can determine which one provides the optimal fit between the task at hand and the strategies used to accomplish that task.

The medical model of rehabilitation could be stated as:

$$B = f (O \times p)$$

Behavior (adjustment) of the spinal injured person (B) is the result of treatments dispensed to the organic (O) variables (skin, bladder and bowel, paralysis, lack of sensation, respiratory function, etc.) unless hindered by underlying personality (p) problems (lack of motivation, depression, low self-esteem, anxiety, anger, frustration, dependency). In this case, units of treatment will be dispensed to the (p) variables in the form of counseling and psychotherapy.

In contrast to the medical model is the educational model of rehabilitation, the learning approach. In this instance, rehabilitation is viewed as the process of teaching the person to live with the disability in his or her own environment. The person must be an active participant in this process, and the program must be designed by the staff with and not for the person, to meet his or her individual needs and goals. These will be determined by an assessment of the person's unique personality style, desires, preferences, and the environment to which he or she will return. If rehabilitation is the process of teaching the person to live with the disability, then the principles of learning and the multiple factors that influence behavior become the concern of everyone on the rehabilitation team, not just the psychologist. Thus, the learning or educational model of rehabilitation can be summarized as:

$$B = f (P \times O \times E)$$

Behavior (adjustment) is a function of the interaction of person variables, organic variables, and environmental variables. Person (P) variables would include habits, locus of control, method of coping with stress, preferences, rewards, self-image, and creativity. Organic (O) variables would include level of injury, age, medical complications, strength, and endurance. Environmental (E) variables would include hospital milieu; stigma value of the disability; family and interpersonal support; financial security; cultural and ethnic influences; access to medical attention, equipment repair, recreational and educational opportunities; architectural barriers; and transportation.

Traditionally we have focused on treating the organic problems and assumed that all responsibility for success or failure rested with the person. That is the essence of the medical model. Perhaps it is most appropriate to use the medical model during the acute phase of treating illness and disability. However, this model is not appropriate during the rehabilitation phase during which a variety of behaviors must be learned that will enable the person to resume a satisfying life as an integrated part of his or her community (adjustment). Using the learning model, $B = f (P \times O \times E)$, we need to pay attention to the multiple factors that influence behavior, particularly the environmental variables that have powerful impacts on the outcome of our rehabilitation efforts. Thus, within this context, the psychological variables are only part of the equation that influences a person's behavior in any given situation. An understanding of the role of psychosocial influences on outcome of rehabilitation efforts is important, and therefore the most important issues will be reviewed.

PSYCHOLOGICAL REACTIONS TO THE ACUTE INJURY

There has been considerable speculation but little research to document the immediate reaction to spinal cord injury. Theorists have proposed a stage theory of adjustment to disability with denial of the physical implications of the injury being the first stage (15, 17, 20, 28). Time spent in an intensive care unit or on an acute surgical ward will reveal that a significant percentage of persons with new injuries ask questions or make statements that suggest that they do not perceive themselves to be paralyzed or the situation to be permanent. They talk about "walking out of the hospital," or ask repeatedly, "When will I be able to move my legs?" However, the question needs to be raised as to whether this constitutes evidence of the psychological defense mechanism of denial or whether there are other explanations for this behavior.

The immediate reaction to spinal cord injury should be examined in terms of the psychological reaction to the injury itself but also to the procedures utilized to ensure the survival of the person during the acute treatment phase. For example, the paralysis restricts movement, and the procedures used to immobilize the spine will further restrict movement for at least 8 weeks. Persons with quadriplegia who have tongs in their head to immobilize the neck have less possible movement than persons with paraplegia. Furthermore, they have a more restricted visual field, looking at the ceiling or floor only. Medications to relax the person, to ease the pain, and to treat associated injuries and medical problems may cloud the sensorium for weeks after the accident. Later in the course of disability it is not unusual for high dosages of valium to be given to control muscle spasms; this can further reduce mental acuity. Anesthesia for surgery, followed by treatment in intensive care units, can add to the deterioration in the quality of mental functioning.

Intensive care units provide little opportunity to rest comfortably because of the frequent interruptions required for medical procedures. In fact, for many months the person with spinal injury will be awakened every 2 hours to be turned in order to prevent skin lesions. Continued loss of sleep will disrupt mental efficiency further. Since there are few cues to identify the passage of time (often no windows and continuous artificial lighting), time and place disorientation can occur.

Loss of sensation associated with the injury is one form of sensory deprivation; the restricted view of the world (ceiling or floor) while in traction is another. The monotony of the hospital routine is certainly a perceptual restriction, in addition to the lack of intellectual challenge that accompanies all long hospitalizations. Consequently, all of the research on the effects of sensory deprivation becomes relevant when trying to understand the behavior of the newly injured person (38). Zubek reports findings that indicate that restriction of movement does produce stress, particularly bodily discomforts and thinking difficulties, but sensory deprivation in addition to restriction of movement is associated with significantly more stress. Physical exercise during periods of perceptual deprivation is associated with significantly less impairment in intellectual and perceptual motor tests and fewer EEG changes in contrast to no exercise at all. Furthermore, 2 weeks of perceptual deprivation is associated with a progressive decrease in mean occipital lobe frequencies on the EEG. The EEG frequencies begin to increase when perceptual stimulation increases, but even after 10 days, they may remain below normal. Correlated with the magnitude of the EEG changes are motivational losses such as an inability to concentrate or to engage in purposeful activity (38).

Newly injured persons have frequently been described as denying their disabilities because they ask what has happened to them, receive an explanation, and act as if they had never received an answer. However, rather than attribute this to deep psychological processes, it seems more appropriate to interpret this "forgetfulness" as a side effect of the sensory deprivation of the acute treatment period.

Harris, Patel, Greer, and Naughton (16) confirm these observations regarding the acute treatment phase and add that pain is a frequent concomitant of spinal injury that interferes with focused thinking. In addition, fear of dying is a realistic concern in many cases, and respiratory complications plus associated injuries may bring survival into question at several points in the immediate recovery phase. Braakman, Orbaan, and Dishoeck (4) report that most of the newly spinal injured persons that they interviewed wanted information on the circumstances of their condition and the implications for the future within a few weeks of their injury. There was no evidence of denial of the disability, and once the intellectually dulling effects of the early treatment procedures had dissipated, the individuals wanted to receive information on what had happened to them.

Nevertheless, even after receiving a complete explanation of the spinal injury, many persons adamantly claim that they will walk out of the hospital. Is this denial or hope? Perhaps we have a semantic problem here. Let us define denial as a nonrecognition of the implications of the injury to such an extent that the person perceives little need to participate in rehabilitation. In other words, they are essentially saying "I am not permanently paralyzed and will not need these rehabilitation therapies because I am going to recover completely." In the author's experience, the number of persons who actually deny the disability in this way and therefore refuse to participate in rehabilitation is small. (These cases have always involved strongly religious people who have viewed participation in rehabilitation as being in conflict with their belief in God's healing power.) However, most of the patients respond to the prognosis of paralysis with an assertion of will and strength; they will prove the physician wrong and walk out of the hospital. It is unfortunate that many professionals view such statements as evidence of a maladaptive coping process (denial) rather than as evidence of the powerful resources on which a person draws in times of adversity (hope).

Caywood (5) believes that information about the disability should be given in such a manner that it does not destroy the patient's hope that things might get better. He believes that hope need not interfere with the rehabilitation process but can provide a motive to keep working despite the many frustrations of a treatment program. He affirms that hope is not the same as denial and should not be placed in the same category as a defense mechanism.

THE STAGE THEORY OF ADJUSTMENT

The stage theory of adjustment has been discussed by many recognized experts in the field (2, 15, 20, 23, 28), but little empirical evidence has been offered to substantiate the assertions of the theory. The stage theory suggests that the first reaction to the onset of disability is denial because of overpowering feelings of anxiety. This denial must be replaced by the second stage, depression, in order for adjustment to occur. This depression, according to the theory, represents a realistic and active mourning for the loss of valued functions and activities and has been considered to be the most important stage. Depression will be replaced by feelings of dependency and hostility that must be worked through in order to reach the final stage, adjustment. It should be noted, however, that no evidence of these stages has been presented in any of the published studies; they represent the clinical impressions of the authors.

To date there is only one research project that has been designed to test the stage theory of adjustment. In his sample Dunn (11) found that there was more variability than similarity in the reactions of 25 persons with spinal cord injury, and thus there was no evidence of stages. Dexter (8) has found no evidence of adjustment stages in a longitudinal study of adjustment to spinal injury.

Since depression is considered to be a key element in the stage theory, research on this variable can shed some light on the validity of the theoretical formulations that have dominated the field for 50 years. Taylor (30) found that his sample of young men, who were within 3 months of onset of injury, displayed Minnesota Multiphasic Personality Inventory (MMPI) profiles similar to uninjured males on any university campus. There was little evidence of depression. Bourestom and Howard (3) found that persons with spinal injury had the most benign MMPI profiles when compared to persons with rheumatoid arthritis and multiple sclerosis. Only mild depression was noted. Dinardo (10) reports that persons with spinal injury who displayed evidence of depression in his study were independently rated as having the poorest adjustment to their disabilities in comparison to those who tended to suppress or repress their feelings. Lawson (22) studied the incidence, severity, and pattern of depression in 10 persons with quadriplegia during their entire inpatient rehabilitation hospitalization. Four measures (self-report, biochemical, ratings by others, and behavioral) of depression were obtained each day on each person from admission to discharge. His results showed that depression was not a major factor in the overall pattern of behavior in his sample. There was evidence of mild depression 3 weeks after admission and just before discharge from the hospital. Otherwise, this sample did not display the pattern of depression that the stage theory predicts. Interestingly, there was a variability among the measures of depression. The self-report, biochemical, and behavioral measures of depression were in agreement and showed few signs of depression except as noted above. However, the staff ratings consistently overestimated the amount of emotionality actually present. Thus, it is not surprising that the patients in this study reported that the most depressing thing was the staff expectation that they should be depressed.

Howell, Fullerton, Harvey, and Klein (18) evaluated 22 patients with spinal injury using a standardized interview and diagnostic process to assess the incidence of depression. All patients were within 6 months of injury. Depression was defined as a sustained and pervasive dysphoric mood accompanied by biological, behavioral, and cognitive symptoms. All interviews were conducted by psychiatrists. Their data showed that no patient suffered a major depressive episode following injury. Five patients showed mild depressive reactions defined as depressed affect that was neither pervasive nor prolonged. Thus, they conclude that depressive disorders affect a minority of patients with traumatic spinal cord injury within the first few months of the accident. It does not appear to be a universal phenomenon, and when it does occur, it does not appear to be as severe or prolonged as expected.

These data should remind us that professionals as well as lay persons are vulnerable to perceiving evidence that is consistent with their expectations. The stage theory has been taught in professional curricula and repeated in most professional books in the section on adjustment to disability. Professional staff members expect to see distress in persons with disability and consistently overreport its incidence and severity (31). Taylor (30) found that the staff members of a highly regarded spinal injury center were no better than college fraternity men at predicting the incidence and severity of emotional reactions to spinal injury; both groups predicted such severe psychological reactions to spinal injury that a diagnosis of psychosis would have been necessary. In actuality, the sample of spinal injured men had MMPI profiles similar to the average man on campus. Rosenthal (24) has documented the existence of expectancy bias and has studied its effect on the results of experimental research. Thus, professionals need to examine some of their assumptions regarding the emotional reaction to disability. The notion that people must get depressed in order for adjustment to occur has not been substantiated. Yet numerous psychologists, counselors, and social workers have encouraged disabled persons to express depressive statements and have labeled any tendency to resist this as denial. That, unfortunately, becomes a diabolical Catch-22: if the disabled person admits to depression, that is a psychological problem that needs treatment; if the person claims not to be depressed, that is denial, a psychological problem that needs treatment.

The requirement of mourning has been described by Wright (35) as the hypothesis that, "When a person has a need to safeguard his values, he will either (1) insist that the person he considers unfortunate is suffering (even when he seems not to be suffering) or (2) devaluate the unfortunate person because he ought to suffer and he does not" (35, pp. 242–243). Wright also describes the requirement of mourning as the need to perceive the succumbing aspects rather than the coping aspects of living with a disability. Furthermore, there may be an expectation discrepancy between the way the disabled person behaves and the way we expect him to behave.

"He (the observer) may, for example, *alter the apparent reality* by doubting the evidence concerning the adequate adjustment of the person with a disability. Thus, he may feel that the person is shamming, simply acting *as though* he were managing, when actually he is not. He (the observer) may suppress evidence regarding the coping aspect of difficulties and high-light evidence bearing upon the succumbing aspects . . . ." (35, pp. 73–74)

Is it possible that some of the publications that professionals have written reflect the "requirement of mourning?" Have professionals seen more distress and psychological difficulty than actually is present? Have professionals uncritically applied terms and theoretical concepts from the field of mental illness to describe the reaction to spinal injury? The onset of spinal cord is not a minimal event in one's life, yet many persons state that it is not the most important thing that has ever happened to them during their lifetime (7). However, admittedly, it must be a most unpleasant experience and one that a person would prefer to avoid if one had the choice. But it seems clear that professionals have stressed the negative emotional aspects unnecessarily and underestimated the strengths and coping ability of people in crisis.

Goldiamond (14) states:

". . . When the professional refers to patients as 'being unaware of,' 'being unrealistic about,' or 'repressing' their problems, it is the *professional* who is often being unrealistic. If I am not discussing pains, problems, and infections to which I am susceptible, it is not because I am unaware, unrealistic, or repressing. At times, I am painfully aware of them, and I mean that literally; I am sure other persons also do not discuss problems when they could. If they do not, in discussions with professionals, 'face up' to these issues, it is because of the same good sense; they are facing, or trying to face, in a different direction, namely one that can help them program attainment of their goals". (14, pp. 119–120)

PERSONALITY AND SPINAL CORD INJURY

One of the fallacies of the stage theory of adjustment to disability was the implicit notion that there would be a sequence of emotional reactions that all persons would go through regardless of preinjury personality style.

Research described in the previous section provides evidence to discredit a theory that assumes a homogeneous response to a disability. Professionals concur that there is no specific personality style or unitary reaction associated with any particular disability (6, 27, 28, 31, 35), yet there is a continuing tendency on the part of rehabilitation staff members to make some global assumptions about the personalities of persons with spinal injury. Unfortunately, this is reinforced by research that attempts to describe the average response of persons with spinal injury to a personality test, such as the MMPI, for example.

There is no one personality style that is associated with spinal injury. According to Wilcox and Stauffer (34):

"Persons with traumatically induced spinal injury comprise a heterogeneous population when they arrive for treatment: age, sex, cultural structure, education, marital status, experience in working and living, are as divergent as human nature itself. They will continue to be a heterogeneous group when they leave the centers, with one obvious difference: they will demonstrate a severe and probably permanent physical impairment (34, p. 115).

However, because a significant proportion of those with spinal injury are males aged 15 to 29, there are certain behaviors often observed such as abuse of alcohol or drugs, physically active lifestyles, a tendency to engage in high risk behaviors, a tendency to prefer spontaneity rather than long-range planning and a tendency to question authority. Such behaviors have a high base rate in the population of males in this age group, and thus, it is not surprising that a subset of them acquire a spinal injury. But to ascribe these behaviors to persons with spinal injury rather than to the population from which they come is fallacious. This group is also only one part of the population of persons with spinal injury, and there is no simple way to characterize the remainder.

There have been several studies that have looked at the average MMPI profile of persons with spinal injury. Bourestom and Howard (3) found that the group with spinal injury was only mildly depressed in comparison to a group of persons with rheumatoid arthritis and multiple sclerosis. The shape of the profile of these three groups was somewhat similar, but the elevation of the profiles of the latter two groups was higher. Taylor (30) found that the average MMPI profile for his group of newly injured young men was similar to fellows on college campuses: slight elevations on scale 4 (Pd) and scale 9 (Ma), indicating independence, assertiveness, and lots of energy. This then is an excellent example of the influence of demographic variables and base rates.

Nevertheless, the question remains: if there is no single response to spinal injury (no spinal injury personality or uniform stages of adjustment), what do we learn from descriptions of the average response on any personality test or assessment device? Why should we anticipate a homogeneous reaction to spinal injury when the one feature these persons have in common is the physical disability? This homogeneity of response is an implicit assumption whenever one considers average MMPI profiles or average scores on other measures. Trieschmann and Sand (32), using terminal renal patients, studied the intellectual and personality response to the process of renal failure. The average MMPI was similar in shape to those in the Bourestom and Howard study (3), and the average profiles showed a very low correlation to measures of kidney function. However, when the MMPI's were sorted according to types of responses to the crisis situation, five different reaction types seemed to occur. It was hypothesized that a person's response to a major life crisis would be similar to one's typical response to severe stress and that people differ in these response styles depending on their precrisis personality. Thus, five different profile types were obtained, none of which was similar to the total group average profile. There were vast individual differences that were obscured by the averaging process, and the total average profile was not descriptive of anyone in the study sample. As a result, the concept of averaging MMPI profiles or other tests of personality for heterogeneous groups of people must be challenged. It would be much more fruitful to study the incidence of a particular personality trait and its association with specific behaviors or to categorize persons according to certain behaviors and study the incidence of certain personality traits.

For example, Fordyce (12) studied a sample of males with spinal injury who had been categorized into two groups: those whose disabilities occurred as a result of their own imprudent behaviors and those whose injuries occurred through accidents with no evidence of imprudence on their parts. He found that the group categorized as imprudent scored higher on scales 3 (Hy) and 4 (Pd) of the MMPI than the prudent group. In a similar study, Kunce and Worley (21) tested two groups on the Strong Vocational Interest Blank (SVIB). One group was composed of those who were active agents in their accidents, and the other group consisted of those who were passive agents. Those who were active agents in their accidents scored higher on the aviator key of the SVIB, which is often interpreted as showing evidence of adventurousness, boldness, and assertiveness. However, the issue of base rates must be considered in both of these studies since the results may reflect the influence of age and sex variables. Nevertheless, they represent an approach to the study of persons with spinal injury that is based on the premise of individual differences.

MOTIVATION

Motivation is an important factor in the process of adjustment to spinal cord injury, and it has received considerable attention in the literature. However, it is a summary term that we use to describe all of those features that determine whether or not the person will incorporate the teachings of rehabilitation into his or her lifestyle. Traditionally, we have assumed that motivation is exclusively a characteristic of the person; recently, however, there has been increasing evidence suggesting that the definition of motivation as an internal drive state is too limited a view of the situation (13). Rather we have evidence that the use of operant techniques on "unmotivated" persons changes their behavior so that it is similar to that of "motivated" persons. Thus, we have begun to look at the environment as a critical element in the assessment of the person's motivation (31). In this approach, the unmotivated person is the one for whom there is no reward sufficient for his work. The focus, external to the person, is on rewards and punishments in the environment.

However, Seligman (26) has proposed that merely having a powerful reward available in the environment may not be sufficient if the person has learned that there is no contingency between his behavior and the outcomes. He calls this learned helplessness. Spinal injury may be a dramatic example of a state in which learned helplessness can occur (31). With the sudden onset of paralysis and the loss of control over life that hospitalization entails, certain people may be very vulnerable to learning to be helpless, to believing that there is nothing that they can do to improve their situation.

There are individual differences in one's susceptibility to the learned helplessness phenomenon, and the locus of control dimension may account for a significant part of the variance. Locus of control is an expectancy or set that one brings into a learning situation and may be defined as the expectation that one can control the rewards that the world has to offer. Those with an internal locus of control believe that their behavior will be rewarded if they work hard, whereas those with an external locus of control believe that fate, luck, and powerful others control the rewards of the world. Seeman and Evans (25) reported that those with an internal locus of control were more interested in gaining knowledge of their disease than those with an external locus of control because the internals saw such knowledge as useful in controlling their lives. Dinardo (10) found that those with an internal locus of control had a better self-concept and were less depressed after spinal injury than externals. Swenson (29) provides the most complete research to date on the relevance of locus of control to spinal injury adjustment. Internals were found to have less time spent in the hospital as a result of preventable medical problems, spent more time in work activities in the home, in educational activities, and in time outside the home, and spent more time in a combination of education, paid employment, and community work. There was no correlation between locus of control and level of disability. Thus, although a person with quadriplegia may have less physical control over life, this does not change the generalized expectancy of control over the rewards and satisfactions of life.

Anderson and Andberg (1) found that those with the highest incidence of time lost because of decubitus ulcers showed the least acceptance of responsibility for care of their own skin. Even with high levels of disability, acceptance of responsibility in a conceptual sense was the paramount factor in prevention of pressure sores, regardless of motor function. Kemp and Vash (19) found that having a large number of goals was highly correlated with productivity and successful adjustment to spinal injury. Although they did not measure locus of control, it is interesting to wonder if internals would report more goals than externals or if the type of goal would differ. The more productive persons in their study reported goals in the vocational and family-interpersonal category, whereas, less productive persons had goals that were avocational and of physical function in nature.

Although management of psychosocial issues will be discussed later, it is important to note that the management of motivational deficits will vary depending upon whether one applies the medical model of rehabilitation or the learning model. Within the medical model, lack of motivation is viewed as the patient's problem, and therefore the psychologist is asked to fix this problem, preferably in the psychologist's office, using counseling or psychotherapy. Unfortunately, these treatments have been unsuccessful at improving motivational level (9). But in the learning model of rehabilitation, motivational deficits are viewed as an environmental problem and the solution is found in modifying the patient-environment interaction (31, 33). This usually means that the rehabilitation staff needs to look at their own behaviors and the operational policy of the team to seek ways to produce the desired behavior from the disabled person. In the medical model, the patient is the failure; in the learning model, the program is the failure. It is important to note that the learning model does not imply that the patient has no responsibility to bring a willingness to cooperate to a therapy program. But it does imply that the issue of motivation is very complex and usually involves an interaction of the person and the environment in which he or she is asked to perform.

MANAGEMENT STRATEGIES

Use of the learning model of rehabilitation requires a recognition that the behavior of persons with spinal injuries will reflect the interaction of the person's personality in response to environmental influences. As a general principle of management, if you are not getting the behavior deemed appropriate, first analyze whether the behavior you want is truly "appropriate." Rehabilitation staff and hospital personnel have a great affection for patient compliance with requests, routines, policies, and orders. It is important to note, however, that compliance may not always be in the best interests of the disabled person in the long run because compliance with externally imposed routines does not teach independence, problem solving, and coping with a disability. Second, if you are not getting the behavior you want, examine the impact of the person's environment and try to assess whether the behavior is in opposition to or agreement with that environment.

An example of behavior in opposition to the environment is the noncompliance with nursing ward routine by young spinal injured men. As a group, they are independent, aggressive, action-oriented, and not overly respectful of authority. Therefore, a rehabilitation routine that emphasizes strict rules and regulations, strictly enforced time schedules, and many prohibitions is the ideal environment to provoke opposition rather than compliance. Naturally every ward needs certain procedures and regulations that hopefully promote the well-being of all patients, but the attitude by which the staff convey these policies can influence the compliance rate. Furthermore, a rehabilitation staff inadvertently may develop such a strict and rigid program for certain "problem" cases that the only way in which the disabled person can exert his or her independence is by not doing what is expected. Such situations lead to an escalation of the conflict with noncompliance leading to further authoritarianism, which leads to further noncompliance.

The resolution of such situations requires a mediator, often the psychologist, who asks the patient and staff to sit down together and to negotiate a new mode of interaction. This usually involves a giving in on both parts and an affirmation of an agreement to work together. As long as the team and the patient agree on the ultimate goal, the maximum function of the patient so that he or she can be discharged from inpatient status, the group can plan steps to accomplish this goal. The confrontation needs to be ended and the personal irritations defused in order to promote cooperation.

An example of behavior in agreement with the environment is the nonparticipation in ADL activities by men who belong to cultures in which women are expected to take care of "incapacitated" individuals. The rehabilitation center may make it perfectly clear that these patients are expected to learn to dress, bathe, groom, and feed themselves. Nevertheless, they may not see the necessity of learning these activites because that is women's work. An associated concept within these cultures is the expectation that disabled persons' productive lives are at an end and their families will take care of them for the rest of their lives. While we may not agree that productivity needs to end at the onset of disability, it is unrealistic to invest great effort in a program that places people in total conflict with their families and culturally defined roles. This is more likely to occur in recent immigrants to North America who have not assimilated western norms and culture, or in much older citizens. Older men frequently do not see the need to expend the energy required to function at their maximal level and will settle for less independence in exchange for assistance.

In such cases, the team needs to make a realistic assessment of the person's culture and what behaviors have a reasonable probability of being continued in the home environment. It is important to understand the goals and wishes of both the disabled person and the family in order to plan an appropriate program.

Young men with spinal injury are action-oriented as a group, and their major way of relating to the world has been markedly changed by the spinal injury. Even if they talk about "walking out of here," this is not necessarily denial and should not be challenged verbally. "To not want to live like this" is not necessarily suicidal ideation but merely a statement of fact, particularly since the newly injured person has no information or understanding as to what life will be like with a physical disability. Only several years of living with the disability will provide information on this, and hopefully a rehabilitation program will be planned that helps the person find meaningful and productive activities to offset the hard work and frustration that disability entails.

Typically, people do not get deeply depressed soon after onset of the injury. Depression should be defined as insomnia, lack of appetite, and psychomotor retardation of at least 3 days duration. In the rare case in which this state occurs, the temporary use of antidepressant medication may help to initiate some of the behaviors needed to fully participate in a rehabilitation program. It should be noted that depression at this stage is not a good prognostic sign, and therefore a counseling and rehabilitation program that emphasizes activity and productivity is certainly indicated. Most persons with spinal injury, however, will be very unhappy about their state of affairs, and loving empathy is the treatment of choice. At the same time, they should not be encouraged to dwell on losses and sad feelings but rather encouraged to look at the assets they still have and to do the best that they can in the program. However, the physical rehabilitation program should be considered as only the first stage in a multifaceted endeavor leading to resumption of a satisfactory life in the community.

Because motor activity has been such a significant part of these patients' lives, the rehabilitation program should seek ways to channel this energy in appropriate directions. In-hospital sports programs and extra physical therapy can help to burn up the emotional tension that sudden onset of disability produces. If these young people have suitable opportunities to expend this energy physically (which is their preferred mode), they are less likely to look for ways to disrupt hospital routine because of boredom. Furthermore, physical fatigue produces a more satisfying sleep than that induced by medication.

Typically, most rehabilitation programs place most emphasis on teaching ADL, bladder and bowel management, and mobility techniques. But these are the skills that the average 5-year-old child has acquired. Successful adult life requires a variety of sophisticated interpersonal skills that the onset of a physical disability makes even more necessary. However, these skills, plus community living skills, receive much less emphasis or are essentially ignored in most rehabilitation centers. Thus, a multistage rehabilitation program is essential with acute injury management, physical restoration, and community living training having equal importance in the long-term program. With such an approach we can assist persons with spinal injuries to live meaningful and productive lives and to be psychosocially integrated into their own communities.

SUMMARY

The population of persons who acquire a spinal injury is predominantly young, male, and action-oriented. These people are in the midst of mapping out the courses that shape their adult lives, and the physical disability serves as a major interruption and a major refocusing of life's activities. There is, however, no evidence of a spinal injury personality, and each person will cope with the disability in a manner consistent with his or her preinjury style of coping with stress.

Although earlier literature emphasized the stage theory of adjustment, current research suggests that people do not go through a reliable sequence of stages but rather follow their unique style of coping. Depression, the evidence demonstrates, does not occur with great frequency and, contrary to the stage theory, is not a necessary precursor to adjustment. On the contrary, there is evidence that early depression is not a good prognostic sign. Depression, however, should be differentiated from unhappiness just as denial should be differentiated from hope.

In order to plan a proper rehabilitation program that seeks to promote independence and successful community living, the models of rehabilitation should be examined to utilize the proper strategy for the proper task. The medical model is appropriate during the acute injury phase but not during rehabilitation. At that point, the learning model should be utilized because it emphasizes the very powerful and pervasive influence of the environment in interaction with the person on the outcome of our rehabilitation efforts.

Suggestions for management of certain psychosocial issues have been given.

REFERENCES

1. Anderson, T., and Andberg, M. Psychosocial factors associated with pressure sores. *Arch. Phys. Med. Rehabil., 60*:341–346, 1979.
2. Berger, S., and Garrett, J. Psychological problems of the paraplegic patient. *J. Rehabil., 18*:15–17, 1952.
3. Bourestom, N., and Howard, M. Personality characteristics of three disability groups. *Arch. Phys. Med. Rehabil., 46*:626–632, 1965.
4. Braakman, R., Orbaan, J., and Dishoeck, M. Information in the early stages after spinal cord injury. *Paraplegia, 14*:95–100, 1976.
5. Caywood, T. A quadriplegic young man looks at treatment. *J. Rehabil., 49*:22–25, 1974.
6. Cook, D. Psychological aspects of spinal cord injury. *Rehabil. Counseling Bull., 19*:535–543, 1976.
7. Corbet, B. *Options: Spinal Cord Injury and the Future.* National Spinal Cord Injury Foundation, Newton Upper Falls, Massachusetts, 1980.
8. Dexter, W. Personality factors associated with adjustment to disability. Paper presented at American Psychological Association, Los Angeles, August, 1981.
9. Diamond, M., Weiss, A., and Grynbaum, B. The unmotivated patient. *Arch. Phys. Med. Rehabil., 49*:281–284, 1968.
10. Dinardo, Q. Psychological adjustment to spinal cord injury. Doctoral dissertation, University of Houston, 1971.

11. Dunn, D. Adjustment to spinal cord injury in the rehabilitation hospital setting. Doctoral dissertation, University of Maryland, 1969.
12. Fordyce, W. Personality characteristics of men with spinal cord injury as related to manner of onset of disability. *Arch. Phys. Med. Rehabil., 45:*321–325, 1964.
13. Fordyce, W. Behavioral Methods in Rehabilitation. In: *Rehabilitation Psychology.* Edited by Neff, W. American Psychological Association, Washington, D. C., 1971.
14. Goldiamond, I. Coping and adaptive behaviors of the disabled. In: *The Sociology of Physical Disability and Rehabilitation.* Edited by Albrecht, G. University of Pittsburgh Press, Pittsburgh, 1976.
15. Gunther, M. Emotional Aspects. In: *Spinal Cord Injuries.* Edited by Reuge, D. C.C. Thomas, Springfield, Ill., 1969.
16. Harris, P., Patel, S., Greer, W., and Naughton, J. Psychological and social reactions to acute spinal paralysis. *Paraplegia, 11:*132–136, 1973.
17. Hohmann, G. Psychological aspects of treatment and rehabilitation of the spinal injured person. *Clin. Orthop., 112:*81–88, 1975.
18. Howell, T., Fullerton, D., Harvey, R., and Klein, M. Depression in spinal cord injured patients. *Paraplegia, 19:*284–288, 1981.
19. Kemp, B. and Vash, C. Productivity after injury in a sample of spinal cord injured persons: a pilot study. *J. Chronic Dis., 24:*259–275, 1971.
20. Kerr, W., and Thompson, M. Acceptance of disability of sudden onset in paraplegia. *Paraplegia, 10:*94–102, 1974.
21. Kunce, J., and Worley, B. Interset patterns, accidents, and disability. *J. Clin. Psychol., 22:*105–107, 1966.
22. Lawson, N. Significant events in the rehabilitation process: The spinal cord patients' point of view. *Arch. Phys. Med. Rehabil., 59:*573–579, 1978.
23. Mueller, A. Psychologic Factors in rehabilitation of paraplegic patients. *Arch. Phys. Med. Rehabil, 43:*151–159, 1962.
24. Rosenthal, R. *Experimenter Effects in Behavioral Research.* Appleton-Century-Crofts, New York, 1966.
25. Seeman, M., and Evans, J. Alienation and learning in a hospital setting. *Am. Sociol. Rev., 27:*774–782, 1962.
26. Seligman, M. *Helplessness: On Depression, Development, and Death.* W. H. Freeman and Company, San Francisco, 1975.
27. Shontz, F. Physical Disability and personality. In: *Rehabilitation Psychology.* Edited by Neff, W. American Psychological Association, Washington, D. C., 1971.
28. Siller, J. Psychological situation of the disabled with spinal cord injuries. *Rehabil. Lit., 30:*290–296, 1969.
29. Swenson, E. The relationship between locus of control expectancy and successful rehabilitation of the spinal cord injured. Doctoral dissertation, Arizona State University, 1976.
30. Taylor, G. Predicted versus actual response to spinal cord injury: A psychological study. Doctoral dissertation, University of Minnesota, 1967.
31. Trieschmann, R. *Spinal Cord Injuries: The Psychological, Social, and Vocational Adjustment.* Pergamon Press, Elmsford, N.Y., 1980.
32. Trieschmann, R. and Sand, P. WAIS and MMPI correlates of increasing renal failure in adult medical patients. *Psychol. Rep., 29:*1251–1262, 1971.
33. Trieschmann, R., and Willems, E. Behavioral programs for the physically dsabled. In: D. Glenwick and L. Jason (Eds.), *Behavioral Community Psychology: Progress and Prospects.* Edited by Glenwick, D., and Jason, L. Praeger Publishing Corporation, New York, 1980.
34. Wilcox, E., and Stauffer, S. Follow-up of 423 consecutive patients admitted to the spinal cord center, Rancho Los Amigos Hospital, 1 January to 31 December, 1967. *Paraplegia, 10:*115–122, 1972.
35. Wright, B. *Physical Disability—A Psychological Approach.* Harper and Row, New York, 1960.

36. Young, J., Burns, P., Bowen, A., and McCutchen, R. *Spinal Cord Injury Statistics: Experience of the Regional Spinal Cord Injury Systems.* Good Samaritan Medical Center, Phoenix, 1982.
37. Young, J. Personal communication, February 7, 1984.
38. Zubek, J., editor. *Sensory Deprivation: fifteen years of research.* Appleton-Century-Crofts, New York, 1969.

13

Physical Therapy in Spinal Cord Injury

M. DECKER
A. HALL

In this chapter the physiotherapy management of the spinal cord injured patient is reviewed in relation to range of motion (ROM), spasticity, muscle strength, cardiorespiratory and muscle endurance, and gait and wheelchair ambulation (wheelchair skills). The first section looks briefly at each of these topics in the context of the total rehabilitation process. The second section explores theoretical and practical aspects of assessment and training in relation to each topic. Technical information of a "how to" nature, already available in a number of comprehensive texts (22, 61), is not included in this chapter.

OVERVIEW OF MOTOR REHABILITATION

The rehabilitation process begins with the patient's admission to the hospital and ends with successful community reintegration. It consists of four phases that may vary depending on factors such as the level of the spinal cord injury, the presence of associated injuries, and the medical complications. Key aspects of this process, from a physiotherapy perspective, are described.

Phase One

Following spinal cord injury, loss of function occurs as a result of neurological damage and immobilization. Although the period of immobilization has been greatly reduced with improved methods of vertebral stabilization and general medical care, it is not uncommon for the patient to be bedridden for 2 to 6 weeks or longer (40, 142). This results in deterioration of the musculoskeletal and cardiorespiratory systems (54, 70, 75, 118, 133). It is estimated that complete immobilization in healthy individuals can result in up to 20% loss of muscle strength per week (133) and in significant loss in joint mobility (75).

One of the principal aims of physiotherapy in this phase of rehabilitation is to minimize the negative effects of immobilization. This is accomplished through the early institution of a controlled exercise program (22, 57, 61, 106, 108, 121, 133). The type and intensity of exercise used in this phase is limited by the stability of the fracture site, the confines of the physical setting, the patient's general medical status, and the adaptability of equipment. These considerations generally prevent active training of the cardiorespiratory system in this phase beyond what can be accomplished through breathing exercises. Treatment emphasis is therefore initially on maintenance of range of motion (ROM) and muscle strength. Precise exercise protocols for this phase have yet to be established and evaluated as to their relative safety and effectiveness.*

Phase Two

Phase Two commences when the patient is able to sit out of bed. Specific long-term functional goals are developed, and exercise programs aimed at achieving these goals are initiated. For the majority of patients, wheelchair independence is an important goal. Training in basic wheelchair skills (or wheelchair ambulation) is, therefore, started as soon as possible so that the patient can quickly become independent within the hospital setting.

As patients tolerate longer periods of sitting and increased levels of activity, strength training is intensified and cardiorespiratory training is begun. Strength and endurance training become increasingly important since low levels of fitness may interfere with optimal participation in the rehabilitation program (74). For some patients, training may continue to be limited with respect to the type and intensity of exercise permitted, particularly if there are ongoing medical problems.

Spasticity often emerges during this phase as spinal shock wanes. With severe spasticity, there is increased risk of developing contractures and increased interference with function. ROM must be carefully monitored and exercise programs adapted as necessary to ensure maintenance of mobility.

Gait training may begin in a limited fashion. This involves preliminary orthostatic training in standing using the tilt table and balance training in the parallel bars. If required, patients may be fitted with braces.

Phase Three

The third phase of rehabilitation involves intensive training of strength, endurance, and functional skills prior to discharge. Patients are encouraged to participate in appropriate community activities and home visits so their

---

* Prevention and treatment of respiratory complications is an important part of physiotherapy management in this phase of rehabilitation. Since this topic is dealt with in detail in Chapter 3, it is not discussed here.

developing skills can be applied in everyday situations. These outings frequently provide a focus for further functional training.

Specific advanced skills, such as wheelchair ambulation and gait, receive increasing emphasis. Walking candidates and patients expected to master advanced wheelchair skills require high levels of fitness.

Various sports activities are often introduced as a means of maintaining fitness levels following discharge. This can be an important aspect of in-hospital rehabilitation (56, 137).

Phase Four

The postdischarge or community reintegration phase is the most challenging and important part of the rehabilitation program. In this phase, the physiotherapist plays a supportive role, providing information and periodic consultation. Reassessments provide an opportunity for exchange of information and monitoring of patient-family progress. Patients requiring continued training in specific problem areas may receive outpatient or home-care services.

Maintenance of achieved gains in all areas is essential for the long-term success of rehabilitation. Nilsson et al (104) recommend that specifically designed exercise programs be continued indefinitely after discharge. Although some community resources, such as fitness centers, have recently begun to modify their facilities so that they can be utilized by the disabled, there is, in general, a lack of appropriate facilities. This lack, coupled with transportation and financial problems, often makes it difficult for spinal cord injured patients to maintain continuity in their training (92). Continued interest in sports for the disabled—particularly at the competitive level—may have a positive impact on future development in this area.

ASPECTS OF ASSESSMENT AND TRAINING

Range of Motion

Adequate range of motion (ROM) or mobility is essential for the performance of everyday activities. Following spinal cord injury, minor limitations in ROM (due to soft tissue contractures) can result in critical loss of functional potential and prolonged hospitalization (22, 41, 57). The two key aims of ROM programs are: (a) to prevent the development of contractures, and (b) to achieve and maintain a target ROM.

Adaptive shortening or soft tissue contracture occurs when normal joint motion is restricted (10, 75, 76). Actual changes in connective tissue architecture develop when the restriction is prolonged. If the restriction persists unopposed, a significant loss in ROM can be seen within one week (75, 76). Further restriction may result in the development of "fixed" contractures, leading to permanent deformity (75, 76).

The spinal cord injured patient is at risk for the development of contractures, not only as a result of loss of voluntary movement but also as a consequence of muscle imbalance (i.e., loss of the normal agonist-antagonist relationship). Muscle imbalance occurs when spasticity in one muscle group acts unopposed on a joint or when there is a significant difference in the strength of opposing muscle groups acting on a joint. Patients with mid-cervical injuries, for example, may develop elbow flexion but lack control of extension (41, 57). Similarly, high-level quadriplegics often develop soft tissue contractures in their hands as spasticity in the finger flexors is unopposed by voluntary finger extension (57). In all patients, factors such as sensory loss, edema, and impaired circulation may contribute to the development of contractures (75).

Because it is easier to prevent the process of adaptive shortening than it is to restore ROM once a contracture has developed, prevention is a treatment priority (75, 76). Once a contracture has developed, relatively large forces must be applied to restore ROM (75). The forces required to overcome a contracture could result in a bone fracture, particularly in patients with osteoporosis (a common complication in spinal cord injury).

The second aim of the ROM program is to achieve and maintain a target ROM for each joint. The target or optimum range is determined on an individual basis depending on the patient's anticipated functional needs and patterns of residual muscle activity. In some cases, this range may be greater or less than that considered normal. In the C6 quadriplegic, for example, a slight degree of soft tissue shortening in the finger flexors is encouraged as it permits the development of a functional tenodesis grip. Attempts to achieve normal mobility of the wrist and fingers would, in this case, have a negative impact on function. Greater-than-normal mobility in the hamstrings, on the other hand, is often considered desirable in paraplegics because this allows certain functional skills, such as dressing, to be performed with greater ease.

Assessment

An initial assessment of ROM is carried out in the first phase in order to establish a baseline measure of mobility. Subsequent assessments are carried out at varying intervals in order to monitor the effectiveness of the ROM program.

Joint range is commonly measured as degrees of motion using tools such as the goniometer or Leighton flexometer. In some cases, however, visual "guesstimation" alone is used, as problems related to patient positioning and handling of spastic or flaccid limbs limit the practical usefulness of other methods.

Although the ability to develop appropriate and effective ROM programs depends partly on the ability to measure ROM accurately, none of the current methods of measurement has been studied to determine its reliability in the spinal cord injured population. Studies involving other patient groups suggest that reliability varies according to which joints are being measured and by whom (19, 37, 83).

ROM Exercises

Management of ROM involves the use of appropriate positioning techniques (including splinting) and ROM exercises (1, 22, 48, 57, 61, 81). Both of these are generally instituted as soon as possible following injury.

ROM exercises may be active, passive, or assisted movements, depending on the presence (or absence) and relative power of voluntary muscle activity. When voluntary control is inadequate to move the joint through the desired range, passive movements are used. In the initial phase of rehabilitation, these are carried out by members of the rehabilitation team or by the patient's family following instruction. During Phases Two and Three, paraplegics learn to carry out their own ROM exercises while quadriplegics may require some degree of assistance indefinitely.

The guidelines for performing ROM exercises evolved on the basis of clinical experience and have changed little over the past 25 years. It is generally recommended that they be performed two to three times daily in the acute phase and once daily thereafter (1, 22, 48, 57, 61, 81). This involves movement of all limb joints through a full ROM (i.e., within the limits permitted by the level of injury and stability of the fracture site).

In recent years, the use of ROM exercises in the acute phase has been questioned by some authors. These authors suggest that early, intensive ROM exercises may be a precipitating factor in the onset of heterotopic ossification (24, 131). Although it has been suggested (50) that this risk can be minimized by using a cautious, gentle approach whenever the paralyzed limbs are handled, there have been no clinical studies exploring this issue or validating the traditional ROM exercise regime.

Stretching to Increase ROM

If soft tissue shortening occurs or contractures develop, it may be necessary to stretch the involved areas. Several stretching techniques exist, including ballistic or small bouncing movements and slow static stretch (96, 122). In patients with spasticity, slow static stretching is most often used because it is less likely to result in damage to soft tissues or to stimulate further increases in spasticity (107). Studies involving flexibility in the able-bodied have shown slow static stretching to be the safest and most effective method of increasing ROM (33, 76, 122).

Spasticity

Our understanding and management of spasticity have improved in recent years*; however, spasticity continues to be a significant problem for many spinal cord patients. If severe, it can result in the development of contrac-

---

* See Chapter 10 for a detailed discussion on the neurophysiology, drug therapy and surgical management of spasticity.

tures and can interfere with many aspects of function, including gait. Although easily recognized in the clinic, there is no universally accepted definition of spasticity. Spasticity has been described as: (a) hyperactive tonic stretch reflexes (125), (b) hyperactive phasic stretch reflexes; and (c) clonus (16, 35).

In Phase One, spasticity is not often a problem as the patient is likely to be in a state of spinal shock, during which time deep tendon reflexes and stretch reflexes are absent. During Phase Two, flexor spasticity (thought to be mediated by flexor reflex afferents) may begin to appear (16, 93). Extensor spasticity (thought to be mediated by the muscle spindles) may develop in Phases Two or Three, and it often becomes predominant (16, 93).

In general, spasticity is treated only if it is severe enough to interfere with function or prevent maintenance of ROM. Severity appears to be related to: (a) the type of spasticity (108); (b) the completeness of the lesion; and (c) the level of the lesion. In addition, the degree of severity may vary from day-to-day depending on the presence of nociceptive sensations such as urinary tract infections, decubiti, bowel impactions, muscle tears or strains, heterotopic ossification, deep vein thrombosis, or contractures. Simple everyday irritations such as tight clothes, leg bags or condoms, improper body position, or improperly inflated cushions, may also increase spasticity (93).

Measurement

Spasticity is usually evaluated subjectively in the clinical setting. This involves testing and grading of stretch reflexes and assessment of the response of specific muscle groups to various stimuli, including passive movement. Simple classification systems such as that described by Merrit (93) (i.e., spasticity is: (a) observable; (b) moderately troublesome; (c) discomforting; or (d) a major obstacle) are widely used. Although there are limitations to the validity and reliability of subjective measurement, no clinically useful alternatives have yet been developed. Many researchers have attempted to assess spasticity objectively by measuring resistance to passive motion using electrogoniometers, potentiometers, torque meters, and strain gauges. In a review article Bajd and associates (4) noted that the equipment seems to be overly complex and of limited usefulness. Other objective measurement systems that have been investigated include polarized light goniometry and myotonometry (60). The latter is a system that permits quantitative measurement of static and dynamic muscle spindle activity during muscle elongation (60). This method may be useful in some specific clinical settings but is not widely applicable.

Treatment Methods

The lack of an adequate means of measurement has impeded attempts to evaluate the effectiveness of various forms of therapy used in spasticity management. Of the many interventions currently used by physiotherapists to reduce spasticity, none has been conclusively demonstrated to have a significant and lasting effect. Very often a combination of different treatment techniques is used. Some of the interventions used in patients with complete spinal cord injuries include:

1. Prolonged stretching. This is done manually or through the use of equipment such as the tilt table. Stretching is thought to decrease the gamma bias of the muscle spindle, resulting in reduced sensitivity of the muscle to stretch (16). Odeen and associates (107) recently reported a 32% reduction in resistance to passive movement at the ankle following an hour on the tilt table with the ankle held in 15° of dorsiflexion. The effect lasted only 2 to 3 hours, which might be adequate time to practice or perform functional maneuvers.

2. Cooling. Prolonged application of ice to spastic muscle groups is thought, by some, to depress sensitivity of the muscle spindle, thereby reducing gamma activity (2, 34). Knuttson, however, has suggested that cooling facilitates the alpha motor neuron and may, in fact, increase alpha spasticity (73).

3. Postural changes. Simple postural changes may be effective in decreasing spasticity for brief periods of time. Reasons for this are unknown but may have the effect of stretching spastic muscle groups or altering a nociceptive sensation.

4. Functional Electric Stimulation (FES). FES elicits contractions in extrafusal muscle fibers but not in higher threshold intrafusal fibers. This may result in "unloading" of the muscle spindles (73) such that strong contractions of spastic muscles may be followed by periods of reduced spasticity (12).

In addition to these interventions, the following methods are sometimes used in treating patients with incomplete spinal cord injuries: reciprocal activation, proprioceptive neuromuscular facilitation (hold-relax techniques) (72), and high or low frequency mechanical vibration (8, 15).

Generally, a trial and error approach is used to find the most effective interventions. In the pyramidal approach to spasticity management described by Merrit (93) (Fig. 13.1), conservative approaches, such as prolonged stretching, are attempted first. Treatments indicated at the higher levels of the pyramid are used only when lower level interventions are ineffective. Spasticity management must include practical consideration of long-term control, particularly during Phase Four. For example, time-consuming stretching programs may be an unrealistic long-term solution for some patients but a viable option for others.

Muscle Strength

Muscle strength is a critical factor in functional outcome following spinal cord injury. In order to maximize the patient's full potential, optimal strength levels must be achieved as early as possible and then maintained.

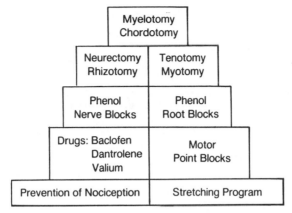

Figure 13.1. Conceptual approach to the management of spasticity. (after Merrit (93))

Preliminary strength training generally begins in a limited fashion in Phase One, as soon as it is medically safe to do so. The aim, in this phase, is to minimize strength loss while the patient is on bed rest. During Phases Two and Three, training is progressively intensified as the patient's condition permits. In Phase Four the emphasis is on long-term maintenance of achieved gains.

In spite of the importance of strength training for spinal cord injury patients, there has been very little research carried out in this area. Principles and methods of training are based primarily on work involving the able-bodied. Special problems, such as training of partially denervated muscles and training of patients with different levels and types of injuries, have not been fully explored.

Assessment

An initial evaluation of the patient's muscle strength is carried out in Phase One. The purpose of this evaluation is to determine whether individual limb muscles are functioning within normal limits and to provide an estimate of strength of innervated and partially innervated muscles. This information is used in planning the strength training program and provides a basis for monitoring neurological recovery in patients with incomplete lesions. Subsequent evaluations are carried out at regular intervals in order to monitor patient progress.

Accuracy and reliability of muscle strength assessment in the spinal cord injured patient may be affected by several factors including limitations in positioning the patient, limitations in the level and type of resistance that can be applied (particularly in the initial phase), and limitations in the patient's ability to cooperate with testing due to pain, fear, and sensory impairment. These issues and the actual methods used to assess strength in spinal cord injured patients have been poorly researched.

The method of strength assessment used most widely in the clinical setting is the manual muscle test (88, 111). This is an inexpensive (i.e., no equipment), easily applied test that involves subjective evaluation of individual muscles or groups of muscles. The strength of contraction is scored using a 0 (absent) to 5 (normal) rating scale (British MRC system). The limitations of this test include the fact that it has not been shown to be either valid or reliable, and it does not provide a means of assessing change within each level (88, 120).

In a recent review of strength testing in the lower-limb disabled, Davis and associates (31) include repetitive weight lifting, static cable tensiometry, hand grip dynamometry, and isokinetic testing in a list of techniques used to evaluate strength. These authors state that isokinetic testing is "probably the best available technique for the assessment of muscle function (31)." This method is becoming increasingly popular in strength testing as it permits objective, quantitative measurement and recording of muscle function (i.e., torque and angular velocity), and eliminates many of the problems associated with other measurement techniques (38, 95). Unfortunately, the cost of isokinetic equipment is high, and it is, therefore, not yet available in most clinical settings.

Strength Training Methods

Principles. In order to increase strength, the neuromuscular system must be subjected to an overload, that is, a stimulus greater than that provided by everyday activity (33, 79, 99, 130). This results in physiological changes or a training effect within the neuromuscular system. These changes include increased cross-sectional area of muscle fiber (specifically type II fibers) (3, 118, 120), increased metabolic capacity (i.e., increased concentration of ATP and CP) (51), and increased myofibrillar proteins (3, 79, 118). An increase in muscle bulk (hypertrophy) also occurs (49, 51). As the system adapts to each new level of demand, a progressively greater stimulus must be applied in order to achieve increases in strength. The expected rate of strength gain during training is related to the intensity, frequency, and duration of training, the type of training undertaken, the muscle groups being trained, and the strength of the muscles at the onset of training.

Neural adaptation (or learning) accounts, in part, for the strength gains achieved during training (33, 79, 98, 123). At advanced levels of strength training, programs must be geared specifically to the skills to be performed in order to optimize the training response associated with neural adaptation.

Type and Intensity of Training. Various types of exercise regimes can be used to increase strength, assuming that the basic principles of training are followed. Factors influencing the type and intensity of training undertaken during spinal cord rehabilitation include the specific goals to be achieved, the site and stability of the lesion, the muscles being trained, the presence of complicating factors (i.e., osteoporosis, spasticity), and the availability or adaptability of equipment. Although strength training methods have been extensively studied in the able-bodied, there have been no comprehensive investigations of these methods in the spinal cord injured population. As a result, our ability to prescribe safe and effective exercise programs for patients in each phase of rehabilitation may not be optimal.

Strength training methods can be classified as static, dynamic or isokinetic depending on the type of muscle contraction involved (135). Each method has its own particular advantages and disadvantages in terms of effectiveness, time required for training, equipment required, and associated risks (79). Static and dynamic training tend to be used most extensively in spinal cord rehabilitation since the cost of isokinetic equipment, as noted previously, is high. Static training methods are often used in the early stages of rehabilitation as a means of maintaining strength and are used in neck and trunk strengthening during the period of vertebral immobilization. Daily performance of a few, brief, submaximal contractions is reported to be effective in preventing muscle atrophy during bed rest (3, 33). It can be difficult to ensure that a safe and effective training level is achieved, since the intensity of contraction can only be estimated.

To increase strength using static contractions in training, progressively higher workloads must be used. Daily performance of several static contractions at 50% to 70% of the maximal static strength is reported to be an optimal training level for untrained individuals (3). A stimulus as low as 35% of maximal strength, however, is reported to be adequate to achieve a training effect initially (33). Advanced training, using static contractions, involves performance of a series of single maximal contractions of a few seconds duration (33, 97, 123).

Dynamic strength training can involve many different combinations of intensity and repetitions. Opinions vary as to which is the most effective approach (13, 43, 109, 123, 135). The progressive resistance exercise (PRE) system developed by DeLorme and Watkins (32) in 1948 for training disabled soldiers is widely used today. This system requires the individual to perform three sets of exercises, each consisting of 10 repetitions. The first set is performed at ½ 10 RM*, the second at ¾ 10 RM, and the third at 10 RM. The resistance used is progressively increased so that no more than 10 repetitions can be performed. Determination of an individual's 10 RM is basically a matter of trial and error.

Another approach to dynamic strength training is the program described by Berger (13). This involves performance of three sets of four to eight maximal contractions. Variations of this system and the PRE program are

---

* 10 RM—the maximum weight that can be lifted ten times.

often used in spinal cord rehabilitation. A program described by Ofir and associates (108) requires paraplegic patients to perform three sets of six contractions at ⅔ 1 RM**, three times weekly in the initial stages of training and five times weekly as training progresses. Once per week, an additional 1 RM contraction with a 5 second static hold is also performed. Resistance is increased by 1.25 pounds per session where strength permits. In a recent paper Chawla and associates (26) describe a weight training program for paraplegics consisting of a series of exercises performed in sets of three with six repetitions per set. Although the authors do not state the exact intensity used (i.e., the percentage of the patient's maximum effort), they state that a gradual increase in resistance and decrease in repetition rate is used to provide a progressive overload.

Recent studies involving the able-bodied suggest that strength training at advanced skill levels should resemble the skills to be performed as closely as possible with respect to type of muscle contraction, velocity of contraction, force of contraction, pattern, and repetition rate (123). Sale and associates (123) suggest that failure to be specific in training can lead to wasted effort and inappropriate development of muscle mass; this can actually interfere with performance of skilled activities. In spinal cord injury rehabilitation the concept of specificity is applied to a certain extent during routine training of functional skills. Comprehensive analysis of the strength requirements of key functional tasks performed by spinal cord injured patients would improve our ability to match training and function with greater specificity.

Once adequate strength levels have been achieved, training programs to maintain strength can be carried out at a less intense level. However, everyday activity alone is not adequate to maintain strength. Ofir and co-workers (108) suggest that a weekly or biweekly exercise program, in addition to everyday activity, is adequate for strength maintenance in the spinal cord injured patient. Variation in everyday activity levels, however, may influence the type of long-term program required. Since low levels of strength and endurance have been reported in wheelchair users (30, 74, 104), it seems appropriate that the area of long-term maintenance be investigated more closely.

Resistance. Various methods are used to provide resistance in static and dynamic strength training programs. In patients with severe weakness, friction from a supporting surface or the resistance of gravity may provide an adequate training stimulus. These patients often train using slings or pulleys.

Manual resistance is commonly used early in rehabilitation when physical limitations prevent the use of other methods. Standard weight training equipment such as springs, free weights (including dumbbells, barbells,

---

** 1 RM—the maximum weight that can be lifted only once.

sandbags), and weighted pulleys are widely used, particularly in Phases Two, Three, and Four. Other devices frequently used include latissimus dorsi bars and sitting push-up blocks. The latter device trains muscle groups in a manner that simulates their functional use.

Electromyographic Biofeedback. Electromyographic (EMG) biofeedback is sometimes used in strength training programs for spinal cord injury patients. It is thought to enhance conventional training by increasing the patient's awareness of activity in specific muscles, particularly those with only partial innervation (9, 23, 101, 124, 140, 141).

Unfortunately, there is little objective information concerning the scope of application and effectiveness of biofeedback training in the spinal cord injured population. The literature is limited to a few case reports (23, 101, 124) and anecdotal accounts (7, 9, 140) that suggest a positive effect but are by no means conclusive.

In a recent case report, Nacht and associates (101) discuss some possible benefits of EMG biofeedback training during the acute phase of spinal cord injury. These authors suggest that it may contribute to the patient's psychological well-being by facilitating early, active participation in the rehabilitation process. They also hypothesize that strength levels may be better maintained during the period of immobilization if patients are made more aware of muscle activity through biofeedback. Baker and co-workers (7) add that in the acute phase of rehabilitation, EMG biofeedback helps to maintain patient interest in performing routine exercises, thereby facilitating efforts to maintain strength.

Electrical Stimulation in Strength Training of Paralyzed Muscles. In recent years investigators have attempted to use electrical stimulation as a means of restoring functional movement in the paralyzed muscles of patients (see section on gait) (6, 47, 78, 82, 116, 134). One of the early problems encountered in this area was that electrically stimulated muscles were unable to generate and maintain sufficient force to be functional (112). Physiological changes associated with prolonged disuse are thought to account for this (112, 134).

In order to improve the capacity of paralyzed muscles for functional contraction, special strength training programs involving prolonged electrical stimulation have been developed. Although work in this area is still in the developmental stages, preliminary results suggest that improvements in the strength and endurance characteristics of paralyzed muscles can be achieved (6, 55, 78, 112, 116, 132). This has been done using a variety of stimulation parameters and exercise protocols, none of which, as yet, has been compared in relation to effectiveness, safety, and long-term outcome.

In a recent article Gruner and associates (55) discuss the use of resistance in electrical training of paralyzed muscles and note that blood pressure control and thermoregulation require special consideration in this type of training.

Endurance

Endurance training for the spinal cord injured patient is directed at both the cardiorespiratory system and spared peripheral musculature. Both types of training are functionally oriented (30). The goal of endurance training is to increase the amount of work the patient can perform before fatiguing. Assessment and training methods are modeled after those used in the able-bodied population but have been adapted to the unique physical limitations of the spinal cord injured population (30). In this context they remain largely untested. Despite this, the benefits of endurance training for the spinal cord injured patient are significant enough that programs should be included in increasing intensity in each of the four phases of rehabilitation.

Physiological Background

Cardiorespiratory and peripheral endurance training involve training the energy systems of the body. These energy systems include the ATP-CP system (anaerobic, aerobic), the lactic acid system, and the oxygen system (aerobic) (3, 16, 79, 90, 126). Cardiorespiratory endurance training is aimed at improving the efficiency of oxygen transport, i.e., the ability of the heart to deliver oxygenated blood (heart rate and stroke volume). Peripheral endurance training is aimed at increasing the ability of the muscle to extract oxygen from the blood (maximum oxygen uptake, hereafter referred to as $\dot{V}O_2$ max.) (3).

Due to the nature of the disability in spinal cord injury, endurance can also be limited by reduced ventilatory capacity or weakness in spared peripheral musculature (3). Specific muscle endurance training for the involved muscles (diaphragm and arm musculature) is necessary. The most limiting factor must be identified and trained first. For example, endurance and strength training of the arm musculature of the spinal cord injured patient must occur before these muscles will be able to work long enough and at loads great enough to produce training effects in the cardiorespiratory system.

Assessment

In Phase One, endurance training will be directed at improving muscle endurance and will consist of breathing exercises, incentive inspirometry and arm exercises. In Phase Two, the patient is assessed to establish the present level of endurance and to identify limiting factors. Initially, upper extremity training programs will be a skill-learning experience until arm muscle endurance has increased to a point where training changes can occur. Cardiorespiratory endurance training is only effective if it is carried out at 75% to 80% of the anaerobic threshold or the point at which the maximum amount of oxygen is being extracted from the blood and an oxygen debt begins to accumulate ($\dot{V}O_2$ max.) (3, 85, 86, 90, 126). At this point there should be significant increases (50% greater than resting rates) in both heart rate and ventilation of low paraplegics and incomplete spinal cord injured patients, and to a lesser extent in high paraplegics and quadriplegics. In the able-bodied, an endurance training level can be established in the laboratory by measuring $\dot{V}O_2$ max. during a stress test or by measuring blood lactate levels (both will indicate anaerobic threshold), and then calculating a level at 75% to 80% of the anaerobic threshold (3). In the clinic, $\dot{V}O_2$ max. can be calculated from the Astrand nomogram or read directly off a chart derived from the nomogram (3). It can also be calculated with the three point or PWC-170 (physical work capacity) test (3). These test methods can be used for paraplegics if $\dot{V}O_2$ max. can be reached, but it may not be possible using only the small muscles of the upper extremities unless the paraplegic is already well-trained in muscle endurance and strength.

$\dot{V}O_2$ max. is a reliable assessment parameter, but the actual cardiorespiratory endurance training program will be monitored by the more easily used and fairly reliable measure of heart rate (3). The training heart rate range should be equivalent to a sub max. $\dot{V}O_2$ (75% to 80% of $\dot{V}O_2$ max.). For paraplegics, training heart rate can be calculated using maximum heart rate and the Karvonen formula (71, 85). It can be read from available tables of approximate values for the able-bodied or the following rule of thumb can be employed: training heart rate = 170 bpm (beats per minutes)–age. This latter method is the least accurate. Endurance training for paraplegics would be more accurate if a chart of approximate training heart rate values could be derived for this population.

Endurance training for the quadriplegic is further complicated by a compromised autonomic nervous system. Due to the lack of sympathetic control over the heart, maximum attainable heart rates for quadriplegics will be around 110 to 120 bpm; therefore, heart rate is a poor parameter for testing or monitoring cardiorespiratory endurance training programs (104, 139). For instance, the training heart rate for an able-bodied 20-year-old $(170 - 20 = 150 \text{ bpm})$ cannot be attained by the same 20-year-old quadriplegic. The lowered heart rate of a quadriplegic, in fact, may not allow the heart to be stressed adequately to produce changes in the cardiorespiratory system (30). However, it could be possible that, although we are unable to increase the heart rate beyond a certain level, changes may be occurring in the stroke volume. To date we are unable to measure such changes clinically if they do occur (30).

In the area of muscle endurance training, we are able to measure improvements in ventilatory capacity and can improve endurance characteristics of muscle (55, 132). Clinically we measure improvements in endurance by measuring increased time and work load.

Training

Type. Endurance training in spinal cord injured patients is primarily limited to the use of the upper extremities. This presents some unique problems because the cardiorespiratory system adapts only to the working muscles. In the able-bodied, exercising the large, well-vascularized muscles of the lower extremities will put enough stress on the cardiorespiratory system to achieve a training effect. In spinal cord injured patients, muscles below the level of the lesion are not under voluntary control and cannot be used for training. The relatively small-bulk, poorly vascularized muscles of the upper extremities, which are under volitional control, are able to do less work and produce less stress on the cardiorespiratory system. It is, therefore, more difficult to achieve training changes (65, 74). In the quadriplegic patient, even fewer muscles are available for use and the ability to stress the cardiorespiratory system through exercise decreases as the level of the lesion rises.

There are a number of reasons why the arm muscles cannot effect good training changes. The most significant are: (a) these muscles work well at high intensity for a short duration only and fatigue quickly; and (b) blood pooling in the nonworking lower extremities limits cardiac output that could potentially pick up and remove lactic acid from the working muscles. When lactate concentrations rise, the muscle fatigues (86).

Researchers are looking at the effectiveness of electric stimulation of the loaded quadriceps muscles of paraplegics and quadriplegics to elicit enough stress to produce changes in cardiorespiratory endurance (55, 113). This may become an effective training method in the future.

Cardiorespiratory and muscle endurance training programs for spinal cord injured patients are generally limited to the use of upper extremity modalities such as arm ergometers, wheelchair ergometers, free-wheeling, or rowing (30). Brattgard (20), Hildebrandt, and Marincek (87) have claimed that arm cycle ergometry is the most efficient method of increasing cardiorespiratory endurance. Glaser, Gandee (36), Beiner and Lundberg (84) claim that wheelchair ergometry is equally effective. Wicks (138) and Glaser (44, 45) have shown that for improvements to carry over to the task of wheeling, the training must be task specific. It therefore follows that, to be effective, endurance training should be carried out on a wheelchair ergometer for wheelers and on an arm ergometer for those who use a wheelchair unicycle for mobility.

Intensity. Activities of daily living have been shown to be inadequate to maintain the endurance level of a trained paraplegic (46, 66, 70) as it taxes only 15% to 24% of aerobic capacity (46, 66). To maintain endurance requires work at 50% to 60% of aerobic capacity; to effect changes requires 70% to 80%. Activities such as paraplegic ambulation with crutches (64% to 69% of aerobic capacity), vigorous basketball (46, 66), swimming (110), uphill wheeling (75%), and intensive distance wheeling will maintain trained levels (46, 66).

Frequency and Duration. The choice of continuous training or interval training depends on the goal to be achieved and the level of injury. The continuous training method would be preferable to train the O_2 transport system to pump larger quantitites of blood to the muscles in the able-bodied and in low thoracic and lumbar paraplegics. Training regime would be at 75% of $\dot{V}O_2$ max. on a daily basis (86). To increase the ability of the muscle to extract O_2 from the blood, the interval training method is superior. Training is at 90% of $\dot{V}O_2$ max. every second day (86). However, quadriplegics and high thoracic paraplegics will be limited to interval training due to fatigue of peripheral muscles, reduced vital capacity, and a compromised sympathetic nervous system (decreased heart rate and venous return). Interval training also more closely approximates activities of daily living. The goal of endurance training should be to improve the previously measured level or functional goal—not to reach predicted chart values or to compete with another individual.

Endurance training, for both muscle and cardiorespiratory systems, should be intensified in Phases Three and Four and may include sport as a training activity. Following discharge, endurance training should be continued indefinitely (104).

Summary of Endurance Training in the Spinal Cord Injured Patient. Low level paraplegics and incomplete cord injured patients are able to train using either the continuous (aerobic) or interval (anaerobic) training method.

The preferred method of cardiorespiratory and muscle endurance training for a quadriplegic or a high thoracic paraplegic is interval training. This is so because this method best meets the needs of the small muscles of the upper extremities that are solely available for use. Because lactic acid develops rapidly in these muscles, the patient will require longer and more frequent rest periods than an individual using the muscles of his legs. Anaerobic activity also more closely approximates the high intensity, short duration functional activities of the patient. Cardiorespiratory training of the quadriplegic and high paraplegic is also limited by lowered vital capacity of the lungs and lowered exercise heart rate. Over time, interval training will improve vital capacity and FEV1. This can be measured by spirometry. At present, we are unable to easily measure changes in stroke volume, but training may still be occurring. Improvements in muscle endurance are measured in time and work load. Subjectively, quadriplegics will complain of less shortness of breath and will be able to wheel themselves for longer distances and so will have achieved their functional goals (30, 31).

Ambulation

Theoretical Considerations

"Will I ever walk again?" is probably the first question asked by most new spinal cord injured patients. Stauffer (128) states that some patients regard the ability to walk, with or without mechanical assists, as successful rehabilitation. Successful rehabilitation would better be described as the achievement of functional and vocational independence, whether it be in a wheelchair or in braces. The physiotherapist, when faced with the question "Will I ever walk again?", must decide if walking is a realistic goal for the patient. Literature on the subject of ambulation for the spinal cord injured divides patients into the following categories:

1. Nonambulators,
2. Standing used only as an exercise,
3. Household ambulators, and
4. Community ambulators (69, 128).

The criteria for successful community ambulation has remained relatively unchanged since Munro (100) defined it in 1948 as pertaining to a patient who can wear his braces all day, can walk 1000 yards nonstop, can climb and descend stairs, and is independent in activities of daily living. A literature review shows that patients with lesions at T2 and up fall into the category of nonambulators, while patients with lesions from T3 to T11 use braces for exercise or occasional walking only. With lesions from T12 to L2, patients may fall into either the household or community ambulator categories, depending on age, spasticity, contractures, endurance, pain, upper body strength, determination and the need to walk (22, 61, 69, 119). Stauffer and Hussey (129) have provided the following key to ambulation:

1. A patient who has pelvic control, i.e., back extensors (quadratus lumborum) and abdominals (rectus abdominis), may walk using long leg braces and crutches.
2. A patient with some control of muscles crossing the hip joint (iliopsoas, adductors, sartorius, gluteus maximus) should walk a limited amount.
3. A patient with control of muscles crossing the knee joint (quadriceps) should walk all the time with short leg braces, perhaps with crutches or canes, and will not need a wheelchair.
4. A patient with control of muscles crossing the ankle joint (tibialis anterior and posterior) or hip extension (gluteus medius, gluteus maximus) should ambulate full time with short leg braces or no braces.

Based on these criteria the most successful ambulators will be patients with cauda equina injuries or those who have incomplete lesions with sensorimotor sparing (129).

North American follow-up studies (91, 102) indicate that, while many patients (74%) (102) are successfully trained in ambulation during rehabilitation, very few (7% to 16%) (94, 105) continue to walk following discharge. According to Rosman and Spira (119), there is an essential difference between walking in the low-stress rehabilitation environment, and walking while faced with the problems of everyday life.

It is of interest to note that European follow-up studies have not found such a high drop-out rate among their paraplegic ambulators. A recent report (136) indicates that 33% of their patients continue to walk after discharge. There are no immediately obvious reasons for this difference given that the equipment and training methods are similar; however it is possible that different social expectations and vocational needs are a factor (91).

Paraplegic ambulators cite the following reasons for discontinuing walking after discharge: (a) it is not practical, wheelchair use is easier; (b) the gait is too slow; (c) braces are too hard to put on; (d) braces do not seem to be safe; and (e) the energy cost is prohibitive (11, 28, 52, 67, 94, 103, 119). Most brace users (95%) felt that they should have had the opportunity to try crutch-walking for psychological value, but most agreed that the prescription of permanent braces should not automatically follow (28). Stauffer agrees with trial walking, stating that patients can always find someone who will brace them if their rehabilitation center will not, and that there are valid reasons to do so (28).

Energy cost and speed of walking appear to be the primary reasons that paraplegics do not continue walking after discharge. Benes compared a 15-yard walk for a paraplegic using braces and crutches to a sharp 4 minute run for an able-bodied individual (11). Walking from the car to the office has been compared to a vigorous game of squash (11). Gordon and Vanderwalde reported the rate of swing-through gait, in a study carried out in parallel bars, was 88 to 282 feet per minute compared to 264 to 484 feet per minute in the able-bodied. Energy requirements were found to be eight times the basal metabolic rate (BMR) (53). Cerny and Gordon demonstrated that paraplegic walking reaches only half the velocity of normals but requires a 50% increase in VO_2 and a 28% rise in heart rate over normals (52, 136). This means that paraplegic crutch-walking very quickly becomes a fatiguing, anaerobic activity. At the same time, wheeling for paraplegics compared favorably with the energy cost of walking in normals. Huang and associates (67) have published a literature survey of a number of studies indicating that the total energy cost of paraplegic crutch-walking rises from three times the BMR at a speed of 14 meters per minute to five times the BMR at 27 meters per minute (53). Physiologically, the work load of the arms during crutch-walking was calculated to be about 351 kcal/hr or the equivalent of a very heavy work load (36). The energy requirements of walking are directly proportional to the level of the spinal cord injury and increase significantly with inadequate bracing and advancing age (17).

Other than the ability to walk, a number of advantages have been attributed to attaining the upright, weight-bearing position. These advantages include maintaining the integrity of the long bones and preventing osteoporosis, reduced incidence of decubiti, reduced incidence of urinary tract infections and urinary calculi, reduced incidence of shoulder complications secondary to wheelchair use, improved vocational expectations, increased level of independence, and improved psychological outlook (5, 21, 27, 28, 39, 46, 69, 91, 102, 136). Despite these claims there have been no well-controlled studies to show that standing, in fact, does result in all of these benefits.

Assessment and Training

Once the physiotherapist and the patient have agreed that ambulation is a realistic goal, very specific training is required to achieve that goal. In Phase Two of the rehabilitation program, the patient will begin pregait activities to strengthen the arms and upper body and to improve balance and coordination in preparation for standing and walking (25, 102). In Phases Two or Three the patient will be fitted with long-leg braces or other bracing as may be necessary. Proper fitting braces and shoes are absolutely essential for successful ambulation. The patient wearing long-leg braces should be able to stand and balance without assistance of any kind if the alignment of the braces is correct (68). Braces should not damage the skin. The type of long-leg braces most suitable for paraplegic gait continues to change with advancing orthotic technology (62–64). In 1984, plastic molded braces with enclosed side struts and sophisticated knee-locking mechanisms are being used. The most popular crutch is the lightweight aluminum forearm crutch with a molded adjustable hand grip.

When the braces fit correctly, the patient will learn in sequence the following activities:
1. putting on and adjusting braces,
2. parallel bar activities,
   –standing balance including head, trunk and pelvic control
   –rising and sitting
   –timing, balance and technique for swing-to, four-point, and swing-through gaits
3. all of the activities in 2. are repeated outside of the parallel bars,
4. side-stepping,
5. backward-stepping,
6. ambulation on uneven surfaces,
7. stairs (the ability of the patient to tilt his pelvis allows him to negotiate stairs),
8. ramps, curbs, doors, car transfers,
9. safe falling,
10. rising from the floor or ground (22, 69, 100, 139).

It is not likely that patients will continue walking after discharge unless they are able to use their braces for 8 hours a day (including stairs) and can ambulate nonstop for 500 meters (28, 102).

In recent years, gait training has generally occurred in Phase Three of rehabilitation. While this is appropriate for the incomplete or cauda equina patient, training the paraplegic to crutch-walk may be more successful 1 or

2 years after discharge from the hospital. The disadvantages of a late ambulation program are primarily physiological. Osteoporosis, muscle shortening, and ligamentous stretching may have developed and could impede training. However, by this time a paraplegic is stronger, better acquainted with his physical capabilities, more realistic regarding the need to walk for vocational or other purposes, and fully cognizant of the cost in time, energy, and money. The result of training at this stage seems to be that patients become better crutch-walkers in a shorter period of time and, more importantly, that they continue to walk over longer periods of time.

The most controversial issue regarding ambulation for the spinal cord injured patient is who should have braces and crutches prescribed for walking. The literature agrees on the probable advantages of standing and walking and on the physical capabilities required to learn to walk. There is also agreement that the percentage of persons who continue to ambulate following discharge is extremely low, even lower in North America than in Europe. From that point it appears that two distinctly different rationales for prescribing braces have evolved. One rationale states that most or all patients who could theoretically learn to crutch-walk should be given the opportunity to try, even though they may subsequently give it up (28, 91, 102, 129). The opposing viewpoint argues that too many braces are prescribed, given the high cost in man-hours and money expended, and the low percentage of successful community ambulators (91, 94). They state further that there are no generally accepted criteria for prescribing braces (94). Each spinal cord rehabilitation unit is probably resolving this highly debatable issue on an individual basis.

Functional Electric Stimulation

The use of functional electric stimulation, briefly mentioned in the discussion on strength, has been used to assist gait retraining for years. Bajd and associates (5, 6) have used two- and four-channel stimulators for standing and walking paraplegics. Brindley (21) implanted electrodes on the femoral nerve and ambulated patients using a finger switch. Turk (132) reported changes in the properties of muscle following a program of intermittent, isotonic contractions at low frequency. Kralj and Bajd (77) have paraplegics walking who are using self-controlled hand switches to successfully trigger four or six channels of electric stimulation. They have demonstrated how preserved reflex mechanisms of the transected spinal cord can be incorporated with electrical stimulation into functional gait (77).

However, the combination of electrical stimulation and microprocessor technology (neural prosthetics) is an exciting field, which, over the past 10 years has introduced a new concept of paraplegic and quadriplegic ambulation. Petrofsky and Phillips (114, 115, 117) have been developing a five-stage walking system. Their work is based on the assumption that the peripheral nervous system is intact and muscle is healthy, though atrophied from disuse. Their five-stage program consists of:

Stage 1: the development of a closed-loop feedback ambulation control system. This includes a means of sensing movement, and a connection of that movement to the thought process.

Stage 2: the development of free balance and smooth walking.

Stage 3: the development of an obstruction-clearance, anti-trip system.

Stage 4. the development of a portable system.

Stage 5. the development and testing of implantable systems.

Training equipment to improve the condition of bone and muscle has already been developed and is commercially available to patients and rehabilitation centers. Testing is being carried out to evaluate stress and conditioning effects on the muscles and long bones of long-standing spinal cord injured persons (55, 77).

Marsolais and Kobetic (89) have developed an implantable, multichannel, programmable microprocessor-controlled stimulator for walking. They have successfully ambulated patients using implanted electrodes that have been maintained for up to 2 years. These patients ambulate using walkers, and are able to climb and descend stairs using two railings.

While present approaches to electrically stimulated ambulation are encouraging, Coburn suggests that research in this field is just now beginning to utilize the full potential of preserved neurophysiological mechanisms (27).

Wheelchair Ambulation

During rehabilitation the patient learns to handle and maneuver a wheelchair in various settings. The level of independence achieved is related to the patient's level of injury, strength, endurance, age, and motivation. In addition, environmental factors related to wheelchair accessibility affect independence.

Patients generally begin to learn wheelchair skills in Phase Two. Initially, training focuses on acquisition of sitting balance and basic skills such as handling brakes and moving the chair in an area relatively free of obstacles. The patient learns how to relieve pressure over the ischial tuberosities and how to move within the chair without loss of balance (22). All of these skills differ subtly depending on the level of the injury and the type of wheelchair being used. Relatively low levels of strength and endurance in this phase usually limit acquisition of more advanced skills.

In most cases, the decision to select either a manual or electric wheelchair is made in Phase Two. This is not always a clear-cut process. Long-term use of manual wheelchairs by some patients, for example, has been associated with an increased incidence of shoulder joint dysfunction (103). On the other hand, manual wheelchair use is reported to have a positive effect on the cardiorespiratory system and may help to maintain patient fitness (30). In determining whether a manual or electric wheelchair will be used, consideration must be given to these issues and to other equally important factors such as energy expenditure, accessibility of home, car, and place of work, monetary expense, and overall functional requirements of the patient.

By Phase Three strength and endurance have improved, allowing the patient to learn more advanced skills. For quadriplegics this includes as many as possible of the following skills: car transfers, bed-to-chair and chair-to-bed transfers, getting into upright sitting, and handling the armrests, armrest locks, caster locks, foot straps, and foot plates. In addition to these skills, paraplegics (and some low-level quadriplegics) learn to fall in the chair without falling out or causing bodily injury, to perform "wheelies," to maneuver in the "wheelie" position over smooth and rough ground, and to ascend and descend curbs and inclines. Patients generally learn more than one technique for these more difficult skills. Some quadriplegics may learn flips, enabling the wheelchair to be moved over low objects. Prior to discharge, paraplegics learn to perform chair-to-floor and floor-to-chair transfers, to right the chair and get back in after a fall, and to jump-shift the chair. Young, active paraplegics may learn to descend four or more stairs independently in their chairs. All patients learn the proper procedure for one or two able-bodied persons to transport them, in their chair, up and down a flight of stairs. It is important that patients understand simple wheelchair maintenance such as lubricating and maintaining wheels and bearings in good condition and proper alignment. Most paraplegics are capable of carrying out simple maintenance independently.

Following discharge, patients continue to refine and improve their wheelchair skills. There is little objective information available concerning either optimal wheeling techniques or the adaptation of wheelchair skills to changing wheelchair designs (127). Therefore, the experience of previous patients is often a valuable source of practical information to both in-patients and therapists. Interaction between in-patients and discharged patients is encouraged in order to capitalize on this.

Recent interest in wheelchair design, reflected in journals such as "Paraplegia News" and "Sports 'N' Spokes," has evolved (in part) out of the growing interest in sports for the disabled. Wheelchairs designed specifically for use in sports, such as racing and basketball, are increasingly in demand (42, 80). As well, the design of everyday wheelchairs has undergone considerable change in recent years. The primary changes include the move to ultra-light weight and improved functional design. Increased availability of different types and styles of chairs has increased the difficulty involved in selecting a chair. Presently, this is basically a matter of subjective judgment and individual preference. However, one comprehensive study is attempting to compare functional design and efficiency among five commercially available wheelchairs (18).

REFERENCES

1. Abramson, A. S. Exercise in paraplegia. In: *Therapeutic exercise*, Third Ed. Edited by Basmajian, J. V. Williams & Wilkins, Baltimore, 1978, p. 307–324.
2. Arnell, P., and Beattie, S. A discussion on the physiological basis for and clinical appreciations of heat and cold in the treatment of hypertonicity. *J. Can. Physiother. Assoc., 24;(2):*61–67, 1972.
3. Astrand, O., and Rodahl, K. *Textbook of Work Physiology. Physiologic Basis of Exercise.* McGraw-Hill, New York, 1977, p. 339–353.
4. Bajd, T., and Bowman, B. Testing and modelling of spasticity. *J. Biomed. Eng., 4:*90–95, 1982.
5. Bajd, T., Kralj, A., Sega, J., Turk, R., Benko, H. and Strojnik, P. Use of a two-channel functional electrical stimulator to stand paraplegic patients. *Phys. Ther., 61:(4):*526–527, 1981.
6. Bajd, T., Kralj, A., Turk, R., Benko, H., and Sega, J. The use of a four-channel electrical stimulator as an ambulatory aid for paraplegic patients. *Phys. Ther., 63:*1116–1120, 1983.
7. Baker, M., Regenos, E., Wolf, S. L., and Basmajian, J. V. Developing strategies for biofeedback. Applications in neurologically handicapped patients. *Phys. Ther., 57:*402–408, 1977.
8. Barolat-Romana, G., and Davis, R. Neurophysiological mechanisms in abnormal reflex activities in cerebral palsy and spinal spasticity. *J. Neurol. Neurosurg. Psychiatry, 43:* 333–342, 1980.
9. Basmajian, J. V. Biofeedback in rehabilitation: a review of principles and practices. *Arch. Phys. Med. Rehabil., 62:*469–475, 1981.
10. Bassett, C. Effect of force on skeletal tissues. In: *Physiological Basis of Rehabilitation Medicine.* Edited by Downey, J. A., and Darling, R. C. W.B. Saunders Co., Toronto, 1971, pp. 283–316.
11. Benes, V. *Spinal Cord Injury.* Baillière Tindall, London, 1961.
12. Benton, L., Baker, L., Bowman, B., and Waters, R. *Functional Electrical Stimulation–A Practical Clinical Guide.* Rancho Los Amigos Rehabilitation Engineering Center, Rancho Los Amigos Hospital, Downey, California, 1981.
13. Berger, R. A. Optimum repetitions for the development of strength. *Res. Quart., 33:*334–338, 1962.
14. Bishop, B. Vibratory stimulation, Part I. *Phys. Ther., 54(12):*1273–1282, 1974.
15. Bishop, B. Vibratory stimulation, Part III. *Phys. Ther., 55(2):*139–143, 1975.
16. Bishop, B. Spasticity: it's physiology and management. *Phys. Ther., 57(4):*371–401, 1977.
17. Blessey, R. L., Hislop, H. J., Waters, R. L., and Antonelli, D. Metabolic energy cost of unrestrained walking. *Phys. Ther., 56(9):*1019–1024, 1976.
18. Bloch, R., and Sutton, J. *The Ergonomic Efficiency of Five Different Commercial Wheelchair Models.* Chedoke-McMaster Hospitals, Chedoke Hospital Division, Hamilton, Ontario, in preparation.
19. Boone, D., Azen, S., Lin, C., Spence, C., Baron, C., and Lee, L. Reliability of goniometric measurements. *Phys. Ther., 58:*1355–1360, 1978.
20. Brattgard, S. O., Grimby, G., and Hook, O. Energy expenditure and heart rate in driving a wheelchair ergometer. *Scand. J. Rehabil. Med., 2:*143–148, 1970.
21. Brindley, G. S., Polkey, C. E., and Rushton, C. N. Electrical splinting of the knee in paraplegia. *Paraplegia, 16(4):*428–435, 1979.
22. Bromley, I. *Tetraplegia and Paraplegia. A Guide for Physiotherapists.* Churchill Livingstone, Edinburgh, 1976.
23. Brudny, J., Korein, J., Grynbaum, B., Friedmann, L., Weinstein, S., Sachs-Frankel, G., and Belandres, P. EMG feedback therapy: review of treatment of 114 patients. *Arch. Phys. Med. Rehabil., 57:*55–61, 1976.
24. Chantraine, A., and Minaire, P. Para-osteo-arthropathies. *Scand. J. Rehabil. Med., 13:*31–37, 1981.

25. Chantraine, A. et al. Analysis of compensatory muscles during walking in paraplegic patients. *Scand. J. Rehabil. Med.*, 7:9–12, 1975.
26. Chawla, J. C., Bar, C., Creber, I., Price, J., and Andrews, B. Techniques for improving the strength and fitness of spinal injured patients. *Paraplegia*, 17:185–189, 1979–1980.
27. Coburn, B. Paraplegic ambulation: a systems point of view. *Int. Rehabil. Med.*, 6:19–24, 1984.
28. Coghlan, J. K., Robinson, C. E., Newmarch, B., and Jackson, G. Lower extremity bracing in paraplegia—a follow-up study. *Paraplegia*, 1:25–32, 1980.
29. Corston, R. N., Johnson, F., and Godwin-Austen, R. B. The assessment of drug treatment of spastic gait. *J. Neurol. Neurosurg. Psychiatry*, 4:1035–1039, 1981.
30. Davis, G. M., Kofsky, P. R., Kelsey, J. C., and Shephard, R. J. Cardio-respiratory fitness and muscular strength of wheelchair users. *C.M.A.J.*, 125:1317–1323, 1981.
31. Davis, G. M., Shephard, R. J., and Jackson, R. W. Cardio-respiratory fitness and muscular strength in the lower-limb disabled. *Can. J. Appl. Sport. Sci.*, 6:159–165, 1981.
32. DeLorme, T. L., and Watkins, A. L. Technics of progressive resistance exercise. *Arch. Phys. Med.*, 29:263, 1948.
33. deVries, H. A. *Physiology of Exercise for Physical Education and Athletics*, Third Ed. William C. Brown Company, Publishers, Dubuque, 1980, pp. 388–408.
34. Dietz, V., Quintern, J., and Berger, W. Electrophysiological studies of gait in spasticity and rigidity: evidence that altered mechanical properties of muscle contribute to hypertonia. *Brain*, 104:431–449, 1981.
35. Dimitrijevic, M. R., Nathan, P. W., and Sherwood, A. M. Clonus: the role of central mechanisms. *J. Neurol. Neurosurg. Psychiatry*, 43:321–332, 1980.
36. Dreisinger, T. E., and Londeree, B. R. Wheelchair exercise—a review. *Paraplegia*, 20(1):20–35, 1982.
37. Eckstrand, J., Wiktorsson, M., Oberg, B., and Gillquist, J. Lower extremity goniometric measurements: a study to determine their reliability. *Arch. Phys. Med. Rehabil.*, 63:171–175, 1982.
38. Elliott, J. Assessing muscle strength isokinetically. *J.A.M.A.*, 240(22):2408–2410, 1978.
39. Farmer, I. R., Poiner, R., Rose, G. K., and Patrick, J. H. The adult orlau swivel walker—ambulation for paraplegics and tetraplegics. *Paraplegia*, 20:248–254, 1982.
40. Flesch, J. R., Leider, L. L., Erickson, D. L., Chou, S. N., and Bradford, D. S. Harrington instrumentation and spine fusion for unstable fractures and fracture-dislocation of the thoracic lumbar spine. *J. Bone Joint Surg.* 59A:143–153, 1977.
41. Freehafer, A. Flexion and supination deformities of the elbow in tetraplegics. *Paraplegia*, 15:221–225, 1977–1978.
42. Gibson, B., Marshall, K., Smith, W. B., and Crase, N. The selection of sports wheelchairs: a survey of 1983 sports wheelchairs. *Paraplegia News*, 25:37, 1983.
43. Gillam, G., McKenzie. Effects of frequency of weight training on muscle strength enhancement. *J. Sports. Med. Phys. Fitness*, 21:432–436, 1981.
44. Glaser, R. M., and Collins, S. R. Validity of power output estimation for wheelchair locomotion. *Am. J. Phys. Med.*, 60(4):180–189, 1981.
45. Glaser, R. M., Foley, D. M. Laubach, L. L., and Suryaprasad, A. G. An exercise test to evaluate fitness for wheelchair activity. *Paraplegia*, 16(4):341–349, 1979.
46. Glaser, R. M., Sawka, M. N., Durbin, R. J., Foley, D. M., and Suryaprasad, A. G. Exercise programme for wheelchair activity. *Am. J. Phys. Med.*, 60(2):67–75, 1981.
47. Glenn, W. W., Holcomb, W. G., McLaughlin, A. J., O'Hare, J. M., Hogan, J. F., and Yasuda, R. Total ventilatory support in a quadriplegic patient with radiofrequency electrophrenic respiration. *N. Engl. J. Med.*, 286:513–516, 1972.
48. Goff, B. Physiotherapy in spinal cord lesions. In: *Neurology for Physiotherapists*. Edited by Cash, J. Faber and Faber, London, 1974, pp. 197–235.
49. Goldberg, A. L., Etlinger, J. D., Goldspink, D. F., and Jablecki, D. Mechanism of work-induced hypertrophy of skeletal muscle. *Med. Sci. Sports.*, 7:248–261, 1975.

50. Goldman, J. Heterotopic ossification in spinal cord injuries. *Physiotherapy, 66:*219–220, 1980.
51. Gonyea, W., and Sale, D. Physiology of weight lifting exercise. *Arch. Phys. Med. Rehabil., 63:*235–237, 1982.
52. Gordon, E. E. Physiological approach to ambulation in paraplegia. *J.A.M.A., 161(8):*686–688, 1956.
53. Gordon, E. E., and Vanderwalde, H. Energy requirements in paraplegic ambulation. *Arch. Phys. Med. Rehabil., 37:*276–285, 1956.
54. Greenleaf, J. E., and Kozlowski, S. Physiological consequences of reduced physical activity during bed rest. In: *Exercise and Sport Sciences Reviews.* Edited by Terjung, R. L. The Franklin Institute, Philadelphia, 1982, pp. 84–119.
55. Gruner, J. A., Glaser, R. M., Feinberg, S. D., Collins, S. R., and Nussbaum, N. S. A system for evaluation and exercise-conditioning of paralyzed leg muscles. *J. Rehabil. R. D. 20(1):*21–30, 1983.
56. Guttmann, L. *Textbook of Sport for the Disabled.* Oxford, Aylesburg: HM and M, 1976 from NLMCC, 1978, p. 897.
57. Guttmann, L. *Spinal Cord Injuries. Comprehensive Management and Research.* Blackwell Scientific Publications, Oxford, 1982, pp. 533–576.
58. Hagbarth, K. The effect of muscle vibration in normal man and in patients with motor disorders. In: New Developments in Electromyography and Clinical Neurophysiology, Desmedt, J. E., ed., Basel, New York, Karger, 1973, *3:*428–443.
59. Hagbarth, K. E., and Eklund, G. The muscle vibrator: a useful tool in neurological therapeutic work. *Scand. J. Rehabil. Med., 1:*26–34, 1969.
60. Halpern, D., Patterson, R., Machie, R., Runck, W., and Eyler, L. Muscular hypertonia: quantitative analysis. *Arch. Phys. Med. Rehabil., 60:*208–218, 1979.
61. Hanak, M., and Scott, A. *Spinal Cord Injury: An Illustrated Guide for Health Care Professionals.* Springer Publishing Co., New York, 1983.
62. Heizer, D. Brace design for flaccid paralysis. *Phys. Ther., 47:*816–817, 1967.
63. Heizer, D. Long leg brace design for traumatic paraplegia. *Phys. Ther., 47(9):*824–826, 1967.
64. Henshaw, J. T. Walking appliances for paraplegics and tetraplegics. *Paraplegia, 17:*163–168, 1979.
65. Hjeltnes, N. Oxygen uptake and cardiac output in graded arm exercises in paraplegics with low level lesions. *Scand. J. Rehabil. Med., 9:*107–113, 1977.
66. Hjeltnes, N., and Vokac, Z. Circulatory strain in the everyday life of paraplegics. *Scand. J. Rehabil. Med., 11:*67–73, 1979.
67. Huang, C. T., Kuhlemeir, K. V., Moore, N. B., and Fine, P. R. Energy cost of ambulation in paraplegic patients using Craig-Scott braces. *Arch. Phys. Med. Rehabil., 60(12):*595–600, 1979.
68. Huitt, C. T., and Gwyer, J. L. Paraplegia ambulatory training using Craig-Scott orthoses. *Phys. Ther., 58(8):*967–978, 1978.
69. Hussey, R. W., and Stauffer, E. S. Spinal cord injury: requirements for ambulation. *Arch. Phys. Med. Rehabil., 54:*544–547, 1973.
70. Itoh, M., and Lee, M. The epidemiology of disability as related to rehabilitation medicine. In: *Handbook of Physical Medicine and Rehabilitation.* Edited by Krusen, F., Kotke, F., and Ellwood, P., W. B. Saunders, Co., Toronto, 1971, pp. 879–897.
71. Karvonen, M. J. Effects of vigorous exercise on the heart. In: *Work and the Heart.* Edited by Rosenbaum, F. F., and Belknap, E. L. Hober Med Div., Harper and Row, Publishers, Inc., New York, 1959.
72. Knott, M., and Voss, D. *Proprioceptive Neuromuscular Facilitation Patterns & Techniques.* Hoeber Medical Division, Harper & Row Publishers, Inc., New York, 1965.
73. Knutsson, E. Physiotherapy techniques in the control of spasticity. *Scand. J. Rehabil. Med., 5:*167–169, 1973.

74. Knutsson, E., Lewen Haupt-Olsson, E., and Thorsen, M. Physical work capacity and physical conditioning in paraplegic patients. *Paraplegia, 11:*205–216, 1973.
75. Kottke, F. J. Therapeutic exercise to maintain mobility. In: *Krusens Handbook of Physical Medicine and Rehabilitation.* Third Ed. Edited by Kotke, F. J., Stillwell, G. K., and Lehman, J. F. W. B. Saunders, Toronto, 1982, pp. 389–402.
76. Kotke, F., Pauley, D., and Ptak, R. The rationale for prolonged stretching for correction of shortening of connective tissue. *Arch. Phys. Med. Rehabil., 47:*345–352, 1966.
77. Kralj, A., Bajd, T., Turk, R., Krajnik, J., and Benko, H. Gait restoration in paraplegic patients: a feasibility demonstration using multichannel surface electrode FES. *J. Rehabil. R. D., 20(1):*3–20, 1983.
78. Kralj, A., and Grobelnik, S. Functional electrical stimulation of paraplegic patients. *Bull. Prosth. Res.,* Fall, pp. 75–102, 1973.
79. Lamb, D. R. *Physiology of Exercise. Responses and Adaptations.* Macmillan Publishing Co., New York, 1978, pp. 121–153.
80. LaMere, T. J., and Labanovich, S. The history of sport wheelchairs, Part 1. *Sports 'N' Spokes, 9(6):*6–24, 1984.
81. Long, C. Congenital and traumatic lesions of the spinal cord. In: Krusen F, Kotke, F., Ellwood, P., eds. *Handbook of Physical Medicine and Rehabilitation.* Edited by Krusen, F., Kotke, F., and Ellwood, P. W. B. Saunders Co., Toronto, 1971.
82. Long, C. L., and Masciarelli, V. D. An electrophysiological splint for the hand. *Arch. Phys. Med. Rehabil., 44:*499–503, 1963.
83. Low, J. L. The reliability of joint measurement. *Physiotherapy, 62(7):*227–229, 1976.
84. Lundberg, A. Wheelchair driving. Evaluation of a new training outfit. *Scand. J. Rehabil. Med., 12:*67–72, 1980.
85. Lunsford, B. M. Clinical indicators of endurance. *Phys. Ther., 58(6):*704–709, 1978.
86. MacDougall, D., and Sales, D. Continuous vs. interval training: a review for the athlete and the coach. *Can. J. Appl. Sport Sci., 6(2):*93–97, 1981.
87. Marincek, C. R., and Valencic, V. Arm cycloergometry and kinetics of O_2 consumption in paraplegics. *Paraplegia, 15:*178–185, 1977–1978.
88. Marino, M., Nicholas, J. A., Gleim, G. W., Rosenthal, P., and Nicholas, S. J. The efficacy of manual assessment of muscle strength using a new device. *Am. J. Sports Med., 10:*360–365, 1982.
89. Marsolais, E. B., and Kobetic, R. Functional walking in paralyzed patients by means of electrical stimulation. *Clin. Orthop., 175:*30–36, 1983.
90. Mathews, D., and Fox, E. *The Physiological Basis of Physical Education and Athletics.* W. B. Saunders, Philadelphia, 1976, pp. 9–69, 239–308.
91. McAdam, R., and Natvig, H. Stair climbing and ability to work for paraplegics with complete lesions—a sixteen year follow-up. *Paraplegia, 18(3):*197–203, 1980.
92. McDonell, E., Brassard, I., and Taylor, A. W. The effects of an arm ergometer training programme on wheelchair subjects. *Can. J. Appl. Sports. Sci., 5:*4, 1980.
93. Merritt, J. L. Management of spasticity in spinal cord injury. *Mayo Clin. Proc., 56(10):*614–622, 1981.
94. Mikelberg, R., and Reid, S. Spinal cord lesions and lower extremity bracing: an overview and follow-up study. *Paraplegia, 19:*379–385, 1981.
95. Moffroid, M., Whipple, R., Hofkosh, J., Lowman, E., and Thistle, H. A study of isokinetic exercise. *Phys. Ther., 49:*735–746, 1969.
96. Moore, M., and Hutton, R. Electromyographic investigation of muscle stretching techniques. *Med. Sci. Sports. Exerc., 12:*322–329, 1980.
97. Morehouse, C. Development and maintenance of isometric strength of subjects with diverse initial strengths. *Res. Quart., 38:*449–456, 1967.
98. Moritani, T., and deVries, H. Neural factors versus hypertrophy in the time course of muscle strength gain. *Am. J. Phys. Med., 58:*115–130, 1979.
99. Muller, E. Influence of training and of inactivity on muscle strength. *Arch. Phys. Med.*

Rehabil., *51:*449–462, 1970.

100. Munro, D. Rehabilitation of veterans paralyzed as a result of injury to the spinal cord and cauda equina. *Am. J. Surg.*, *75:*3–18, 1948.

101. Nacht, M. B., Wolf, S. L., and Coogler, C. E. Use of electromyographic biofeedback during the acute phase of spinal cord injury. *Phys. Ther.*, *62:*290–294, 1982.

102. Natvig, H., and McAdam, R. Ambulation without wheelchairs for paraplegics with complete lesions. *Paraplegia*, *16(2):*142–146, 1978.

103. Nichols, P. J., Norman, P. A., and Ennis, J. R. Wheelchair user's shoulder. shoulder pain in patient's with spinal cord lesions. *Scand. J. Rehabil. Med.*, *11(1):*29–32, 1979.

104. Nilsson, S., Staff, P. H., and Pruett, E. D. Physical work capacity and the effect of training on subjects with long-standing paraplegia. *Scand. J. Rehabil. Med.*, *7:*51–56, 1975.

105. O'Daniel, W. E., Jr., and Hahn, H. R. Follow-up usage of the Scott-Craig orthoses in paraplegia. *Paraplegia*, *19(6):*373–378, 1981.

106. Odeen, I. Early mobilization of paraplegic patients after traumatic spinal cord injuries. *Physiother. Can.*, *31:*75–83, 1979.

107. Odeen, I. Evaluation of the effects of muscle stretch and weight load in patients with spastic quadriplegia. *Scand. J. Rehabil. Med.*, *13:*117–121, 1981.

108. Ofir, R., and Hofkosh, J. M. The role of the physical therapist in treatment of the spinalcord injured patient. In: *Physical Medicine and Rehabilitation Approaches in Spinal Cord Injury.* Edited by Cull, J. G., and Hardy, R. E. Charles C Thomas, Publisher, Springfield, Illinois, 1977, pp. 174–202.

109. O'Shea, P. Effects of selected weight training programs on the development of strength and muscle hypertrophy. *Res. Quart.*, *37:*95–107, 1966.

110. Pachalski, A., and Mekarsk, T. Effect of swimming on increasing cardiorespiratory capacity in paraplegics. *Paraplegia*, *18:*190–196, 1980.

111. Parry, A. *Physiotherapy Assessment.* Croom Helm, London, 1980, p. 48.

112. Peckham, P. H., Mortimer, J. T., and Marsolais, E. B. Alteration in the force and fatigability of skeletal muscle in quadriplegic humans following exercise induced by chronic electrical stimulation. *Clin. Orthop.*, *114:*326–334, 1976.

113. Petrofsky, J., and Glaser, R. Bicycle ergometer for paralyzed muscle. Submitted to Journal of Clinical Engineering. In Review. National Center for Rehabilitation Engineering, Wright State University, Dayton, Ohio.

114. Petrofsky, J., and Phillips, C. Computer controlled walking in the paralyzed individual. *J. Neurol. Orthop. Surg.*, *4(2):*153–154, 1983.

115. Petrofsky, J., and Phillips, C. Computer control of walking in paraplegic subjects. National Center for Rehabilitation Engineering, Wright State University, Dayton, Ohio (unpublished).

116. Petrofsky, J. S., and Phillips, C. A. Active physical therapy: A modern approach to rehabilitation therapy. *J. Neurol. Orthop. Surg.*, *4:*165–173, 1983.

117. Petrofsky, J. S., Phillips, C. A., and Heaton, H. H. Feedback control system for walking in man. National Center for Rehabilitation Engineering, Wright State University, Dayton, Ohio (unpublished).

118. Rose, S. J., and Rothstein, J. M. Muscle mutability. General concepts and adaptations to altered patterns of use. *Phys. Ther.*, *62:*1773–1787, 1982.

119. Rosman, N., and Spira, E. Paraplegic use of walking braces: a survey. *Arch. Phys. Med. Rehabil.*, *55:*310–314, 1974.

120. Rothstein, J. M. Muscle biology. Clinical considerations. *Phys. Ther.*, *62:*1823–1830, 1982.

121. Rusk, H. *Rehabilitation Medicine*, Fourth Ed. C. V. Mosby, St. Louis, 1977, pp. 326–355.

122. Sady, S., Wortman, M., and Blanke, D. Flexibility training: ballistic, static or proprioceptive neuromuscular facilitation? *Arch. Phys. Med. Rehabil.*, *63:*261–263, 1982.

123. Sale, D., and MacDougall, D. Specificity in strength training: A review for the coach and athlete. *Can. J. Appl. Sports. Sci.*, *6:*87–92, 1981.

124. Seymour, R. J., and Bassler, C. R. Electromyographic biofeedback in the treatment of incomplete paraplegia. *Phys. Ther.*, *57:*1148–1150, 1977.
125. Shambes, G. M. Influence of the muscle spindle on posture and movement. *Phys. Ther.*, *48(10):*1094, 1102, 1968.
126. Shephard, R. *Endurance Fitness.* University of Toronto Press, Toronto, 1977.
127. Spooven, P. Technical characteristics of wheelchair racing. *Sports 'N' Spokes*, *7(4):*19–20, 1981.
128. Stauffer, E. S., Hoffer, M. M., and Nickel, V. L. Ambulation in thoracic paraplegia. *J. Bone Joint Surg.*, *60A(6):*823–825, 1978.
129. Stauffer, L. S. Do you recommend long leg braces for patients with paraplegia? If so, what type of bracing do you prefer? *Phys. Ther.*, *51(7):*823–824, 1971.
130. Syrotiuk, D., and Mendryk, S. Principles of athletic conditioning. *Can. J. Appl. Sport. Sci.*, *1:*229–231, 1976.
131. Therbizan, A. T. Physiotherapeutical mistakes in the early stages after SCI. *Paraplegia*, *16:*233–235, 1978–1979.
132. Turk, R., Kralj, A., Bajd, T., Stefancic, M., and Benko, H. The alteration of paraplegic patients muscle properties due to electrical stimulation exercising. *Paraplegia*, *18:*386–391, 1980.
133. Vallbona, C. Bodily responses to immobilization. In: *Krusens handbook of physical medicine and rehabilitation*, Third Ed. Edited by Kotke, F. J., Stillwell, G. K., and Lehmann, J. F. W. B. Saunders Co., Toronto, 1982, pp. 963–976.
134. VanderMeulen, J. P., Peckham, P. H., and Mortimer, J. T. Use and disuse of muscle. *Ann. N.Y. Acad. Sci.*, *228:*177–188, 1974.
135. Walmsley, R. P., and Swann, I. Biomechanics and physiology of muscle strengthening. *Physiother. Can.*, *28:*197–200, 1976.
136. Waters, R., Hislop, H., and Perry, J. Walking and wheelchair energetics in persons with paraplegia. *Phys. Ther.*, *60(9):*1133–1139, 1980.
137. Weiss, M., and Beck, J. Sport as part of therapy and rehabilitation of Paraplegics. *Paraplegia*, *11:*166–172, 1973.
138. Wicks, J. R., Lymburner, K., Dinsdale, S. M., and Jones, N. L. The use of multistage exercise testing with wheelchair ergometry and arm cranking in subjects with spinal cord lesions. *Paraplegia*, *15(3):*252–261, 1977–1978.
139. Wolf, E., and Magora, A. Orthostatic and ergometric evaluation of cord-injured patients. *Scand. J. Rehabil. Med.*, *8:*93–96, 1976.
140. Wolf, S. L. EMG biofeedback applications in physical rehabilitation: an overview. *Physiother. Can.*, *31:*65–72, 1979.
141. Wolf, S. L. Neurophysiological factors in electromyographic feedback for neuromotor disturbances. In: Basmajian JV, ed. Biofeedback Principles and Practice for Clinicians, Second Ed. Williams & Wilkins, Baltimore, 1983, pp. 5–22.
142. Yosipovitch, Z., Robin, G. C., and Makin, M. Open reduction of unstable thoracolumbar spinal injuires and fixation with harrington rods. *J. Bone Joint Surg.*, *59A:*1003–1015, 1977.

14

Occupational Therapy in the Treatment of Spinal Cord Injuries

A. VAUGEOIS

"So he with difficulty and labour hard
Moved on, with difficulty and labour he."

Milton's "Paradise Lost"

From a clinical point of view, damage to the spinal cord expresses itself in a loss of motor power, sensation, and autonomic function. The true burden of disease is the inability to care for oneself, to move, or to pursue vocational and avocational activities.

Occupational therapy concerns itself with narrowing the gaps between an individual's neurological function and the activities that the patient wishes to perform. It is a challenging and complex task that requires the therapist to serve as a supportive resource while the patient restructures his life goals and tasks. The therapist helps maximize the physical restoration, analyzes functional elements, enhances performance, and retrains or adapts techniques as necessary. The therapist performs three functions (assessment, training, and planning) in four strata (Table 14.1).

Common to all four strata is the need for an accurate assessment of the patient's current functional level and his desire and need to perform given activities. Collaborative goal setting is essential to allow the patient to use his problem-solving, coping, and decision-making skills (19). It is interesting to note that in a study by Taylor a need was identified for closer collaboration between the occupational therapist and the patient. Treatment priorities of the therapist were not the same as those identified by the patient. "Success or failure of a treatment may depend upon resolution of a fundamental conflict of values between the patient and the caregiver (9)." Other studies have identified the therapist's feelings of impotence when

Table 14.1.

	Assessment	Training	Planning
Functional substitution	X	X	
Technical aids	X	X	X
Environmental modification	X		X
Personal assistance	X	X	

dealing with such severely handicapped patients, resulting in overzealousness to provide goals to the patient, inevitably resulting not only in failure but in anger and frustration for both the therapist and the patient (3). System analysis and problem solving are vital elements in structuring a treatment program. Often the therapist will be required to act as a teacher, making the patient aware of alternative methods of function, and suggesting (although not prescribing goals) and implementing strategies to substitute for lost function. Also significant to the degree of success is motivation for achievement of independence, attitude towards the treatment program in terms of achievement and benefits, premorbid personality, education, occupation, and interests. Consequently, patients with the same neurological deficits will demonstrate a wide variance of achievement at the end of their rehabilitation process.

FUNCTIONAL SUBSTITUTION

Functional substitution makes use of the fact that many activities can be performed by changing one's technique to substitute residual function for function lost, such as in the tenodesis grip. Patients will often invent functional substitution on their own, with the therapist's role being that of a change agent, facilitating the growth and development of the patient.

UPPER EXTREMITY FUNCTIONAL EVALUATION

The therapist must establish a clear picture of joint limitations, functioning muscles and their strength, and sensory deficits.

The importance of positioning, prevention of contractures, and maintenance of range of motion cannot be overemphasized. It must begin immediately following injury and be maintained on a regular basis. It is upon this rigid regime that all functional performance hinges. A careful and complete initial evaluation of the patient's physical and neurological status is essential as a change in the neurological level by one or two segments is not uncommon, due most often to a change in the status of the edema surrounding the cord (24). The assessment must be recorded to include active and passive ranges of motion, sensory dermatomes (touch, temperature, position sense, and two-point discrimination), spasticity, muscle strength, and dexterity, and could be done in conjunction with the physiotherapist to avoid duplication of assessments and to better provide a comprehensive and graded treatment program.

ADL EVALUATION

The scope of activities of daily living (ADL) is unlimited and can include such activities as homemaking, child care, and life skills. When evaluating patients in this area, they can be divided into two groups—C4 and C5 individuals without functioning carpi radialis muscles, and C6 and C7 persons who do have active wrist extensors and are capable of achieving higher levels of functional independence with less equipment. All functional evaluations must include the expectations of the patient, his family, and the medical team. Consideration must be given to safety, practicality, available help, age, degree of preinjury physical fitness, energy consumed, time factors, and life-style involved. It may be easier for family and attendants to do some activities for the patient rather than to encourage independence. Dressing of the lower extremities for example is a particularly time-consuming and difficult task for the quadriplegic individual. It requires considerable time, training, and effort to achieve an independent level, and may be impractical, particularly if the patient wishes to return to the community and pursue a vocation. It is vital therefore, for the therapist and patient to consider the home and discharge plans when developing treatment strategies.

Despite all interventions, an individual may still require assistance in some specific activities. It is important for the therapist to clearly identify these activities, as well as the activities that can be performed independently. Excessive attention to one specific aspect may result in overdependence in others or to frustration. If assistance is to be provided, it is equally important that the assistant be instructed in the proper technique.

Based on experience with patients who have sustained injuries at various spinal levels, one can predict with fair confidence the degree of independence a patient is expected to achieve (Table 14.2).

ENVIRONMENTAL EVALUATION

Beyond functional substitution and technical aids, it is often necessary to modify a patient's home or work environment. Accessibility to and within a building may require ramps, elevators, or other architectural changes. The therapist must therefore be able to communicate with architects and builders, and have a good knowledge of relevant standards, designs, and bylaws that may affect modification designs. A home visit should be made as soon as appropriate to determine what changes will be needed, on a short-term or temporary basis, to allow for weekend or day passes from the rehabilitation setting as well as to assess requirements for discharge. This is a very sensitive area and the therapist must be well-attuned to the needs of all the family members, and in particular to the patient's wishes, goals, and expectations. Financial resources will vary tremendously from one patient to another and must be carefully investigated. Availability of funding varies with different health care systems, insurance policies and procedures, policies and eligibility of agencies such as the Department of Veteran's Affairs, Workmen's Compensation Board, and Vocational Rehabilitation Services. Once a resource and a sum of money have been identified, modifications, equipment purchases, and long-term planning can commence.

COMMON TREATMENT APPROACHES AND MODALITIES FOR FUNCTIONAL TRAINING

Splinting, aids, and adaptations can often meet with resistance, causing anger, embarrassment, and frustration, and need to be introduced carefully. Their cosmetic appearance must be acceptable and the patient allowed time to practice with them. When possible, all splinting and aids should be kept to the bare essentials. Most aids will need to be customized to suit the individual patient but many are commercially available. When developing an aid, it is important to keep the patient's neurological level and needs in mind, and to keep it simple, small, functional, and easily fitting. One of the most inconspicuous and acceptable aids is the universal cuff to which several utensils and aids can be attached (Fig. 14.1).

Follow-up studies have indicated that the level of self-care achieved during hospitalization is generally maintained on discharge, and that at least some assistive devices continue to be utilized, although it has been suggested that these are few and tend in general to be the larger items such as ramps, technical devices, and home modifications (4, 15, 16, 21). The reasons for discord have been indicated in a United Kingdom study as:

1. The aid did not do what it was intended to do.
2. It was an unacceptable solution to the problem.
3. It was unsuitable for the person and his environment.
4. The person's condition had changed.

It is equally important that family members or significant others also understand the use and applications of splints and devices and that they accept the importance of allowing the patient the opportunity of independent functioning.

Treatment can be divided into four phases. Phase One begins in the intensive care unit with the introduction of the role of the occupational therapist, provision of resting splints, and, for high quadriplegic patients, an environmental control unit to provide at least the ability to call the nurse. A lengthy immobilization period results in a negative adaptation or detraining effect. (See Chapter 11.) Prism glasses may be acceptable at this time, and other activities that begin during this period include maintenance of range of motion, strengthening of unaffected muscle groups, increase of sitting tolerance and balance (graduating to 90° sitting), and bed mobility. Functional skills such as eating and personal hygiene can be initiated while the patient is still in bed. However, it must be remembered that halo traction, vests, braces, and intravenous tubing's hinder movement, causing increased anger and frustration, and with pressure to perform, may lead to a reluctance to pursue these activities at a later date.

Table 14.2.
Possible Outcomes of Functional Skill

	C3, C4	C5	C6	C7	C8
Eating	D Some may achieve S with a balanced forearm orthosis (may have fear of choking and prefer assistance when eating)	S—with aids and devices	I—should require minimal aids with a tenodesis splint or univer- sal cuff	I—no aids Will learn technique to substitute for lost function in all activi- ties	I—no aids
Personal hygiene	D	S—facial care with aids and de- vices A—for other activi- ties using aids and adaptions (aids may include razor cuff, padded handles, adapted deodorant con- tainer)	I—teeth, shaving, hair, deodorant A—washing above waist	I—some aids	I—no aids
Dressing	D	D—for below waist A—above waist with adapted clothing	I—possible with adapted cloth- ing, good bed mobility, and sit- ting balance (this activity is usu- ally done on the bed, and is time- and energy-con- suming for all pa- tients.)	I—no aids above waist, adaptions to below waist garments	I—a few simple clothing adap- tions may be appropriate
Transfers	D—Hoyer or two- man lift (transfers to and from commode are much more difficult)	A—when sitting balance is satis- factory a one- man transfer can be done	A—one-man slide transfer usual I—slide transfer possible to bed, car	I—slide transfer	I—slide transfer

of pulleys may be used for wheelchair to/from bed

Bathing	D	A—will be able to do some above-waist washing with aids D—below waist	A—with aids and adaptations will be able to shower in a stall (aids could include mitts, long sponges, temperature controlled shower, shower seats; shower stalls are simplest to use)	I—with aids and adaptations in a shower	I—as in C7
Toileting	D—bladder: intermittent catherization, condom, or bowel programs easiest done on side lying down	D—bladder: condom or intermittent catheterization D—bowel: anal stimulation, can use a commode (all patients benefit from modified bathrooms and commode chairs)	A—bladder: aids to open and drain bags, aids for condom application, intermittent catheterization A—bowel: assistance for toilet or commode, aids for stimulation	A—as in C6 —Crede method for bladder emptying, some able to do intermittent catheterization A—as in C6	I—same methods and aids as in C6 and C7 I—should achieve I in anal stimulation
Bed mobility	D—side to side A—electric bed can be used to position long sitting	D—able to help with roll from supine to side A—with straps, may achieve long sitting	I—may achieve long sitting with aids A—needs assistance to position pillows when going supine to side, benefits from ropes or	I—roll from supine to side I—long sitting, benefits from aids as in C6	I

Key—I = Independent
A = Assisted
S = Supervision/Setup
D = Dependent

Table 14.2—Continued

	C3, C4	C5	C6	C7	C8
Wheelchair management	I—uses a power wheelchair with chin control or puff blow mechanism	I—uses power wheelchair	overhead bars to change positions I—may use power wheelchair for long distance —could use regular wheelchair with rim projections for upper extremity strengthening and short distances	I—regular wheelchair	I—regular wheelchair
Writing Typing Reading	D I—using mouthstick or environmental control I—using page turner, mouthstick, or prism glasses (positioning of equipment needs consideration)	S—with adaptations but may not be functional if a lot is necessary I—using environmental control or mouthstick & electric typewriter as in C3 and C4 can also use pencil in cuff I—uses pencil in cuff to turn pages	I—using adaptations I—using adaptations & electric typewriter I—as in C3, C4, and C5, but should not require prism glasses	I—padded pen practice for speed and accuracy I—using adaptations I—minimal adaptations	I—as in C7 I—as in C7 I—as in C7
Driving	will need to be transported in an adapted vehicle	D—can be transported in a car (some C5 patients have achieved driving independence in	I—could drive an adapted vehicle with controls —would need assistance to get	I—uses controls, can use a two-door car and manage own wheelchair	I—as in C7

		an adapted vehicle)	a wheelchair into a car		
Educational	I—possible to continue using computers, word processors and printouts, and tape recorders (accessibility, endurance, sitting tolerance to be considered to all levels)	I—as in C3 and C4	I—possible as in C3, C4, and C5 Less reliant on an E.C.U. but definitely advantageous	I—as in C3, C4, C5, C6, and C7	I—as in C3, C4, C5, C6 and C7
Vocational	I—desk job using E.C.U. possible, using E.C.U.'s (accessibility issues to be considered—see Chapter 13 for more details)	I—desk job using E.C.U.	I—desk job or non-manual labor —Some homemaking, child care	I—desk job or non-manual labor	I—desk job or non-manual labor
Recreational	I—using computer, mostly homebound activities	A—for activities outside home	I—can consider some wheelchair sports	I—can be achieved in some selected activities	I—same as C7
Independent living environment	Needs care full time I—manager in homemaking, parenting, budgeting, family management	A—needs attendant care and homemaking assistance	A—needs some attendant care and homemaking assistance A—can perform some meal preparation and some simple homemaking with adaptations	A—needs some attendant care and homemaking A—can perform meal preparation and some simple homemaking tasks with aids and adaptations	S—needs monitoring only A—needs assistance with heavy house cleaning

Key—I = Independent
A = Assisted
S = Supervision/Setup
D = Dependent

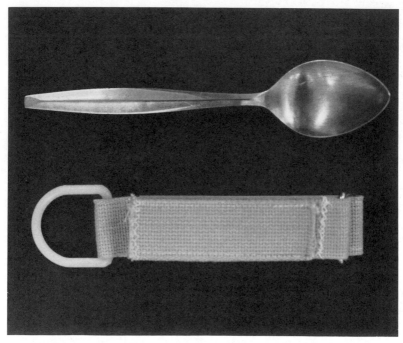

Figure 14.1. The universal cuff is easily manufactured in an occupational therapy department. The volar pocket allows insertion of such utensils as cutlery, toothbrush, and comb for functional use.

Phase Two begins as soon as the patient is able to be out of bed (6). He must be positioned in an appropriate wheelchair with attention given to back and neck support and adequate cushioning. Sitting tolerance and balance are gradually increased and wheelchair mobility introduced. Activity levels are also increased. The selection of an optimal wheelchair cushion is largely based on personal experience at this time. Dry flotation cushions appear effective in reducing the incidence of skin breakdown with prolonged sitting. Higher level self-care skills such as dressing, transfers, and bed mobility using ropes or pulleys to achieve long sitting where necessary can be introduced (22, 23). Wheelchair propulsion can begin in conjunction with the physiotherapy program when sitting balance, muscle tone, strength, mobility, endurance, and dexterity are satisfactory. When the patient masters these skills, the treatment program begins to focus on long-term functional needs and potential.

In Phase Three of treatment, more complex skills will be introduced. At this time the patient will be more agile, having gained strength in remaining muscle groups. Endurance and tolerance to treatment programs will have significantly increased. Medical issues such as continence and orthostatic hypotension will no longer be immediate concerns. Bowel and bladder management can be addressed in close conjunction with nursing staff.

Although several aids and adaptations are available to allow the patient to achieve independent management of these areas, careful selection must be made in order to prevent additional problems from improper use. Some authors suggests that C6 female quadriplegics can successfully master self-catheterization (11). However, our experience has shown that this is rarely achieved. Long-term, postdischarge plans must be considered: where, when, and how this program will be done for the safety and convenience of the patient.

Transfers to and from the commode and bathtub are considered to be the most difficult and require a great deal of practice both by the patient and his assistant. Emphasis must be placed on skin protection during these transfers, and regular skin inspection is encouraged.

These three phases take place during the rehabilitation process in the institution. The final phase of occupational therapy, however, involves reintegrating the patient into the community. There is a large and important role for a community therapist to help the patient adjust to community living. The therapist can direct the patient toward advocacy groups, self-help groups of other similar patients, and recreational facilities. It is also important for this therapist to become involved on boards of agencies that are involved with community planning, access, and transportation for the disabled. She must be able to direct the patient to the appropriate agency when situations or problems arise.

PREDICTED OUTCOMES OF SOME FUNCTIONAL ADL SKILLS (Table 14.2)

Diaphragm, Trapezius (C3, C4)

Technical aids are particularly appropriate for these patients, allowing them some freedom of mobility, control of the environment, and opportunities to pursue vocational, educational, and recreational activities. Mouthsticks have also been used successfully to perform such activities as typing, page turning, painting, and the operation of some electrical devices (7). The degree of success is largely dependent on at least fair strength in the neck musculature and the patient's acceptance of technology. Energy factors must also be considered together with the amount of respiratory control. The patient will remain dependent for all self-care skills.

Deltoid, Biceps, Supinator, Brachioradialis (C5)

These patients will be able to perform some self-care skills and remain dependent for others. They may also benefit from environmental control systems. A powered wheelchair is mandatory for functional mobility.

Extensor Carpi Radialis (Longus & Brevis), Pectoralis Major (C6)

With active wrist extensors and tenodesis splint, a much higher level of independence in self-care skills is possible for these patients. Driving aids may be considered and assessed at this level. This assessment will include the appropriate hand control, the type of vehicle to be driven, access to and from the vehicle, and the costs involved. Should a patient wish to achieve total driving independence, getting the wheelchair in and out of the vehicle becomes a major issue. A van with an adapted seating arrangement or a Ricon or similar lift may become necessary.

Triceps, Extensor Digitorum Communis (C7)

Independence in all self-care skills can be achieved with a minimum of aids for these patients. A standard chair is appropriate, and driving can be achieved in a car with hand controls. Wheelchair management in and out of the car can also be done independently.

Intrinsics (Including Thumb), Ulnar Wrist Flexors and Extensors (C8)

These patients can achieve independence in self-care with more speed, dexterity, strength, and endurance.

Paraplegics

The patients can achieve a totally independent life-style as they have no upper extremity limitations.

SPLINTING

Having completed the assessment, fabrication of splints for the quadriplegic patient will be necessary to allow for maximal upper extremity function (12). There are two schools of thought regarding splinting: one that uses very little splinting and allows for a functional contracture to develop, and the second that favors both static and dynamic splinting to enhance functional performance. Splints are available commercially but can be rather costly. They can be custom-made by an orthotist or more cheaply fabricated by a therapist. It is essential that the splint be cosmetically acceptable, well-fitting, easy to apply, and in the case of dynamic splinting, be of assistance to the patient in a functional capacity or it will quickly be rejected (10). Two basic types of splints are commonly used: (a) static splints stabilize weak joints and prevent deformities; and (b) dynamic splints correct a deformity and facilitate functional use. There are several types of static splints used basically for the maintenance of a good functional position or to allow, as mentioned, for a functional contracture. The desired position for a temporary static splint is with the wrist in a neutral position or up to 30° of dorsiflexion. The thumb should be rotated at the carpometacarpal joint and abducted in the plane of flexion. There should be slight flexion of the metacarpal and proximal interphalangeal joints to 45° and the distal interphalangeal joints to 15°. This position is desirable to achieve three-point prehension, or a pinch grip.

The long opponens splint is worn when there are no active wrist extensors, and it holds the hand in position for a prehension grip (Fig. 14.2 to 14.4).

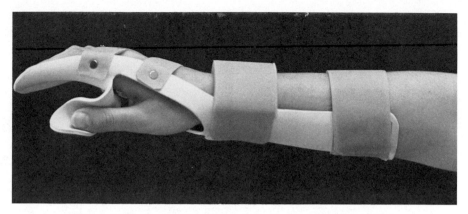

Figure 14.2. Heat-formed thermoplastic long opponens splint.

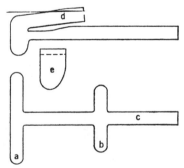

Figure 14.3. Basic long opponens splint (Rancho los Amigos): (a) dorsal extension; and (b) volar support. (From Redford, J. B., and Licht, S. H. *Orthotics Etcetera*, Second Ed. Williams & Wilkins Company, 1980.)

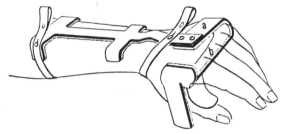

Figure 14.4. Template for basic long opponens splint: (a) proximal tab; (b) wrist extension bar; (c) distal bar; (d) opponens bar; and (e) C-bar. (From Redford, J. B., and Licht, S. H. *Orthotics Etcetera*, Second Ed. Williams & Wilkins Company, 1980.)

The short opponens splint allows for free movement of the wrist while maintaining the hand in position for the prehension grip. The web space of the thumb is maintained, and the metacarpal phalangeal joints are held in flexion (Fig. 14.5). A dorsal wrist splint can also be considered in this category (Fig. 14.6 and 14.7). This splint holds the wrist in extension and can be fitted with utensils or aids to permit performance of functional activity.

An example of a dynamic splint is the tenodesis splint, which brings the fingers into flexion and the thumb into opposition (Fig. 14.8). For effective use of this splint it is first necessary for the wrist extensors to achieve Grade 3 muscle strength (pull against gravity). The C6 and, to a lesser extent, the C7 quadriplegic patients derive most benefit from the tenodesis splint as it will allow them to pick up objects. Considerable practice is needed to gain strength, dexterity, and precision.

Mobile arm supports, allowing movement in the horizontal and vertical planes, are supportive ball-bearing devices that can be balanced to assist weak muscles and substitute for absent power in the shoulder and elbow to

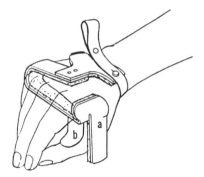

Figure 14.5. Rancho short opponens splint: (a) opponens bar; and (b) C-bar. (From Redford, J. B., and Licht, R. H. *Orthotics Etcetera*, Second Ed. Williams & Wilkins Company, 1980.)

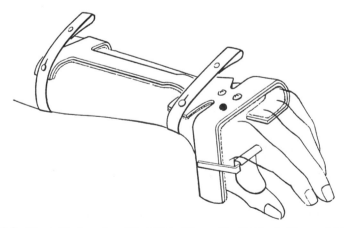

Figure 14.6. Bennett dorsal wrist splint. (From Redford, J. B., and Licht, S. H. *Orthotics Etcetera*, Second Ed. Williams & Wilkins Company, 1980.)

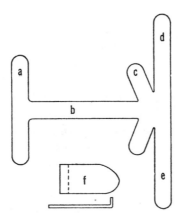

Figure 14.7. Template of Bennett basic dorsal wrist splint: (a) proximal tab; (b) wrist extension bar; (c) distal tab; (d) opponens bar; (e) hypothenar bar; and (f) C-bar. (From Redford, J. B., and Licht, S. H. *Orthotics Etcetera*, Second Ed. Williams & Wilkins Company, 1980.)

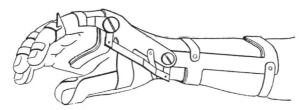

Figure 14.8. Rancho flexor hinge tenodesis splint. (From Redford, J. B., and Licht, S. H. Orthotics Etcetera, Second Ed. Williams & Wilkins Company, 1980.)

counteract gravitational forces. Used in combination with an external power source, e.g. electrical motor, splints and adaptations allow patients to perform such tasks as typing and eating. While most successful with the C5 patient who has poor shoulder flexion and abduction but fair elbow flexion, studies have indicated that few of these devices are used after hospital discharge due to their cumbersome nature and appearance as well as the need for careful set up of the patient before he is able to function at all. Learning to perform functional activities with powered devices requires much patience and practice to achieve precision of movement within reasonable time.

TECHNICAL AIDS

Technical aids range in complexity from a universal splint to a computer-based environmental controller and communication system. Their aim is to augment residual function by technical means. An environmental controller consists of a patient interface, such as switches, mouthstick, etc., a logic control unit, and peripheral actuators that can operate various equipment such as lights, appliances, telephone, radio, and television. The therapist requires a broad knowledge and extensive data base on an ever-expanding wealth of available equipment in order to identify the most effective device for a specific situation. Most commercially available equipment requires field installation, adaptation, and adjustment. Except in major centers, this task usually remains for the therapist. Patients must be carefully assessed, considering their physical and cognitive abilities, their functional needs and desires, financial resources, and the environment in which a complex aid has to function before a prescription can be made. After a device has been provided, the patient and the family require instruction in the use and maintenance of the aid, and where it can be repaired or serviced after discharge. The equipment selected must be evaluated to ensure the fullest development of user potential.

Technical aids can be basically divided into the following categories (5, 16, 18):

1. Environmental controls such as TOSC, ENCO, POSSUM, and PRENTKE ROMICH (Table 14.3).
2. Computers, which can include word processor and printer, are particularly valuable in educational, vocational and recreational activities, but may also function as environmental controllers.
3. Mobility aids such as powered wheelchairs.

Sell & Stratford have shown significant differences in the activity patterns of users and nonusers of technical aids. Their study showed that users spend more time performing educational activities independently. It is also noted that individuals who were exposed to these devices early in their treatment programs were more likely to use them than those who were introduced to the devices later (17, 18).

Cost factors for this type of sophisticated equipment cannot be ignored and must be carefully considered during the assessment process. Close liaison with a biomedical engineering department is an asset in aiding the therapist to become familiar with new designs, research, and development, and in the evaluation of equipment.

ENVIRONMENTAL MODIFICATIONS

Home modifications can vary from simple to complex and will be dealt with in broad terms only; as there are many books and publications dealing with dimensions and layouts that are appropriate for wheelchair dependent persons. (See also Chapter 13). Every design will differ according to the needs and financial resources of individual patients (1, 2, 8, 13).

A pragmatic approach to the process of home modifications may be to consider the following procedure:

1. Determination of minimal and optimal home modifications, based on a patient's physical abilities, expected life-style, present resi-

Table 14.3.
Environmental Controls.

	Splinting/Appliances	Switch/Control types	
TOSC	Tape recorder Telephone Intercom Door unlock Emergency alert Air conditioner Light Fan Television Electric bed control Dictaphone call bell	Button Pneumatic (puff/suck switch) Rocker switch	
ENCO	Television Stereo Ceiling light Radio Fan Lamp Telephone	Pneumatic switch Lever switch Touch switch	
POSSUM	All the above Television channel selector AM-FM radio Automatic telephone dial Household appliances	Microswitch Joystick Pneumatic	
PRENTKE ROMICH	All the above Wheelchair with power recline feature Computer Print outs	Switch Tongue switch Pneumatic Slot control Chin control Joy stick E.M.G.	Combined with a control unit with a feedback display, remote control feature

dence, and the degree of physical assistance available to the patient.
2. Identification of the funding agency.
3. Identification of the contact person within that agency.
4. Identification of the amount of money available for modifications, supplies, equipment, and other long-term needs.
5. A home visit with the patient and the representative of the funding agency where possible. (It is essential that the patient be involved in this problem-solving process.)
6. Monitoring of the progress and relaying of this to the medical team as in many situations discharge from the hospital is dependent on the completion of home modifications.

The process is extremely slow with the many systems involved, and an early start is imperative.

There are three main needs common to all spinal cord injured patients: (a) access into and around the residence, (b) emergency exit from the residence, and (c) access to and functionality of the bathroom.

A fourth area where access is essential for some patients is the kitchen.

If major modifications are necessary, the following must be considered:
1. Zoning bylaws.
2. Present real estate value of the home.
3. Value of modified home and resale potential, and predicted length of stay in this residence.
4. Feasibility of modifications to present residence or relocation.
5. Effects of all of the above on the family unit and their life-style.

SUMMARY

The rehabilitation of the spinal cord injured person is complex and costly, taking from 3 to 12 months, and requires total involvement by the patient and team to achieve a successful outcome. The occupational therapist plays a vital role within this network in directing the patient toward his maximal level of function. Coping behaviors and emotional support must be considered and addressed while planning and working through treatment programs. The therapist assumes the role of educator to the patient and his family, helping the patient to reorganize his future goals and life-style.

Most occupational therapy in the rehabilitation of the spinal cord injury has been based on experience and common sense. Long-range effectiveness of interventions has been difficult to assess since most publications in the field are of a descriptive nature. Assessment methods are rarely evaluated for reliability and validity, and the effectiveness of interventions has seldom if ever been vigorously tested. Different rehabilitation centers use different methods, and many patients living in the community have developed their own tricks and modifications in technique. At this point in time we have very little evidence to help us identify the optimal solution for a given problem. We propose that the occupational therapists in this field direct themselves in the future to validating the clinical effectiveness of occupational therapy treatment.

In order to learn more about efficacy and effectiveness of occupational therapy in spinal cord injury, several steps will be necessary:

1. Establishment and validation of a widely accepted nomenclature of level and degree of neurological deficit.
2. Establishment and validation of a widely accepted and used methodology for functional assessment of the spinal cord patient.
3. Establishment of a widely accepted nosology of treatment modalities.
4. Properly conducted prospective studies, comparing different types of intervention, if not randomized, at least using comparable analytical cohorts.

REFERENCES

1. Cary, J. R. *How to Create Interiors for the Disabled.* Pantheon Books, Inc., Random House, New York, 1978.
2. Chasin, J. *Home in a Wheelchair.* Paralyzed Veterans of America, Washington, D.C. 1978.
3. Clark, P. N. Human development through occupational theoretical frameworks in contemporary O.T. practice. *Am. J. Occup. Ther., 33(8):*505–515, 1979.
4. De Jong, C., and Hughes, J. Independent living methodology for measuring long-term outcomes. *Arch. Phys. Med. Rehabil., 63(2):*68–73, 1963.
5. Environmental Control Systems and Vocational Aids for Persons with High Level Quadriplegia. Rehabilitation Monograph No. 55. Institute of Rehabilitation Medicine, New York University Medical Center, New York, 1979.
6. Ford, J. A., and Duckworth, B. *Physical Management for the Quadriplegic Patient.* F. A. Davis Company, Philadelphia, 1974.
7. Garcia, S., and Greenfield, J. Dynamic protractible mouthstick. *Am. J. Occup. Ther., 35(8):*529–530, 1981.
8. Goldsmith, S. *Designing for the Disabled,* Third Ed. Royal Institute of British Architects, London, 1976.
9. Lobitz, C., and Shepard, K. Effect of compatibility on goal achievement in patient-physical therapist dyads. *Phys. Ther., 63(3):*319–324, 1983.
10. Malick, M. H., and Meyer, C. *Manual on Management of the Quadriplegic Upper Extremity.*
11. McGuire, E., and Savastano, J. A. Long-term followup of spinal cord injury patients managed by intermittent catherization. *J. Urol., 129(4):*775–776, 1983.
12. Nickel, V. H. *The Total Care of Spinal Cord Injury.* Little, Brown & Company, Boston, 1977.
13. Barrier-Free Site Design. Office of Policy Development and Research, U.S. Dept. of Housing and Urban Development, Washington, 1975.
14. Rogers, J. C., and Figone, J. J. Psychological parameters in treating person with quadriplegia. *Am. J. Occup. Ther., 33(7):* 432–439, 1979.
15. Rogers, J. C., and Figone, J. J. Traumatic quadriplegia: follow-up study of self-care skills. *Arch. Phys. Med. Rehabil., 61:*316–321, 1980.
16. Roy, O. Z. Research and technology for the disabled in Canada. *Rehabilitation Digest, 13(2):* 2–5, 1982.
17. Sell, G. H., Stratford, C. D., Zimmerman, M. E., Youdin, M., and Milner, D. Environmental and typewriter control systems for high-level quadriplegic patients, evaluation and prescription. *Arch. Phys. Med. Rehabil. 60:*246–252, 1979.
18. Sell, G. H., and Stratford, C. D. Typical disabilities. *Int. J. Rehabil. Res., 4(1):*66–67, 1981.

19. Symington, D. C., O'Shea, B., Batelaan, J., and White, D. Independence through Environmental Control Systems. Canadian Rehabilitation Council for the Disabled, 1980.
20. Taylor, D. P. Goals for quadriplegic and paraplegic patients. *Am. J. Occup. Ther.*, *28(1)*: 22–29, 1974.
21. Trombly, C. A., and Scott, A. D. *Occupational Therapy for Physical Dysfunction.* The Williams & Wilkens Company, Baltimore, 1977, pp. 305–311.
22. Turner, A. *The Practice of Occupational Therapy. An Introduction to the Treatment of Physical Dysfunction.* Churchill Livingstone, Edinburgh, 1981.
23. Willard, H., and Spackman, L. *Occupational Therapy*, Fifth Ed. J. B. Lippincott Company, Philadelphia, 1978.
24. Young, J. S., and Dexter, W. R. Neurological recovery distal to the zone of injury in 172 cases of closed traumatic spinal cord injury. *Paraplegia, 16(1)*:39–49, 1978.

15

The Living Environment

PAMELA J. CLUFF
JEANETTE KEENAN

Any severe trauma to the spinal column, either through injury or disease, will cause a loss of sensation and concomitant loss of voluntary motion below the level of the injury. When the injury occurs in the cervical vertebrae, the individual is likely to become quadraplegic. If the injury is lower, the individual is likely to be paraplegic, with losses of function in the lower extremities. Since the functional ability of the individual will vary dependent upon the level of the injury, some will be able to manage a wide variety of activities while others may be heavily reliant upon life-support systems and considerable assistance with the activities of daily living.

There is however one condition shared by all spinal cord injured persons: the need for an accessible and supportive living environment. This does not mean that all such persons will require the same degree of access or support since their coping skills will vary considerably when confronted by similar problems or barriers. However, it is fair to assume that many injured persons will experience similar problems with those elements that require the use of physical ability, dexterity, endurance, or strength, although this too will vary depending upon the role that individual expects to perform in society.

The most significant dilemma to date, however, has been consideration of each disabled person as an individual with personal need and preferences. These may involve very different needs for safety, privacy, and personal space, plus their social complements of risk taking, social interaction and integration. A new approach is therefore required in planning for the future. Disabled persons, due to both greater life expectancy and better health services, will generally occur in the following distinct grouping:

1. Those who can manage independently.
2. Those who need some supportive or personal care.
3. Those who need some personal or nursing care.
4. Those who need full supportive care.

In designing physical solutions for these persons we must recognize at least the first three groups that every attempt should be made to maintain and optimize their capabilities to manage their environments and actions, thereby retaining the right to self-determination for as long as possible.

Designing shelter or work settings for those suffering from physical losses presents a relatively simple problem in many cases. Studies in ergonomics and anthropometrics have broadened to a point where no one should still be making the simple mistake of designing buildings with physical barriers or inadequate provisions for personal safety. However, greater acknowledgement of the psychological needs and stresses affecting disabled persons still needs to be addressed.

In the first instance, inappropriate selection of sites and housing locations can contribute significantly to the many frustrations and psychological pressures already experienced by those with injuries. Leon Pastalan of Ann Arbor, Michigan, has undertaken considerable research into *life space* as it affects older persons. This same concept can be directly related to the experiences of disabled persons. To explain this concept simply, life space includes the space, area, or region in which any individual can cope while undergoing a series of physical and psychological losses. For many disabled persons, this range may be extremely limited to a short radius from their homes unless they have independent transportation. Such information can provide us with locational criteria for new housing sites with easy access to needed social and public services such as shopping, churches, doctors' offices, community centers, work, and recreation. Pastalan has also demonstrated that as the nature and scope of their disabilities increase, affected individuals are able to cope less and less with complex environments. We need therefore to consider also the scale and number of units built in one location, the complexity of the interior design, and the social context within which the housing is created to ensure that the environment created is manageable in all aspects.

While disability and incapacity are useful epidemiological factors in creating new or in retrofitting existing housing for the disabled, a more personal and positive approach would be to assess the particular individual's functional ability to manage the normal activities of daily living:

1. Getting in and out of bed.
2. Transferring and toileting.
3. Getting washed and bathed.
4. Preparing and eating meals.
5. Moving about the apartment or house.
6. Getting in and out of the building.
7. Negotiating the public environment, garden, or site.
8. Utilizing public facilities and work settings.
9. Interacting socially and utilizing recreational opportunities.
10. Communicating with friends and others.

Any design solution should then compensate for physical losses by enhancing the environment to allow that individual to manage independently.

Since the most effective form of rehabilitation is often self-directed, those things that disabled persons learn to do for themselves are frequently far more important than those done for them by others. Self-dependence, even in small measure, assists individuals in preserving their senses of dignity and personal worth while dependence on others tends to deprive them of their initiative and self-esteem. Moreover, those who do not learn to cope as much as possible for themselves are likely to compound their frustrations. Their disabilities can indeed become handicaps rather than limitations to be managed.

In addition to an accessible and appropriate physical and social environment, many disabled persons rely heavily upon other aids and devices in order to pursue an independent life-style. Such adaptive equipment can be of considerable assistance in the promotion of independent living. The range of assistive devices now available embraces all facets of daily living and can resolve many of the physical and psychological issues listed previously. Appropriate housing design should make provision for the inclusion or utilization of a wide variety of these aids, including not only those that are appropriate specifically to the individual but those that are germane to all with spinal cord injuries.

In addition to accessible housing design and appropriate physical and social locations, many nonambulatory persons require other support services in order to live independently in the community. These might include homemaker services, meals-on-wheels, visiting nurses, home care, attendant or personal care, or respite care for families. In addition, many of these people also require financial assistance in obtaining technical aids or maintaining costs of living, vocational rehabilitation and counseling, physiotherapy, home adaption assistance, and transportation. Often a combination of these supports is necessary for full optimization of potential. However, the coordination and organization of such services remain an individual and collective problem.

HOUSING ADAPTION PROGRAMS

There exists in Canada a significant disabled population requiring special housing appropriate to their specific needs in a variety of housing contexts. However, as a consequence of low personal income levels, many disabled persons need to rely heavily on social housing programs, congregate living settings, or their own families, where some financial support may be available to offset the high costs of special accommodation or home modification.

While there are funding programs sponsored by all levels of government for the purpose of adapting housing units, the degree to which these programs have been utilized by disabled persons appears to be very dependent upon the income eligibility of the individual as well as the costs of the required adaption, the location, sponsorship, and life-style appropriateness.

For instance, the Residential Rehabilitation Assistance Program (RRAP) is a federal program available through Canada Mortgage and Housing Corporation (CMHC) under Section 34.1 of the National Housing Act (NHA). This program offers low interest loans and grants to homeowners and landlords who wish to make repairs or alterations to existing substandard housing in designated areas. Recent amendments to the program allow disabled persons to take advantage of this program to make their homes more accessible.

Under the program, loans of up to $10,000 are available to qualified individuals. A maximum of $3,750 of this may be forgiven where the adjusted family income is $9,000 or less. Recently proposed changes may increase these amounts to a $13,000 loan with a maximum of $6,500 forgivable where the family income is $13,000 or less. Persons with higher incomes may also be eligible but the grants will be prorated accordingly. In order to apply, the person seeking the loan must own and live in the home, be disabled or have a disabled person living with them, need specific repairs or alterations to make the home accessible for the disabled person, and meet the CMHC and RRAP standards for the work.

The forgivable portion of the loan is based upon the adjusted family income, the cost of renovations and repairs, and the continued ownership and occupancy of the home. RRAP funding may be made available to both public and private nonprofit groups and cooperatives where funding for repair or modification of existing buildings is required. There is some advantage in applying for such RRAP funding at the time of purchasing an existing building. The calculation of assistance under Section 56.1 of the NHA is based solely on the agreed-upon cost of the project, including the cost of rehabilitation. The forgivable portion of the RRAP is then subtracted from the repayable portion of the loan. This effectively reduces the loan amount and decreases the mortgage payments for occupants of renovated projects rather than new buildings.

Canada Mortgage and Housing Corporation has demonstrated ongoing concern with the provision of accommodation to meet the needs of special groups such as the disabled. To meet these needs, CMHC has commissioned considerable research on the housing needs and costs that affect disabled persons. While the primary focus of this research has been in the development of design criteria and barrier-free environments, other research activity has been directed at the development of policy options and new programs for barrier-free housing and communities.

Recent amendments to the National Housing Act have shifted the financial responsibility for the majority of social housing programs to the provinces themselves. At the national level, Canada Mortgage and Housing Corporation (CMHC) maintains an important role in insuring loans, developing and administering programs and policies, and researching the housing market. Similar programs exist in many other countries. The provision of suitable housing alone, however, still leaves unanswered many basic questions involving mobility and other factors:

1. The selection of sites: needs to be determined by such questions as access, transportation, travel distances, location of essential services, etc.
2. The design or context of the solution: low-rise or high-rise choices are frequently a factor of zoning, related neighborhood development, and land costs. In urban settings, high-rise buildings may be a very satisfactory answer, providing there is easy access to garden or recreational areas at ground level. However, prevailing attitudes regarding fire safety often inhibit the use of such solutions.
3. The social context of the solution: segregation or integration of the disabled is a difficult problem. A high level of user satisfaction has been observed in settings that are integrated into coherent neighborhoods where there are no perceivable boundaries between types of housing.

DESIGN GUIDELINES FOR DISABLED PERSONS

Optimum design of housing units for those with spinal cord injuries, whether in apartments or single family dwellings, should address 13 principle design criteria.

PRIMARY ENTRANCES AND VESTIBULES

Where the accessible unit is in an apartment building all primary entrances should be located at or be accessible from ground level. Where this is impractical, appropriate ramps no steeper than 1:12 should be provided. Such entrances should be wide enough to permit access by those in wheelchairs with little or no level change at the threshold. A minimum of 810 mm clear space between the open door face and the door jamb is required, and entrance doors should be operable by a simple and single effort. Where there is a vestibule, space must be provided to permit wheelchair maneuverability. Where doors are opposite each other in sequence, the dimension between doors should be a minimum of 2000 mm; minimum dimensions in other directions should be 1500 mm.

Elevators

Apartment building elevators should comply with the appropriate local safety standards for elevators, escalators, and moving walks, such as CSA and Underwriters, and should be accessible to the main points of entry. They should serve all major areas and floors of the building, including storage and underground parking.

Elevator door openings should permit safe and easy access by persons in wheelchairs and should open and close by automatic means. All doors should be provided with an automatic reopening device to ensure that the car door and the hoistway door will reopen automatically if obstructed by an object or person. In addition, each car should be provided with a self-levelling feature.

The interior floor space of the cab should be large enough to permit a person in a wheelchair to maneuver in addition to accommodating an attendant or other passengers as necessary.

All elevator call buttons in lobbies should be within reach of persons in wheelchairs with the center line of buttons not more than 1200 mm from the floor surface.

The interior cab controls should be useable by both wheelchair users and any other persons with varying disabilities such as sight impairment. Standard symbols should be used to identify all controls with the highest control being positioned no higher than 1200 mm from the floor surface to its center and no lower than 750 mm. In addition, an emergency two-way communication system should be provided from the elevator to a controlled location in the building. The highest operable part of the emergency system should also be at a maximum of 1200 mm from the floor surface and no lower than 750 mm with its location identified by an adjacent raised or incised symbol. Where the system is connected to the building's power supply it should transfer automatically to a source of emergency power within 10 seconds of normal power failure, and should ensure two-way communication and lighting for a minimum of 4 hours.

Handrails should be provided on all sides of the elevator cab and should be positioned 810 mm to 900 mm from the floor and 40 mm from the wall. Interior illumination should be a minimum of 250 lux at 900 mm and 50 lux at floor level.

Corridors

Corridors should permit easy access by persons in wheelchairs, providing a clear width of 900 mm to 1500 mm. Changes in level should be avoided wherever possible, or ramps should be provided that conform to acceptable criteria.

In order not to cause an obstruction for the seeing-impaired, care should be taken to ensure that fixed objects do not project into the corridor unless mounted higher than 2250 mm. Below this height, objects should be recessed and identified by color or textural change.

Exits

While significant concentration is frequently given to issues of access, insufficient attention is generally given to emergency exit. Design solutions should therefore ensure that all exit routes from a building are accessible to and useable by disabled persons in an emergency situation such as fire. Exit and access corridors should be designed to be easily seen, understood, and utilized by all persons, including those with varying disabilities.

All doors leading into fire stairs, exit corridors, or exits should be equipped with hardware distinguished by a change in texture. Supplementary illuminated emergency exit signs should also flash as visual emergency alarms with a frequency not exceeding 5 Hz in addition to audio alarm signals. All visual emergency alarm devices should be located in such a manner that the signal or reflection can be seen anywhere in the area served by the alarm. Where such systems use a permanently installed electrical power source they should be on the same circuit as the audible emergency alarms and be transferable to emergency power systems if not wireless and portable. The height at which fire alarm pulls or buttons are located should not exceed 1000 mm to 1200 mm from the floor to the center of the alarm within easy reach of persons in wheelchairs and the elderly with limited reach.

Ramps

Ramps should be provided to ensure a simple and direct sloped transition where level changes are unavoidable. The ramp itself should not exceed 1:12 in order that wheelchair disabled persons can easily and safely negotiate the level change. A wheelstop/guard measuring 76 mm to 101 mm high and 152 mm wide should be provided where the ramp is not flush with the adjacent level. In addition, all ramps should be equipped with appropriate handrails and guardrails to ensure that disabled persons can negotiate them safely. The approach to the ramp should be clear and level for an area of 1500 mm by 1500 mm to permit a person in a wheel chair to maneuver on or off the ramp easily. The width of the ramp should accommodate two-way pedestrian flow where possible, with the minimum width being 914 mm. Where ramps exceeding 9750 mm in length are unavoidable, landings should be provided between segments at 9000 mm intervals. Such landings should measure at least 1500 mm long or be the same width as the ramp if wider than 1500 mm. All interior and exterior ramp surfaces should be nonslippery under all conditions to ensure the free movement of wheeled traffic.

FLOOR SURFACES

Design solutions should ensure that all floor finishes and patterns are unambiguous in design and color for those with sight impairments. These surfaces should contrast significantly with adjacent vertical surfaces in color or tone. Floor surfaces should also be nonslippery under both wet and dry conditions and be easy to clean and maintain. Where carpets are laid on floors or ramps they should be securely attached to the subfloor, be of a dense weave and low loop pile, and have only the minimum underlay, if any at all.

Doors and Doorways

All doors should be operable by a single effort with the door-opening pressure low enough to ensure that persons with limited arm strength can open them safely and easily. For example doors should be balanced to require a minimum of 53 newtons (N) for exterior hinged doors and 22 N for interior hinged, sliding, or folding doors. In addition, delayed action door closers should permit the door to remain in an open position for a minimum of 5 seconds before beginning to close. This ensures a further delay of a minimum of 3 seconds before the door finally closes from an open position of 70°. Where sliding doors are used, they should be useable from both sides.

The floor surfaces on the inside and outside of each doorway should be level for a distance of 1500 mm from the door in the direction of the door swing and extend 300 mm beyond each side of the door. Wherever possible level changes should be avoided at door thresholds. Where this is not possible, thresholds should be bevelled, not exceed a height of 13 mm, and be sloped to facilitate the easy passage of wheelchairs. Thresholds accommodating a vertical change in level should not exceed 19 mm.

Door Hardware

All manual door openers should be of a horizontal lever design or a shape that is similarly easy to operate and grasp with a simple downward pressure. These are easier to manipulate than knobs or push-and-pull handles. Such hardware should be mounted 910 mm to 1000 mm from the floor surface to the center of the actuating portion, and there should be knuckle clearance of at least 60 mm between the handle and the door surface. In addition, door hardware should be designed without sharp corners or edges to reduce the risk of catching clothes.

Mail Boxes

Mail boxes in entrance lobbies and doors should be mounted at a height that ensures their easy access and use by persons in wheelchairs. They should be equipped with locks and opening mechanisms easily operable by persons with limited hand dexterity. The level of lighting at communal mail boxes should be at least 250 lux.

Accessible Bathrooms

Toilets

Toilets should be mounted at a height that ensures that the seat is level with the seat of a wheelchair, positioned in such a manner that enough space is provided at the side and in front to permit either a lateral or frontal transfer from a wheelchair. Grab rails should be provided on an adjacent wall within easy reach of a person seated on the toilet. Toilet paper dispensers and any emergency call system also should be reachable from this position. The toilet seat should be open-fronted and of a material that is easily cleaned. In addition, the flushing mechanism should be of the lever type, mounted on the tank or at the rear of the stall above seat level.

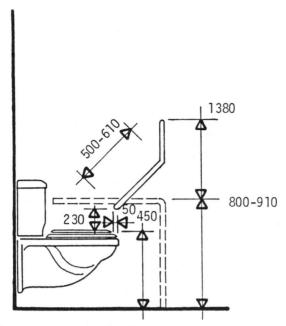

Figure 15.1. Alternate grab bars adjacent to toilet. Many alternatives are possible. (From Cluff, P. *Nursing Homes and Hostels with Care Services for the Elderly*. Canada Mortgage and Housing Corporation, 1979.)

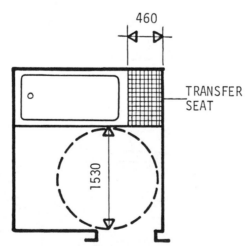

Figure 15.2. Bathroom. (From Cluff, P. *Nursing Homes and Hostels with Care Services for the Elderly*. Canada Mortgage and Housing Corporation, 1979).

Bathtubs

Domestic bathtubs should be raised to 450 mm and provided with a rim that can be grasped easily by disabled persons and used for leverage or support. In addition, a flat surface or transfer seat should be provided at

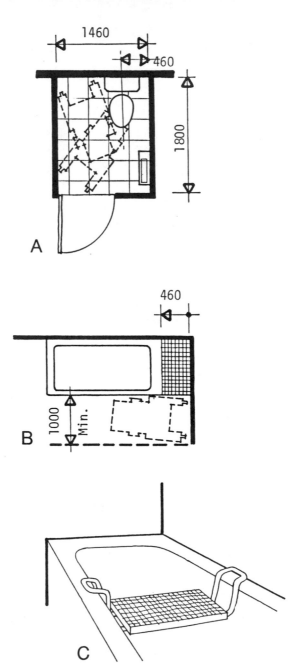

Figure 15.3. (*A*) A small compartment for wheelchair users. (*B*) Built-in transfer seat. (*C*) Removable transfer seat. (From Cluff, P. *Nursing Homes and Hostels with Care Services for the Elderly*. Canada Mortgage and Housing Corporation, 1979.)

the head of the tub at the same height as the wheelchair seat to facilitate transfer.

Bathroom Accessories

All bathroom accessories should be easily used by disabled persons and should be mounted at an appropriate height.

Grab Bars

Grab bars should be provided adjacent to bathtubs, toilets, and showers as both transfer and security aids. In some instances a variety of grab-bar arrangements may be appropriate. Such grab bars should be mounted at an appropriate height, be a minimum of 30 mm in diameter, and be located no further than 40 mm from the adjacent wall surface. Grab bars should be securely mounted and capable of supporting an individual's weight in an emergency situation.

Special Washrooms and Bathing Areas

Individuals requiring assistance with bathing may also need options in bathing and toileting accessories, depending on their disability. Solutions may include the following alternatives, used alone or in conjunction with

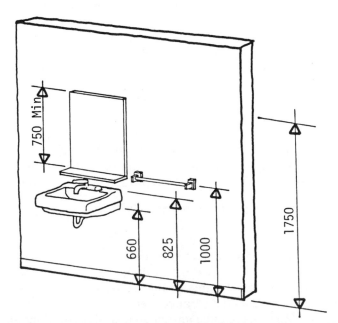

Figure 15.4. Washroom fixture and accessory arrangement. (From Cluff, P. *Nursing Homes and Hostels with Care Services for the Elderly*. Canada Mortgage and Housing Corporation,1979.)

others:

1. A raised standard bath with transfer seat at one end and grab rails to permit partly assisted bathing.
2. A special tub with mechanical transfer seat, portable lift, or a hydraulic lifting post with integral seat.
3. Flexible hose and shower, useable in a variety of positions or hand-held and located in a wheelchair shower or over a bathtub.
4. Automatic thermostat and temperature control on hot water supply.
5. Raised toilet or adjustable toilet seats at 450 mm maximum, suitable for lateral or frontal transfer.

Showers

Wheelchair shower stalls should be designed to permit easy access and safe use by a person in a wheelchair and wide enough to accommodate an attendant if and when necessary. Shower heads over bathtubs or in special wheelchair showers should be of the adjustable telephone head type, and water temperature should be controllable to prevent accidental scalding. Access to the shower stall should be direct and level, with sufficient floor drainage provided to ensure easy run-off of water. All floor and wall surfaces should be easily maintainable.

Grab bars should be provided that allow a standing or seated person adequate security. A demountable seat of nonslip material may be desirable, but the location of such a seat should not inhibit wheelchair access to the shower stall. Space adjacent to the shower stall should be provided for personal clothing and for changing.

Faucets

Faucets in washrooms and kitchens should be of the lever or blade type since these are more easily manipulated by persons with limited hand movement or strength. Hot and cold faucets should be clearly marked and mounted wide apart to allow for easy identification and handling by disabled persons. A single-action faucet is preferred where its use is appropriate.

Maneuverability

Wheelchairs

There are a wide variety of manually propelled or electrically powered wheelchairs on the market today that are designed to accommodate various types of disabilities. When chosing a wheelchair, attention should be given to the overall dimensions and clearances required.

Wherever wheelchair use can be anticipated, design solutions should take into consideration the type of wheelchair used, its overall measurements, and, where necessary, enough space should be allowed for an attendant accompanying the wheelchair user.

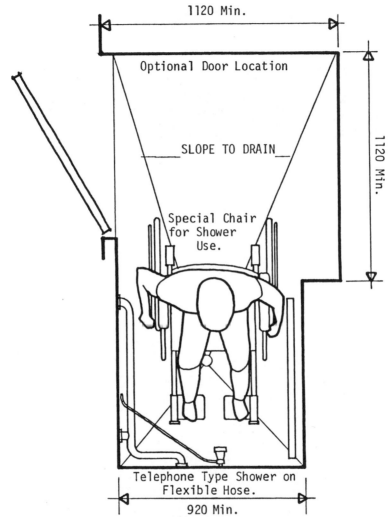

Figure 15.5. Wheelchair shower. There are many alternatives to this solution. (From Cluff, P. *Nursing Homes and Hostels with Care Services for the Elderly*. Canada Mortgage and Housing Corporation, 1979.)

Turning Space

Design solutions should ensure that adequate space has been provided for maneuvering or turning a wheelchair in all rooms and areas accessible to and used by disabled persons. Particular attention should be given to washrooms, bathrooms, kitchens, laundries, entrance ways, and vestibules, as well as bedrooms, living rooms, and storage spaces. Exterior walkways,

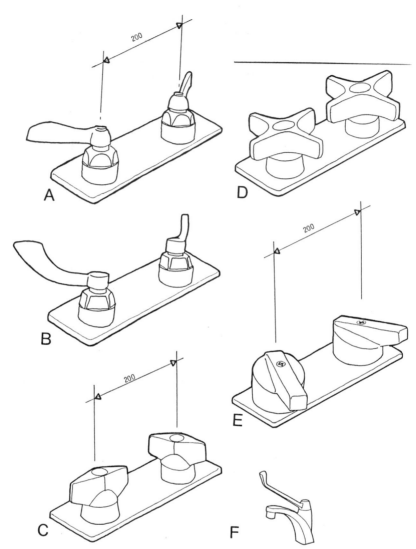

Figure 15.6. (*A and B*) Faucets with blade handle. (*C and D*) Alternate faucets. (*E*) Faucet with lever handles. (*F*) Single lever action. (*A–E* from Cluff, P. *Nursing Homes and Hostels with Care Services for the Elderly.* Canada Mortgage and Housing Corporation, 1979. *F* from Goldsmith, S. *Designing for the Disabled*, Third Ed. R.I.B.A. Publications Ltd., London.)

recreation areas, and balconies should also be considered where use by persons in wheelchairs is anticipated.

Living and Dining areas

Typical living and dining areas should be increased beyond the minimum to permit wheelchair users to maneuver and park their wheelchairs easily

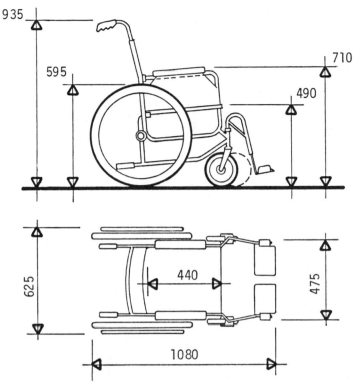

Figure 15.7. Standard wheelchair. Turning radius of a wheelchair is 5 feet (1525 mm). (From Cluff, P. *Nursing Homes and Hostels with Care Services for the Elderly*. Canada Mortgage and Housing Corporation, 1979, and from Goldsmith, S. *Designing for the Disabled*, Third Ed. R.I.B.A. Publications, Ltd., London.)

and safely. A clearance of 1500 mm between walls and furniture should be allowed for circulation and turning, and an area of 813 mm should be provided to accommodate a wheelchair at the table. If a separate dining area is provided, it should be directly accessible from the kitchen. A hatch is recommended, positioned 1000 mm from the floor between the two rooms.

Bedrooms

Bedrooms should be generous in size with design solutions accommodating both use and storage of a wheelchair. Clearance around beds should be based on the need for a 1050–1550 mm wheelchair turning space on one side of the bed and 900–1050 mm in other areas where access or circulation by a wheelchair is necessary. A minimum clearance of 813 mm in all other areas should be provided. The location of bedrooms should ensure direct and convenient access to the bathroom.

Controls

For those persons confined to bed, certain equipment controls may be necessary. These should be positioned within easy reach from a prone or sitting position. A variety of environmental and communication controls are available that may be utilized by disabled persons for operating the telephone, radio, television, two-way intercom system with a remote control unlocking device for the front door, and light switches for the bedroom, bathroom and other areas.

Counters and Vanities

Counters and vanities should be mounted at a height appropriate to a person in a wheelchair with the lower edge of mirrors being preferably 910–1000 mm from the floor surface. In addition, vanity aprons should be designed to permit approach and use by a disabled person with a clearance of 660 mm provided beneath the bottom of the lavatory to a point of at least 250 mm in from the front edge of the vanity.

Kitchen Accessories

Ranges

Ranges should be selected with cooking surfaces and ovens that are easy to use and easily cleaned and maintained. Controls should be located at the front or side of the range where the disabled user can reach them easily without risking burns. Space should also be provided on either side of the range for placing pots, etc.

Refrigerators

Refrigerators should be easy to open, self-defrosting and of an appropriate size for use by a person in a wheelchair. In addition, refrigerators should be located so that the door can be easily opened by a person in a wheelchair with access to counter space for loading and unloading groceries.

Sinks

Sinks should be mounted at a height useable by the wheelchair bound person. Where sinks are located in a vanity or counter, sufficient knee space should be provided. In addition, kitchen sinks should have counter space on either side large enough to accommodate a dish rack or tray, and sufficient knee space clearance and an insulated waste trap below.

Storage

Design solutions should ensure that adequate and accessible storage areas for personal belongings (clothing, housekeeping supplies, food, etc.) are provided, designed to complement the abilities of the disabled person. All

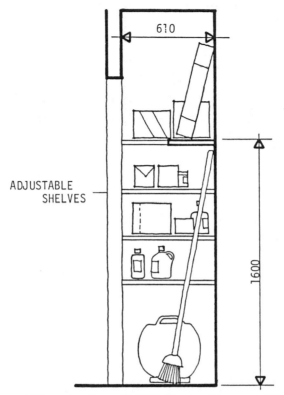

Figure 15.8. General Storage. (From Cluff, P. *Nursing Homes and Hostels with Care Services for the Elderly.* Canada Mortgage and Housing Corporation, 1979.)

storage cupboards should be equipped with sliding or folding doors that are easily opened by persons in wheelchairs or with limited manual dexterity or strength. All shelving, rods, etc., should be adjustable in height.

Laundry

Laundry facilities and accessories should be located in one general area accessible to by persons in wheelchairs or those with limited functioning abilities. It is recommended that space be provided in the laundry area to accomodate a wheelchair or seating that is accessible to the disabled person. Such space should also provide counter space for ironing and folding clothes, and for storing items such as detergents and laundry baskets adjacent to accessible front-loading washers and dryers. In addition, disabled persons should be able to see outdoors from such areas.

All surface finishes should be selected for their easy maintenance and cleaning properties with particular care being taken to ensure that the floor surface will remain nonslippery under all conditions.

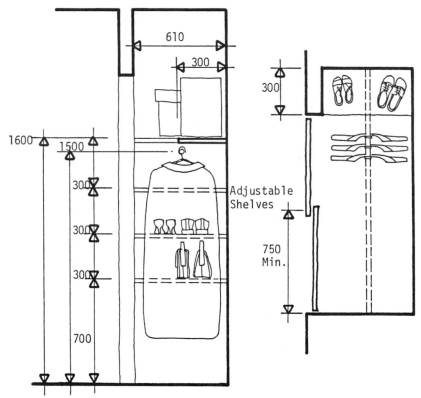

Figure 15.9. Personal storage. (From Cluff, P. *Nursing Homes and Hostels with Care Services for the Elderly*. Canada Mortgage and Housing Corporation, 1979.)

Miscellaneous

Windows

Design solutions should ensure that windows in bedrooms and living areas provide a view to the outdoors that is unobstructed by sills or horizontal transoms at heights that are inappropriate to persons in wheelchairs or lying in bed.

In addition, operating mechanisms and vents should be located where the disabled person can reach them. They should be easy to operate by persons with limited manual dexterity and strength, and should deflect air away from the bed or sitting areas.

Controls, Dispensers and Receptacles

All controls, dispensers, and waste receptacles should be placed in positions that permit easy operation and use by persons in wheelchairs and those with limited dexterity or strength.

Mirrors

Mirrors should be mounted to allow viewing by wheelchair-bound persons, or where a number of mirrors are provided, at least one should be useable by a person in a wheelchair. Lighting at mirror locations should be sufficient for grooming purposes.

Furniture

Special care should be taken in the selection of chairs and tables, lounge furniture, and garden furniture to ensure that the sitting provides good lumbar and lateral support where required.

SUMMARY

It has long been recognized that the design and construction of the home environment together with the use of assistive devices will minimize care needs and maximize the functional independence of disabled persons. However it must be noted that many special design solutions and assistive devices that benefit some disabled persons may not meet the needs of others with similar disabilities since each individual will demonstrate or exhibit different coping mechanisms and skills.

It is recommended therefore that guidance be sought from an occupational therapist prior to initiating any design changes in order to determine the specific needs of the individual person and to obtain an informed assessment of the home environment relative to the specific needs and activities of the disabled occupant.

In particular, the role of the individual in the family unit or the degree to which they will need to perform all functions of daily living for themselves will be a key determinant. The objective throughout should always remain clear, that of optimizing and supporting the skills and abilities of the disabled person and reducing his or her dependence on others.

All drawings appearing in the text are credited to the design document, Nursing Homes and Hostels with Care Services for the Elderly, which was prepared by Associated Planning Consultants Inc. for CMHC in 1979.

SUGGESTED READINGS

1. *Accessible Residential Communities—Issues and Solutions.* Canada Mortgage and Housing Corporation, 1982.
2. *Aids: Decision and Provision—A Systematic Approach To The Selection of Assistive Devices For The Disabled Person.* Community Occupational Therapy Associates, Toronto, 1981.
3. *Aids For The Handicapped.* National Research Council, Biomedical Engineering Reseach Program, Ottawa,
4. *Cost and Design of Housing Disabled Persons—Case Studies.* Canada Mortgage and Housing Corporation, 1982.
5. Foot, S. *Handicapped At Home.* The Whitefriars Press, London, 1977.

6. Goldenson, R. M., Ed. *Disability and Rehabilitation Handbook.* McGraw-Hill Book Company, 1978.
7. Goldsmith, S. *Designing for the Disabled.* R.I.B.A. Publications Ltd., London.
8. *Guidelines: Designing for Wheelchair Handicapped Persons.* COMSOC, 1981.
9. *Housing Disabled Persons.* Canada Mortgage and Housing Corporation, 1982.
10. *Nursing Homes and Hostels with Care Services for the Elderly.* Canada Mortgage and Housing Corporation, 1979.

16

The Resocialization Process After Spinal Cord Injury

ELDON TUNKS
NATALIE BAHRY
MEL BASBAUM

Until relatively recently, long-term survival rates of persons with spinal cord injuries were such that little attention was paid to problems associated with reintegration into the community. By necessity, emphasis was placed upon the needs for improved medical and health care. As the latter began to meet with success and survival rates improved significantly, health professionals have become increasingly concerned with the quality of life following spinal cord injury (7, 33). The process of resocialization involves the reacquisition of social (including familial), recreational, productive, and adaptive functions and roles.

Rehabilitation specialists know there is wide variation in the degree to which their patients are able to make the necessary adaptations following injury, and that in no way is this simply a function of the degree of physical impairment. For the professional, the problem becomes not simply one of predicting the individual's chances for a successful outcome, but it is also one of developing the ability to identify both the specific needs and program structures necessary to enhance the chances of success. To achieve this, one needs some framework that identifies both the factors influencing outcomes and the tools necessary to better assure that successful reintegration occurs.

Cogswell has suggested that while professionals have provided patients with general knowledge on the interpersonal problems they may encounter following discharge, the spinal cord injured have, for the most part, had to discover and solve these problems on their own (5, 6). This she feels is

387

contrary to what should be the socialization process of rehabilitation by which individuals with the assistance of an intervening agent (i.e. the rehabilitation team) will learn new skills, activities, and roles, and in the process, develop a new set of self-definitions.

The purpose of this chapter is to identify those factors influencing outcome and to discuss ways in which the rehabilitation experience can be structured to enhance resocialization. We will consider the meaning of disability in our society, personality factors that may influence outcome, the individual's social context before and after injury, and environmental considerations in terms of both professional interfaces with, and physical needs of, the spinal cord injured persons. We have chosen to present this material in the form of theoretical discussion illustrated with case material because research in this area is still preliminary; there is on the one hand little outcome research dealing with the resocialization process of spinal cord patients postdischarge, while at the same time established clinical practice with spinal cord and other rehabilitation patients permits us still to define what are the major clinical and theoretical issues. Hopefully, new research will not be long in appearing in the literature.

PERSONALITY FACTORS

Recent literature supports the conclusion that there is no typical spinal cord personality (4, 27, 28, 30, 32). Thus it becomes imperative to understand the different personality factors influencing behavior following spinal cord injury, and to recognize that these differences among patients will often require differences in the approach to management. It is also essential to recognize that, while no one personality type exists, certain common factors such as age, sex, and life-style, will require an understanding of cultural influences upon behavior.

Personality variables have been identified as particularly significant in the individual's ability to maximize the learning that is part of the rehabilitation process. These include one's belief in personal control and sense of efficacy, problem-solving styles, and ability to establish and maintain interpersonal relationships.

Belief in Personal Control and Self-Efficacy

The factors of belief in personal control and self-efficacy, are being recognized more and more as key ingredients in successful rehabilitation (2, 11, 29). The concept of *personal locus of control* has been established as a psychological construct; this has to do with the person's belief about the causes of events, and may be assessed on a continuum from internal to external (17). The individual with perceived internal control attributes responsibility for events to himself and his own actions rather than to the environment. "Internals" tend to seek out more information relevant to their goals, are less prone to subtle social influences, can usually laugh at themselves more easily, and exhibit a greater degree of frustration tolerance. "Externals", at the other extreme, will not only be less interested in but may actually avoid information related to their goals, be more prone to subtle social influences, and tend to internalize frustration, which makes coping with stress more difficult.

It should not be assumed from the above that the more internally-directed individual will therefore automatically prove to be the higher achiever following spinal cord injury. Hospitals by their nature have an interest in maintaining control over the patient's activities in order to minimize disruption of the established routine. As a result, regardless where on the continuum a patient may find himself, the danger becomes one of either reinforcing for him the fact that there is little he can do about his situation or creating an adversary situation in which the most internally directed individual will present as the most difficult patient by frequently questioning the routines or acting out against them. The more arbitrary or punitive the staff response to this, the quicker the development of a sense of threat to personal control. For rehabilitation personnel, it becomes essential to not only recognize the patient's need to participate in the problem-solving process but appreciate that each individual will approach the process with more or less conviction that his own effort may lead to a more independent functioning and improvement in the quality of life. The goal therefore cannot be strictly in terms of compliance with treatment, nor should it be assumed that goals cannot be set too high, particularly in the early stages of rehabilitation.

SOCIAL FACTORS

Interpersonal

Cogswell noted that following discharge from rehabilitation, paraplegics go through three distinct stages as part of the process of reestablishing themselves in the community (6). In the first stage, there is a noticeable reduction in the number of social contacts as compared to able-bodied individuals. There is an avoidance of public settings, and paraplegics play a reduced number of roles in the community. This appears to be related to an assumption on the part of injured persons that they have socially devalued roles. Following this first phase, the individual will frequently begin to associate with others who, prior to injury, would have been considered to be of lower social status, whereas relationships with previous friends rarely will be resumed. There is at the same time very careful selection of the settings in which such contacts are made, taking into consideration physical accessibility and the ease with which one can leave the setting. It is only after some time has passed and the individual begins to develop a sense of increased worth and self-esteem that relationships are developed with persons who would have previously been considered to be of equal status. Cogswell identifies this process as one that exists for those who ultimately have made some successful attempt at reintegration into the community. Many spinal cord injured, on the other hand, never successfully complete the process of the two earlier stages and may become stuck.

A.B. was 17 years old at the time of his injury. The second of three children in an upper-middle-class family, his parents refused to acknowledge the permanence of his disability. This attitude served only to reinforce his own fears about the reactions of people to his disability, resulting in his withdrawal from most community activities. Now, 8 years after injury, he describes his initial associates as individuals heavily involved in the drug culture, in which context he himself also encountered frequent problems with the law. Not until 6 years postinjury was he able to form strong social relationships (including heterosexual ones), and return to school. Interestingly, A.B. describes the rehabilitation center as an "ivory tower" approach to treatment in which insufficient effort was made to involve family members or prepare the patient for the realities he would encounter following discharge.

Today, to counteract these difficulties, considerable effort is made to involve family members in the rehabilitation process and to encourage the use of community facilities for social and recreational programming on both an individual and group basis, including the utilization of the existing community transportation system for the disabled.

The patient has come from a society in which the disabled individual is stigmatized and devalued, and therefore may very well perceive himself in a similar fashion. It is essential for rehabilitation workers to recognize that disability cannot be defined strictly in terms of organic and functional impairment, but must also include the losses related to social roles that were an integral part of the individual's life prior to the injury, and must include awareness of the change in self-evaluation. The months of rehabilitation entail a socialization process whereby staff members serve as the agents who assist in the learning necessary for defining new rules, self-concepts, and skills that will be necessary to cope with and hopefully overcome the stigma referred to above. At the same time, the hospital environment is a protective one in which the learning can occur with a minimum threat of failure. It does not, however, duplicate the reality confronting the spinal cord injured person following discharge. This socialization process therefore must continue once the individual has left the hospital, usually with considerably less access to professional resources.

Family

The reactions of families to illness or disability in one of their members and their influence upon rehabilitation outcomes are well-documented for other problems such as chronic pain, and it is reasonable to believe that the same principles apply to other areas of rehabilitation (1, 3, 21, 22, 23, 25, 31). The purpose of this discussion therefore is to consider aspects of family adaptation that may be uniquely relevant to spinal cord injured persons. Rehabilitation naturally concentrates the major part of the therapeutic energies on the patient with the injury. Yet, the injury affects not only the patient but also his family. There is a risk of overlooking the family relationships and interactions because they are less obvious than the problems of the patient, and because they may be observed during visiting hours and days at home when the staff members are not present. The relationships between the patient and staff also have a diluting effect on the patient's interactions until the patient-family interactions are intensified at the time of discharge.

Spinal cord injury most frequently affects males in adolescence or young adulthood, and impacts on families in a manner that is largely dependent upon the social roles typical of these developmental stages. Two major subgroups can be identified: (a) those who still maintain an economic or social dependency relationship with parents, and (b) those who are at an early stage in the development of both a nuclear family system and personal career objectives. It is essential to consider these groups separately. At the end of this section consideration will also be given to patients who form attachments during their rehabilitation hospitalization.

In the first group, parents of the patient are often keenly aware of their responsibility to assist their child to grow and develop in a healthy manner, physically, emotionally, and socially. In the healthy family situation parenting is directed towards building self-esteem, responsibility, competence, and eventual independent maturity. While the manner in which these objectives are played out will vary depending on personal differences and cultural influences, the goals are relatively common in most western societies. Spinal cord injury places the individual in a position of considerable dependency, not only for basic functions but for social and psychological support as well, and interrupts the normal timetable of maturation, autonomy, and leaving home. The potential for regression in the existing role relationships between parents and their son or daughter is not only significant but, in the initial stages, may even be encouraged by a young, legitimately frightened patient, and by family members who, feeling helpless in the face of the injury to their loved one, may try to deal with it by becoming overly protective. The danger exists that, in the process of working with their patients, rehabilitation personnel may pay insufficient attention to the emotional and psychological responses of family members with the potential that, as the spinal cord injured person becomes more self-confident and independent, his attempts to reestablish previous role relationships will be undermined by family members who feel the need to be protective or oversolicitous. The full impact of this situation is often not evident during hospitalization since the difficulties the patient is encountering may be compensated for by relationships that exist between himself, staff, and other patients. Following discharge however, with many fewer social contacts, overprotective attitudes on the part of parents may lead to either acquiescence by the spinal cord injured patient, and resulting adoption of a sick role, or an intensification of normal adolescent conflicts that, if not addressed appropriately, may result in an increased sense of helplessness and hopelessness on the part of family members who may be forced to desert the disabled member.

C.D., a young quadriplegic, and her family had only limited financial resources available to them. Her accident occurred several years after that of A.B. at a time when the community was much more aware of and prepared to provide for the needs of the disabled in terms of housing, education, transportation, and accessibility. Her family's early acceptance of the disability resulted in the expectation that she take responsibility for her life-style, and within obvious limitations, her physical well-being.

If we compare A.B. and C.D., both felt they could not immediately move into full participation in the community, but for C.D., the expectation that this would be required after a brief "time-out" resulted in her being unable to unduly prolong the dependency relationship and forced her to take responsibility for short- and long-term goals.

For the person who has already left his family of origin, the problems are somewhat different. Preexisting heterosexual relationships, whether within marriage or otherwise, were based upon complementary needs of fulfillment, security, and sharing. Such healthy relationships allow for maintenance of one's self-esteem and individuality, and the ability to obtain satisfaction of unique needs. Once again, the initial reactions to the disability may force the establishment of role relationships that are at first mutually desirable and beneficial, but that over the long term are contradictory to the preexisting family system and not likely to be maintained without considerable associated stress.

Two men of about 30 years of age, E.F. and G.H., both sustained injuries as the result of accidents involving alcohol abuse. At the time of their accidents, both men were married with young children and were successfully employed in semiskilled jobs. Both men were discharged to their family homes with their wives as primary care-givers. Although both marriages ultimately resulted in separation, the circumstances surrounding the dissolutions and outcomes following them were significantly different.

During the course of rehabilitation, both men encountered difficulty with hospital routines and procedures, and what they perceived as the attempts to usurp from them control and decision making. E.F.'s approach to the problem included developing rapport with staff members who might be potential advocates, and frequently raising the contentious issues in ward meetings that were being held to resolve problems associated with the milieu. G.H., on the other hand, refused to attend milieu group meetings, used more extreme behaviors such as refusal to eat or participate in therapy, and perceived patients and staff as being either "with him" or "against him," rather than as individuals in the total system who might participate in his problem solving. After discharge, similar behaviors persisted. E.F. acknowledged both his part in the original accident and the part he must play in making the marriage work. Although the couple separated after 3 years of trying, it was with the realization that there was mutual responsibility. The couple remains in contact and shares child-rearing responsibilities. G.H. on the other hand continued to project responsibility for success or failure onto his wife and children. After only 6 months, the marriage terminated, with only minimal contact between him and the other family members.

Rehabilitation staff members must therefore be sensitive not only to the emotional and psychological impact of spinal cord injury on the patient but upon family members as well. Such injury requires both patient and family to reassess preexisting role relationships and to make mutually satisfactory changes. Whether in terms of the healthy promotion of an adolescent's separation from his parents, changes in child-rearing responsibilities and economic roles, or in the sexual relationship, the danger exists that these may take second place to the rehabilitation of physical function alone. While there may be no one set of stages that can be applied to the adaptation process of all families, the presence of some initial distress is not only normal but healthy. The staff must be able to assess families' normal coping mechanisms and as necessary either support these or assist in the new learning that may be required.

To achieve this requires the ability to communicate to family members the sense that their involvement in the rehabilitation process is not only desirable but valued, a recognition that there are emotional needs, not only on the part of the patient but of family members as well, and finally that rehabilitation does not terminate on discharge from the hospital. Rather, rehabilitation is perhaps even more dependent upon the ability to identify social and role stresses that occur when the patient has returned home to the family, and to utilize both their own and community resources in the problem-solving process that must continue following discharge. In addition to family casework, family groups can be employed therapeutically to provide information, serve as support groups, and provide normalizing experiences for the patients with their families (24).

A further frequently encountered situation is that of a young person with spinal cord injury who falls in love during the months of hospitalization and rehabilitation. When the object of the affection is another patient, as it may be, then staff and family members may be faced with some dilemmas. On the one hand, there is the natural instinct to be protective of patients and to be inclined to voice caution or even to intervene, especially if staff members are aware of potential personality problems that have appeared during the extensive hospitalization. On the other hand, there may be an investment in allowing such a relationship to develop; parents may perceive it as a partial solution to the autonomy issue, especially if the object of the affection is more able-bodied. But there may also be some worry that the more able-bodied mate may have heroic or neurotic motives, get into more than was bargained for, and then suddenly pull out, with repercussions all around. What is needed in such situations is the perspective that the rehabilitation time frame involves a relatively large segment of a patient's life, and that it should not be surprising if some patients fall in love; such psychosocial events require the same professional attention and impartial assistance that would be normal for other areas of the patient's life without gratuitously imposing value judgments or taking a laissez-faire attitude.

How Skills and Functions Become Occupations and Roles

If today were the "first day of the rest of your life" as a quadriplegic, you may choose to live "one day at a time." Both of these quotations illustrate the type of coping skills one would require to function throughout the rehabilitation period and then in the community. While spinal cord injured persons must plan and work for a better future, they encounter daily frustrations of dependency, loss of skills, discrimination, and bureaucratic red tape.

Levels of Incapacity and Function

The rehabilitation of these individuals requires that they learn new living skills that allow them to function within a "new body," with a revised values system, and within a new cultural minority group (the disabled). The initial awareness that all activities and movement will have to be relearned must be truly awesome. In order to describe the complex changes that such a person must experience during the rehabilitation process, Kielhofner has described various levels of dysfunction in spinal cord injuries; this will be used for our discussion (15). These levels are arranged in a hierarchy of complexity but remain interrelated. For more details of the levels and a description of the laws governing the relationships between them, please refer to Kielhofner's *Health Through Occupation*, Chapter 2 (16).

At the most basic level, physical integrity is affected by muscle atrophy and bone decalcification; the patient has no control over these processes. At the level of somatic systems, active, normal muscle movement is either absent or disrupted by weakness, contractures, spasticity, or paralysis. The sensory loss from denervated areas poses a threat to the health of the body, since pain signals and the need to relieve pressure are not perceived by the patient. The regulation of body temperature is another feedback system that is disturbed. The individual must thus learn the skill of reading new signals such as spasticity, skin redness, and autonomic dysreflexia in order to be alerted to physical disorders.

In the next level, the previously self-sufficient system of personal functions (in the biological, psychological, or social domain) is no longer self-regulated. The spinal cord injured patient must now learn the skills necessary to perform the functions of emptying his bladder and evacuating the bowels. He must also learn a new method to express his sexuality, which is no longer subject to normal CNS regulation. The usual methods of interaction with one's own body and with others can be greatly compromised with changes in the sense of self-efficacy.

The majority of therapeutic intervention is focused on the next complex level that deals with a revised division of labor for physical functioning. During many months, new skills must be learned for mobility. Paralyzed legs are replaced by the action of arms and equipment as new means for locomotion. For the quadriplegic, the skillful use of hands, splints, aids, and the mouth must be learned to replace the work of fingers. Basic self-care activities may be dependent upon assistance from an attendant, thus losing the personal autonomy the injured person once had. The function of vision becomes expanded to replace sensory loss for body awareness in space, and for the protection against burns or other injuries.

In the next level, previously learned patterns or mental images for performing a skillful movement are no longer valid with the "new body." New ways to perform activities must incorporate a revised repertoire of limited but necessary skills. It becomes more important for the person to interact with people through verbal expression of needs and feelings. Affective communication is an essential skill that should be fostered and perhaps taught in conjunction with assertiveness training techniques. It is also important to develop the cognitive skill of knowing what activities are safe to execute when alone and what measures should be taken in an emergency.

All of these previous levels have an impact upon the symbolic level that focuses on one's sense of life's purpose, goals, and meaning. The individual's previous self-concept and values may have been based upon the occupations and roles he or she can no longer pursue. A psychological need to be independent could be suppressed and replaced by an anxiety about becoming dependent. Community living is a new noninstitutional environment where physical, financial, and employment obstacles threaten the patient's past patterns of functioning. A new productive self-image, based upon adapted skills, must be developed in order to realistically maintain or renew self-esteem in the individual. Previous productive and creative methods of self-expression must be altered to the new physical, cognitive, and social skills that the disability can allow the body to realistically perform. These skills must be integrated initially through meaningful occupations as basic as gaining independence in writing. Such occupations can then be utilized to formulate new roles and a sense of meaning as a homemaker, student, artist, or volunteer. To acquire roles that have personal and cultural significance is very important in developing a new self-image and sense of competency.

Once at home, quadriplegics are faced with more leisure time than in the hospital. Productive use of time becomes a vital goal that can prevent drug abuse, family discord, depression, and suicidal ideation. The occupational therapist should focus on leisure time productivity and creativity for quadriplegics as a natural extension and application of the patient's newly acquired skills.

The final, most complex level places importance on the social roles the person assumes upon discharge as an integral member of the family and society. Previous roles of breadwinner, independent bachelor, parent, or son or daughter are compromised and threatened to become redefined under society's distorted image of an invalid. An altered life-style that no longer includes employment must include new roles that enhance self-esteem by providing opportunity for control, efficacy, creative expression, interpersonal responsibility, and sexual gratification. These are vital in order to compete with and counteract society's deeply entrenched work ethic and the media-fostered ideal of the average young, healthy, and glamorous individual. Taken to the other extreme, very busy quadriplegics who are full-time students, part-time students and parents, or full-time employees may find it difficult to schedule their time to socialize because, once at home, there are still time-consuming self-care routines to complete. A balance of productivity, rest, and play is necessary for everyone.

Moving into the Community Environment

A study by Green and associates attempted to distinguish factors related to the self-concept of 71 spinal cord injured persons who had been injured at least 4 years previously (13). The findings suggested that persons with the highest scores of self-concept perceived themselves to be as independent as physically possible in relation to daily activities and the use of transportation. Greater need for interactions with an attendant, as well as living within suitable, noninstitutional, accessible accommodations, were additional factors relating to a better self-concept. It appears that the level of injury and previous level of education had little significance in the findings. Since the development of a good self-concept is important in our discussions of resocialization, it may be beneficial to focus on those skills and functions of independence that are affected by family and community stresses.

Although function and independence in certain activities can be achieved during rehabilitation, they might not be applied once the person begins to live at home. The optimally strengthened muscles become weaker without the daily use of exercise equipment. Due to this, and probable weight gain, transfers may become more difficult and dependent. Range of motion exercises are forgotten as family care-givers are unable to incorporate them into a daily routine. As a result, increased spasticity and restricted joint motion could restrict some skills that were learned. Intermittent catheterizations have social and employment implications if assistance is required. The wife and mother with young children to care for usually does not find time to catheterize her quadriplegic family member more than twice a day. As a result of these situations, the quadriplegic not only decreases his fluid intake dramatically but may restrict his social outings to very familiar settings only. Another family duty that often is neglected is the need to turn a quadriplegic regularly during the night; this often decreases to once a night, if at all.

The issue of access to independent transportation is an important ingredient for socialization. An individual can only develop his own sense of personal competence among other members of society when he can be present as a peer or coworker. This in turn depends on the possibility of transportation and on overcoming architectual barriers. (It also is important for rehabilitation staff members to be sensitive to such issues while arranging outpatient follow-up visits since the patient may not be inclined to mention the problem.)

The physical equipment and architectural changes required and available for a spinal cord injured person to become independent in the community will vary according to the family situation, finances, and the family's acceptance of such equipment. A health care professional may believe that a patient with more equipment and finances has a greater chance of adjusting to his or her disability. It is important to realize that this is not necessarily the case. In addition to fostering the development of new occupations, the rehabilitation team should focus on other psychosocial issues of equal importance to all spinal cord injured persons, regardless of their financial situations. It is the individual's personality resources, self-concept, and family and social support systems that will sustain him or her in the community. As Green's study suggests, those with greater social interaction through attendants seemed to develop a better self-concept, yet they were the most physically limited. There are many cases of marital separation of well-equipped couples in contrast to couples whose marriages have survived with minimal community support or equipment.

The development of new skills and the acquisition of a good self-concept might not be achieved upon discharge from the institution. They may in fact, take several years to develop while the individual lives in the community.

I.J. was 21 years old when he became C5–6 quadriplegic. He was engaged to be married at the time of his injury but terminated this relationship after several months of living in a chronic care institution. He had not yet formulated a good self-concept that would enable him to feel he had anything to offer in a marriage. The next several years were consumed with activities involving alcohol abuse and a gambling addiction. He socialized within a restricted group of family and friends, and developed transient relationships with several women. Four years after his injury he had the opportunity to be readmitted to a spinal cord rehabilitation center where he acquired many new skills and greater muscle strength. Although he initially had strong suicidal ideations, these subsided as the intense rehabilitation program gave him a new sense of worth. Soon after this "second chance," he was able to establish a serious relationship with a woman and is now living in the community with her. He has the responsibility of managing some household routines and socializes with the neighbors, family, and friends. Some of his activities are associated with a local quadriplegic club as well. The most important fact remains that he is now very content and satisfied with his current life-style.

Thus rehabilitation provides the opportunity to develop skills that are used to perform meaningful functions that are then united and applied toward desired occupations and roles. This process can only fully mature through adaptation and interaction within a cultural and social context. In this way, the community becomes the final stage in the rehabilitation process.

ADAPTATION

Adaptation is a common word but one that it is hard to be precise about. For our purposes here we will say that it is the ability to respond with a reasonable degree of comfort to new situations and problems, and to demonstrate adequate activity and initiative in the areas of productivity (which may include employment or other creative work), recreation, and social and family roles. In anyone, patient or otherwise, adaptation is a relative thing, depending on maturity, skills, resources, severity of stresses, and other factors, and premorbidly patients have adapted well in some cases and not so well in others. Some have been injured at critical times when they were working out some issues relating to maturity. With this equipment for adaptation, such as it is, the patients present with the new liability of spinal cord injury. The explicit task of the rehabilitation professional is to facilitate the patient's adaptation, not just in terms of instrumental aid and physical skills, but also in the social and recreational frameworks mentioned above. Among the many possible factors to consider are the patient's knowledge, evaluation and acceptance of his or her own situation, his or her problem-solving style, personal goals, supports, and psychological assets. Adaptiveness also has to take into account the patient's stage at the time of a given task or goal. For example, after 6 months of rehabilitation one might expect some patients to have developed fairly clear plans for their postdischarge residence; in the first 6 weeks after the injury it would be hasty to expect such planning. Built into the rehabilitation program are multiple opportunities for achieving mastery in small, gradual, and orderly steps. These structured therapeutic experiences have to be managed in such a way that the goals are realistic, considering the patient's assets, stage, and progress. Furthermore it is important that the patient develop a sense of mastery; this cognitive component should be part of all of the instrumental and rehabilitation tasks. This is achieved by being conscious of the patient's need for a sense of control and efficacy, and avoiding being overly controlling, overprotective, or excessively routine.

K.L. is a 20 year old C4 quadriplegic from a family with a long history of poor coping skills, poor employment history, frequent dependence upon public welfare, and the attendant problems in living. Though the family insisted that K.L. was to return home, it was evident to most that this had little chance of success. K.L. was himself aware of this but did not wish to concede to the rehabilitation team that placement in a chronic care facility might be more appropriate; this he would have perceived as giving up, or "the end of the road." With the decision for either discharge or transfer imminent, K.L. suggested going to the chronic care facility for 1 month until the family could make the final arrangements for his return home. This was agreed, and after 1 month in the chronic care facility, he suggested that a second month might be advisable. In the meanwhile, he was making social contacts both within and outside the facility, and after the second month, he gave up the idea of returning home as he felt he would be more restricted there than he felt he was in the chronic care facility. At present, he is attempting to coordinate a community education program for adolescents, emphasizing the prevention of spinal cord injury.

The sort of goals that might be suitable for the spinal cord injured patient may be different from those that would be normal for an uninjured person. For example, it may be unrealistic to expect the majority of such patients to become fully competitively employable, although some will eventually be quite successful. Still, there is a need to develop in all productive, recreational, and social areas. It may be necessary for some to put extra stress on development of recreational pursuits. Some may become productive in managing family affairs, artistic pursuits, or group or service club activities, for example. To achieve the end of good adaptation, the rehabilitation professional has to assess and support the patient's adaptive efforts throughout rehabilitation and help the patient make adequate provisions for aftercare, with the understanding that adaptation is a process that continues lifelong. If the base and the skills are good, future success is more likely.

Employment is an outcome hoped for by many and achieved by some. Part of the vocational-rehabilitation effort may be to return to school after treatment in the rehabilitation center. El Ghatit and Hanson (10) followed-up 745 male veterans with spinal cord injury. About 40% had increased their educational status, and they found that such increases were more frequent in patients who had either married after their spinal cord injuries or who had maintained their marriages intact. Those who increased their educational status after their injuries or those who already had high educational status at the time of injury were more likely to have attained employment. In another study, DeVivo and Fine (9) found that predictors of return to work after a follow-up of 3 years included the factors of being young, white, female (including housewives), having high Barthel score, and having been employed at the time of the original injury. Goldberg and Freed (12) followed up 24 patients for a period of 8 years and found that the best predictors of employment in their group were educational grade attained, the presence of vocational plans and interests, work values, the rehabilitational outlook, and the number of dependents. Employment status did not correlate with marital status, the level of lesion, or severity of impairment. The employment statuses at 4 years and at 8 years were also similar, suggesting that the probability of employment was not increasing as a function of time. Most of the above predictors of future employment are not surprising. Factors such as the stable marital status, drive and capacity to attain further education goals, and work values, for example, are those that would be considered to augur well for an able-bodied prospective employee as well. The importance of such studies may be in pointing this out, leaving us with the suggestion that employability might be improved by supporting some more general objectives such as helping the family unit to maintain its integrity, assisting the patient to set goals, and facilitating the acquisition of further education.

Facilitating the Resocialization Process

Professionals working together in rehabilitation teams direct their attention to complementary areas of expertise. What they all have in common is the task of establishing orderly short- and long-term objectives and focus for therapeutic activity that is coherent with the patients' goals and environments, while being realistic and coordinated with the efforts of other helpers and significant others. These therapeutic activities have to be organized in such a way as to provide mastery experiences. In these endeavors, there is a clear cognitive and interpersonal learning experience involved in instrumental tasks such as learning transfers or using aids, and a clear reality base is involved in psychosocial therapies: all are interdependent. Both are in the context of positive therapeutic relationships between the patient and the team members.

Personality Issues and Psychotherapy

People are amazingly resilient and, with time and support, make adjustments and get on with their lives. In the study mentioned earlier, Green, Pratt, and Grigsby (13) followed up 71 patients who had suffered spinal cord injuries 4 or more years previously. They found that these individuals generally demonstrated good self-esteem and a positive self-concept. This positive view of themselves correlated with factors of perceived independence, provision of one's own transportation, and living with spouses, friends, or family.

On the other hand, in some cases, problematic personality features may be identified; these may include distorting the view of the world as either overly good or bad, externalizing or projecting problems, denying or distorting unpleasant affect, displaying antisocial, mistrustful, impulsive, passive, anxious, fragile, or aloof traits, or having value systems that may clash with those of the middle-class professional team members. If these traits are found, patients are likely to be singled out for referral to psychiatrists, psychologists, or social workers. The tasks of the psychosocial team members are to make an assessment, judge the importance of the traits or problems identified, and set in motion plans for psychosocial intervention. These might be pitched at several levels; in some cases formal psychotherapy is indicated—in others, family therapy, psychotropic drugs, or behavior management programs that concentrate more on staff strategies than on patient insight.

Even more important is the need for supportive psychotherapy as an ongoing process during the rehabilitation. This is the responsibility of many team members. Often patients will themselves single out a particular staff member that they feel close to, not necessarily a member of the psychosocial staff. In such a relationship, there is the capacity to at times clarify misconceptions by providing cognitive input, to allow for the airing of frustrations or anxieties, to obtain the encouragement of a respected person, and to continue to give a familiar face to the complex rehabilitation program. This relationship continues to be important and valuable as the time of discharge nears.

A problem often referred for psychosocial consultation is the appearance of depression early in the course of hospitalization or sometime later when the enormity of the changes occasioned by the injury cannot any longer be denied. Often this represents normal grief and responds to empathic support. In a minority of cases, depression may represent an affective illness for which antidepressant medication is indicated. Always, it signals the need to bring to bear the supportive psychotherapy relationship. Although transient feeling of grief and even consideration of suicide likely has no negative prognostic significance, prolonged depression may possibly be more important. In a small study (which should be replicated), Malec and Neimeyer (18) studied 28 spinal cord injured patients through rehabilitation, at discharge, and at follow-up. They found that depression during hospitalization predicted poorer self-care at discharge and longer hospitalization. Further, they found that self-care at 6 months postdischarge was predicted by self-care at discharge.

Psychotherapeutic intervention is likely to be most effective if the therapist demonstrates knowledge regarding spinal cord injury rehabilitation, ability to be relevant to the patient's goals and concerns, appreciation of appropriate timing in the development of future goals, patience, ability to be sensitive to the patient's need (however expressed) for control, and tolerance of possible negative transference. Learning experiences through psychotherapy during the months of rehabilitation begins to provide some of the equipment that will later be necessary in the process of resocialization. In this sense, resocialization begins at the first staff contact and continues through the multiple levels of skill-acquisition, becoming more obvious toward discharge. The patient during this time needs to progressively develop a new set of definitions of himself based on what he can (rather than cannot) do and based on role relationships with significant others, on a sense of control and personal efficacy, future-oriented goal-directedness, and on a healthy sense of personal worth in respect to others.

Interpersonal

Some authors suggest that the rehabilitation center provides too protective an environment for the spinal cord patient to learn the skills necessary for effective interpersonal relationships following discharge (7, 19, 20, 26, 33). There may be at times some truth in this assumption. However, rehabilitation centers are not inherently unhealthy places (from a psychosocial point of view), and the shortcomings may sometimes be due to the failure to exploit certain unique features of the treatment environment because the spinal cord rehabilitation team's primary focus may be one of physical more than social rehabilitation.

By way of example, consider who are the rehabilitation health professionals. The nature of spinal cord rehabilitation, whether in terms of the physical demands of the job, the inherent behavioral problems that frequently occur, and demographic characteristics of both the spinal cord injured and health care professionals in general, results in a rehabilitation team that is primarily female, young (under 40), and from middle-class backgrounds. Spinal cord injured patients on the other hand tend to be primarily male, under 30, and frequently, in the authors' experience, from a slightly lower-class background. The similarities and differences between the groups are often the source of considerable conflict. However, this need not necessarily be an obstacle, and in fact if appropriately utilized, could serve to enhance the resocialization process. Haney and Rubin (14) studied 18 spinal cord injured males; they arranged for female volunteers (physical therapy students) to visit with these patients, and found that the patients reported improvements in morale, boredom, social skills, and sense of attractiveness to the opposite sex. That this seemed to have been a valuable experience also for the volunteers can be seen in the fact that two-thirds of the volunteers made further visits to the patients.

The similarity in age between spinal cord injured patients and those involved in their rehabilitation is frequently the source of considerable transference and countertransference. There may be anger on the part of the patient because they perceive staff members as able to live their lives as they wish and as not fully understanding the implications of the disability. Conversely, staff members may feel that "there but for the grace of God go I," creating overprotective behaviors motivated by pity. Similarly, the situation of young males being very dependent for treatment, often of a very intimate nature, upon young females leads to a great deal of testing in regard to sexual roles and behaviors. Unfortunately, the nature of such testing may become very threatening to staff members who in turn may become defensive or angry. Finally, where there are differences in social class background, conflicts associated with the staff's heavy cultural investment in achievement-oriented goals frequently dominate. Because of their ages and backgrounds, patients may be more present-oriented and less concerned with high achievement. In establishing rehabilitation goals, this may lead to conflict if the different value structures are not taken into consideration.

DeJong has made a distinction between what he defines as the "rehabilitation" and "independent living paradigms" (7, 8). Rehabilitation institutions, he suggests, attribute problems to the disabled individual by defining them in terms of poor performance (physical impairment, poor psychological adjustment, and lack of motivation and cooperation), which are to be corrected by compliance with treatment regimens and with professionals. Independent living centers, on the other hand, attribute problems to environmental barriers, encouragement of dependency, and lack of provision for social and community supports. Solutions, from the latter point of view, are to be found in encouraging patients in consumerism, providing peer counseling, self-help, and barrier removal. Our opinion is that either approach by itself is simplistic, but the conclusions of the paper are valid— rehabilitation must spend considerable effort on removal of barriers and on encouraging patients toward consumerism as part of their resocialization. DeJong concludes that the final outcome for discharged patients will be a function of the interaction between personal characteristics, environmental factors, and organic variables.

It becomes essential, if one is to assist the patient not only with overcoming functional disabilities but interpersonal stresses as well, to utilize the milieu to its maximum benefit. Central to the conflicts described above are the concepts of control and autonomy. Patients by the very nature of their situation are frequently left with the sense not only of dependency upon the hospital and its personnel but frequently of impotence in their ability to influence the behaviors of others. This perception of a lack of control is focused either upon the individuals around them, who will not allow them to be part of the decision-making process, or upon their own disability, which has made them both different and helpless. If this is in fact accurate, then it is only natural that patients will respond with either severe apathy or, at the other extreme, noncompliant behaviors. The differences and similarities between the patient and staff groups are a given that, while unalterable, can be used in ways that enhance the patients' abilities to regain autonomy and self-esteem. An antidote to the belief that the staff members understand the meaning of disability is accurate empathy that recognizes the transferences that occur and in turn allows patients to test out their relationships with others on a very practical level—not in a condescending or punitive manner but in a way that encourages the development of appropriate life skills.

The nurse who has just had her bottom pinched by a patient may choose to ignore the incident totally, may become angry and respond in a hostile manner, or may indicate a sense of indignation and identify the behavior as inappropriate and indicative of frustration, not solely sexual in nature, but relating more to a sense of impotent frustration created by the disability and the patient's perception that the environment is more concerned with routines than people. All three reactions by that nurse provide behavioral sanctions. However, the educative goal should involve more than a suppression of the unacceptable behavior. The assumption conveyed in the first approach is that, while the behavior is unacceptable, it is also very nonthreatening, coming from someone with a spinal cord injury. However, this also disqualifies the significance of the patient's nonverbal communication. An overtly hostile reaction certainly labels the behavior as unacceptable but also indicates that control of interpersonal relationships, if it is possible for the disabled person, may have to come from acting-out, thus reinforcing behaviors that may ultimately serve to further alienate the individual. The final approach serves to place the problem more in terms of its social context. The nurse in this situation is indicating that there is a recognition of the significance of the disability and dependency for the individual. She does not deny the individual's masculinity and leaves the door open to learning that will assist in the process of self-definition, development of interpersonal skills, and positive self-esteem.

The issue of social class differences may similarly be utilized as part of the learning process. For example, all too often the emphasis by rehabilitation personnel is on the need for the development of an educational or vocational plan. Statistics in regard to vocational outcomes with spinal cord injury certainly suggest that this has been one of the major failures in spinal cord injury rehabilitation. While not entirely related to an overemphasis on such values and certainly influenced by societal attitudes and conditions, it does nonetheless point out the need to deemphasize the conflicts created by value differences and instead to create mechanisms that perhaps will teach patients the skills and values necessary for successful and productive reintegration into the community. A recent development in the authors' setting has been a "milieu group" geared to addressing concerns of both patients and staff about the manner in which the rehabilitation program operates and the difficulties encountered by both groups. The assumption is that there is mutual responsibility for both the problems that exist and the solutions that may be possible. The focus is on the here and now, and issues are therefore meaningful and of concern to both groups. The outcome logically is to enhance the development of appropriate problem-solving skills while at the same time assist in overcoming the natural sense of helplessness and self-depreciation that can accompany major loss of physical function.

Facilitating Adaptation

In the context of structured therapeutic experiences, therapists assist their patients to learn adaptive attitudes and skills, and to acquire the necessary coping tools. Multiple opportunities are offered during the course of rehabilitation to learn and to acquire this necessary equipment, always in small but orderly steps, often in what seems daily routine, but with the outcome that the patient also acquires a sense of self-efficacy and control. This sense of control grows, not suddenly but gradually with each experience, and is not a function of only one kind of learning (such as in learning to use new tools), but rather grows with the whole fabric of the transactions that characterize the rehabilitation process. However, it is not automatic that all patients will acquire an adequate sense of self-efficacy and skills by osmosis during hospitalization, and staff members may vary in their abilities to facilitate the development of a sense of success from a routine exercise. This part of the learning process is best facilitated if the staff appreciates that each day gives the patient the opportunity to learn and acquire some vital tools and experiences that will be the foundation for future adaptation. The cognitive element of a belief in personal success and control comes from three sources, all of which can be influenced and augmented by the staff; (a) recognition of mastery experiences in the rehabilitation setting; (b) factual information that might be provided in respect to the patient's condition and options; and (c) interpersonal learning that involves attitudes toward disability, or more correctly, toward the patient's new capacities. The second item may come from educational sessions with the staff, from service groups, and from some more experienced patients, and the third item results from patient-staff interactions and from the treatment milieu. Not to be forgotten is the need for the family of the patient to acquire new information and attitudes in parallel.

Community-based health care services are very important to utilize in discharge planning for those regions that are fortunate enough to have such government-sponsored programs. A formal method of communication between the community professional (nurse, occupational therapist, physiotherapist) and the rehabilitation center can facilitate future good quality care. New equipment or housing needs may require the assistance of a community-based occupational therapist who can provide a detailed assessment of the person's current abilities and changing environmental situation. Such changes occur when a quadriplegic moves to a new residence or decides to begin educational upgrading a few years later. A marriage separation may provide a new challenge for a C6 quadriplegic to learn how to live alone with assistance from an occupational therapist, daily visits from a nurse, and regular homemaker visits during the week. Likewise, the development of new romantic relationships may result in a move away from the original parental family setting to that of living with a partner who holds a full-time job. Such a move often creates financial difficulties as some disability pensions may be minimized or cancelled. A social worker can be helpful during such a transition.

M.N. was an employed wife and mother of two boys when she became a C5 quadriplegic in her early 30s. With the help of community support services, financed by the government and by her husband's insurance from work, she is receiving several nursing visits daily, health care aids, a visiting homemaker, a physiotherapist for recurrent shoulder pain, and an occupational therapist to primarily assist her with part-time university studies via assessment of equipment needs and accessibility. Family and marital counseling have both been utilized as well to help this family unit to function. In the past 5 years she has received the following new equipment to facilitate her changing needs, via recommendations made by the community-based occupational therapist: a power reclining wheelchair to replace her regular power wheelchair, a new light-weight manual wheelchair to replace her manual reclining wheelchair, a large work desk with two powered rotating discs that hold course material, a typewriter, tape recorder, page turner, personal computer, printer, and telephone, accessibility features such as ramps and lifts for her second home since her injury, expansion of environmental controls throughout the house, and various miscellaneous aids to assist with course work and daily activities. A government program has financially sponsored the above equipment since M.N. is retraining for gainful competitive employment. As a result, the husband has been able to maintain his full-time employment and is anticipating the day when his wife will be employed as well.

In this community, a self-help social club for spinal cord injured quadriplegics has emerged. It offers recreational wheelchair rugby and social events during the year. Initially organized by health professionals and one high-level quadriplegic, this club is now functioning under direction of its members with several able-bodied vounteers. It serves as an important support and information network for those who participate. A self-help support group for wives and girlfriends of quadriplegic males has also developed in this community. These women meet to discuss care-related problems, coping problems, and reasons for staying, loving, or leaving their partners. Spinal cord injured persons in a separate group have interested themselves in the efforts of fund-raising for spinal cord research. Yet again, other quadriplegics may soon participate in a proposed future community-based exercise program to be developed for their specific needs. These and other community services and agencies facilitate health care delivery both within and outside the hospital setting. They also provide a greater opportunity for socialization and the development of support networks for those individuals who have not returned to full-time employment.

In many communities, there exist halfway houses and independent living facilities where the patients can be a step removed from the controlled environment of the hospital but yet obtain specialized assistance. For some, these facilities provide a useful step in the process of return to the community. For others who are psychologically isolated or severely impaired, it provides a compromise between prolonged hospital living and an inaccessible goal of fully independent living. The existence of such facilities is not the magical ingredient in resocialization and independence of spinal cord injured people, even though such resources are valuable. The essential is good management, good facilitation, and adequate and enduring support that extends long into the postdischarge period.

SUMMARY

In a recent paper, Zola (33) discussed the issue of independent living for patients after discharge from rehabilitation centers. A contrast was drawn between independence as it might be seen from the point of view of the patient and the view of the rehabilitation agency. The author gave the example of how, during one period of his life, he attempted to walk rather than use his wheelchair because that was seen to be a universal rehabilitation goal, but consequently when he had to walk longer distances, he was not able to keep up with others. The result was limitation rather than an improvement in social independence. He noted that safety may be a major consideration posed by rehabilitation staff in the management of patients but that patients themselves may see the need for some risk-taking. Patients may not in the long-term assess their needs in the same way as they would be assessed in the relatively short-term by professionals involved in the rehabilitation industry. Patients may for example put a higher value on quality of social life, sense of self-control, and of stability. His summary is completely appropriate here.

"We must expand the notion of independence from physical achievements to psychosocial decision-making. Independent living must include not only the quality of life we lead. Our notion of human integrity must take into account the notion of taking risks. Rehabilitation personnel must change the model of service from doing something to someone to planning and creating services with someone. In short, we must free ourselves from some of the culture-bound and time-limited standards and philosophy that currently exist." (33)

REFERENCES

1. Baekeland, F., and Lundwall, L. Dropping out of treatment: a critical review. *Psychol. Bull.*, 82:738–783, 1975.
2. Bandura, A. Self-efficacy: toward a unifying theory of behavioral change. *Psychol. Rev.*, 2:191–215, 1977.
3. Block, A. R., Kremer, E. F., and Gaylor, M. Behavioral treatment of chronic pain: the spouse as a discriminative cue for pain behavior. *Pain, 9:*243–252, 1980.
4. Bourestom, N. C., and Howard, M. T. Personality characteristics of three disability groups. *Arch. Phys. Med. Rehabil., 46:*626–632, 1965.
5. Cogswell, B. Rehabilitation of the paraplegic: process of socialization. *Sociological Inquiry, 37:*11–26, 1967.
6. Cogswell, B. Self-socialization: readjustment of paraplegics in the community. *J. Rehabil., 34:*11–13, 1968.
7. DeJong, G. Independent living: from social movement to analytic paradigm. *Arch. Phys. Med. Rehabil., 60:*435–446, 1979.
8. DeJong, G. *Environmental Accessibility and Independent Living Outcomes.* Michigan State University Press, East Lansing, Mich., 1980.
9. DeVivo, M J., and Fine, P. R. Employment status of spinal cord injured patients 3 years after injury. *Arch. Phys. Med. Rehabil., 63:*200–203, 1982.
10. El Ghatit, A. Z., and Hanson, R. W. Educational and training levels and employment of the spinal cord injured patient. *Arch. Phys. Med. Rehabil., 60:*405–406, 1979.
11. Friedman, H. S., and DiMateo, M. R. *Interpersonal Issues in Health Care.* Academic Press, Inc., New York, 1982.
12. Goldberg, R. T., and Freed, M. M. Vocational development of spinal cord injury patients: an 8-year follow-up. *Arch. Phys. Med. Rehabil., 63:*207–210, 1982.
13. Green, B. C., Pratt, C. C., and Grigsby, T. E. Self-concept among persons with long-term spinal cord injury. *Arch. Phys. Med. Rehabil., 65:*751–754, 1984.
14. Haney, M., and Rubin, B. Modifying attitudes toward disabled persons while resocializing spinal cord injured patients. *Arch. Phys. Med. Rehabil., 65:*431–436, 1984.
15. Kielhofner, G. *Health Through Occupation: Theory and Practice in Occupational Therapy.* F.A. Davis Co., Philadelphia, 1983, pp. 80–81.
16. Kielhofner, G. *Health Through Occupation: Theory and Practice in Occupational Therapy.* F.A. Davis Co., Philadelphia, 1983, pp. 55–92.
17. MacDonald, A. P. Internal-external locus of control: a promising rehabilitational variable. *J. Coun. Psyc., 18:*111–116, 1971.
18. Malec, J., and Neimeyer, R. Psychologic prediction of duration of inpatient spinal cord injury rehabilitation and performance of self-care. *Arch. Phys. Med. Rehabil., 64:*359–363, 1983.
19. Margolin, R. Motivational problems and resolutions in the rehabilitation of paraplegics and quadriplegics. *Amer. Arch. of Rehabil. Ther., 20:*94–103, 1971.
20. Mikulic, M. Reinforcement of independent and dependent patient behaviors by nursing personnel: an exploratory study. *Nurs. Res., 20:*162–164, 1971.
21. Mohamed, S. N., Weisz, G. M., and Waring, E. M. The relationship of chronic pain to depression, marital adjustment, and family dynamics. *Pain, 5:*285–292, 1978.
22. Painter, J. R., Seres, J. L., and Newman, R. I. Reassessing benefits of the pain center: why some patients regress. *Pain, 8:*101–113, 1900.
23. Roberts, A. H., and Reinhardt, L. The behavioral management of chronic pain: long-term follow-up with comparison groups. *Pain, 8:*151–162, 1980.
24. Rohrer, K., Adelman, B., Puckett, J., Toomey, B, Talbert, D., and Johnson, E. W.

Rehabilitation in spinal cord injury: use of a patient-family group. *Arch. Phys. Med. Rehabil., 61:*225–229, 1980.

25. Shanfield, S. B., Heiman, E. M., Cope, N., and Jones, J. R. Pain and the marital relationship: psychiatric distress. *Pain, 7:*343–351, 1979.
26. Shontz, F. Behavior settings may affect rehabilitation client. *Rehabil. Rec., 8:*37–40, 1967.
27. Taylor, G. P., Jr. Moderator-variable effect on personality-test-item endorsements of physically disabled patients. *J. Consult. Clin. Psychol., 35:*183–188, 1970.
28. Trieschmann, R. B. *Spinal Cord Injuries: Psychological, Social and Vocational Adjustment.* Pergamon Press, Inc., Elmsford, New York, 1980.
29. Turk, D. C., Meichenbaum, D., and Genest, M. *Pain and Behavioral Medicine: A Cognitive-Behavioral Perspective.* The Guilford Press, New York, 1983.
30. Vash, C. The psychology of disability. *Rehabil. Psychol., 22:*145–162, 1975.
31. Violon, A., and Giurgea, D. Familial models for chronic pain. *Pain, 18:*199–203, 1984.
32. Wilcox, N., and Stauffer, E. Follow-up of 432 consecutive patients admitted to the spinal cord center, Rancho Los Amigos Hospital, 1 January to 31 December 1967. *Int. J. Paraplegia, 10:*115–122, 1972.
33. Zola, I. K. Social and cultural disincentives to independent living. *Arch. Phys. Med. Rehabil., 63:*394–397, 1982.

17

Sexual Function in the Spinal Cord Injured

GEORGE SZASZ

In human existence the meaning of sexual life or sexual behavior has certainly gone beyond the description of behaviors that merely precede, accompany, and follow the reproductive act. There seem to be three areas included in these words. The first, implying private experience, genital reactions, and practices that bring about desired sensation, is clear enough. The second area is less obvious. Human beings exist under pressure for pair bonding, however temporary that alliance might be. Culturally, this has a competitive element built into it, creating a need to be "marketable" and available for courting. A marketable or unmarketable person might be defined in various ways according to the subjective view points of people.

Courting, the third area, refers to partner selection activities. In this process one has to present one's best attributes to another person. Some of these attributes might be publicly seen, such as showing oneself off as a potential husband, wife, father, or mother. Other aspects of courting may require promises or demonstrations of performance capability (doing) in the mating act. Marketing, courting, and doing need a great deal of skill, and real or imagined failure in any one may result in self- or public rejection as a desirable man or woman.

In this chapter, sex and sexual will be used in the sense described above pertaining to doing, courting, and marketing. However, the focus will be on the experiences related to doing.

SEXUAL CONSEQUENCES OF SPINAL CORD INJURY

The diagnosis of spinal cord injury is based on physical and neurological examination rather than on seeing the damaged cord. In sex-related work the uncertainty about the precise nature of the injury is important for two reasons. From the patient's point of view in the early stages, a spinal cord injury is a spinal cord injury, with all the negative implications that one can conjure or with a lack of understanding that may be the result of denial (45). In either case poor understanding of the implications of the various types of injuries leads to chaos in the patient's life (16).

From the clinician's point of view, it is important not to make assumptions about sexual functioning potential only on the basis of a report like "complete lesion at the C8-T1 level."

> A 21-year-old man with "complete lesion at C8-T1" was reassured that whatever other problems he might have, he would have strong reflex erections. He was deeply disappointed therefore when he discovered that while he did get momentary erections in response to penile stimulation, they were so short lasting that he could not enter into the act of intercourse.

In this instance health care advisors gave reassurance on the basis of statistical data and not on the basis of the patient's history, physical examination, and consideration of such factors as medication side effects or the effect of recent urological surgery. Information based upon anything other than a proper assessment may lead to lasting negative consequences.

Several identifiable areas are useful in defining the sexual consequences of the cord injury:

1. Sexual response status reflects the physiological ability to experience genital sensations, erection, ejaculation, vaginal lubrication, orgasm, pelvic thrusting, and other responses to stimulation.
2. Sexual activity status indicates the available motor functions that might be used for such activities as embracing, caressing, and intercourse.
3. Sexual interest status reveals the degree to which the person wants to be involved in sex activities.
4. Sexual behavior status gives information about availability of partners and the social interaction skills leading to sexual activities.
5. Sex organ status describes the anatomical integrity of the genitalia and the sexual problems caused by urinary drainage apparatus, genitourinary infections, or surgery.
6. Fertility status reveals evidence of the need or ability to procreate or the nature of contraception desired.
7. Sexual self-view status reflects the person's self-evaluation regarding appeal and desirability as a sexual partner.

Consequences Related to the Sexual Physiology

Space does not permit a review of the sexual response cycle in the able-bodied. Proper understanding of the implications of spinal cord injury requires this information, and the reader is alerted to the many available texts.

Genital Responses in Complete Spinal Cord Injury

Sacral Injuries. In men with complete sacral injuries there is no erection response to tactile stimulation of the penis, and the usual genital sensation is lost. Some swelling and an occasional erection may occur in response to psychological or mental stimuli. The brain seems to "let go," and the released signals arrive at the still intact T11–12 segments. From there sympathetic fibers carry the messages to the cavernous tissues of the penis. The resulting swelling is often short lasting. After a few seconds, drops of sticky prostatic or seminal fluid may appear at the tip of the penis, and the penile swelling usually subsides. The neurological explanation is not clear, but as the T11–12 and L1–2 segments are seemingly related both to erection and seminal fluid secretion, the interaction of the two events is not surprising.

In women with complete sacral injury, the accustomed genital sensation is lost. Mental stimulation does not appear to produce visible changes in the vulva or the vagina. The sacral cord injured woman is able to accommodate the penis in the act of intercourse. The vagina remains moist, even without stimulation, and the preinjury vaginal muscle tone is retained.

Lesions Above T11 Neurological Level. In men with complete lesions above T11, usual genital sensations to touch or caress are lost. However, erection may occur quite reliably in response to any physical stimulus applied to the penis. This reaction is reflex in nature, involving the now-uninhibited reflex arc connecting the penis to the intact sacral segments of the cord.

The stimuli eliciting such a reaction may not be sexually intended at all. For example, tight trousers, applying a condom, or washing the penis may cause a reflex erection. The penis may become elongated and swollen within a matter of seconds. With further stimuli, the penis may become firm, although the tip often remains unengorged. The reflex erection may last from a few seconds to several minutes. Repeated squeezing of the penis usually brings about renewed engorgement of the organ. The capability for reflex erection does not alter noticeably with age or with the time elapsed after the injury. The reflex may be impeded by factors such as the effects of medications or the complications of some types of urological surgery. Muscle spasms may also interfere with the maintenance of reflex erections. Once the penis is inside the vagina, the reflex erection may be lost because of insufficient stimulation.

There is no seminal fluid in response to customary physical or mental stimulation. Vibrator-induced stimulation of the glans penis may, however, cause a reflex ejaculation of seminal fluid with accompanying muscular spasms and visceral sensations reminiscent of the build-up-and-release sensations associated with orgasm.

Accustomed genital sensation is also lost in women with complete lesions above the T11 level. Stimulation of the genitalia, however, may bring about swelling of the lips and clitoral tissues. The vagina is usually moist, even without physical stimulation, and the preinjury tone of the vaginal muscles is retained. Spasms do not close the vaginal opening, and the vagina is able to accommodate the penis in the act of intercourse.

Lesions Between T12 and S1. In complete lesions between the T12-S1 neurological levels, the accustomed genital sensations and usual orgasmic and ejaculatory reactions are lost in men. However, they may experience some penile swelling both to mental stimulation and to physical touch of the penis. These reactions are not coordinated, and the erections are usually poor in quality and often short lasting. Seminal fluid discharge may also occur in this type of lesion. The reason for these reflex reactions is that both the sacral segments and the segments above the T12 area are available for independent responses.

In women with complete lesions in the T12-S1 area, the clinical picture is essentially that occurring in a complete sacral injury.

Extragenital Responses in Complete Spinal Cord Injury

Mental stimulation and physical caressing of the neurologically intact portions of the body may cause momentary increases in respiratory rate, pulse rate, and blood pressure. Skin flush may occur, and perspiration may be noted on the intact areas. Muscle spasms are common. These reactions are similar in both men and women.

Quadriplegic women have reported orgasmic experiences occurring during sleep (35). Men with similar lesions do not seem to have these experiences. Both men and women with various lesion levels have reported that, in the course of active genital stimulation (e.g. using a vibrator), they have experienced buildup of pleasant sensations in the lower abdomen and bladder area, followed by gradual loss of these sensations (51). Others described referred sensations in some sexual situations. Sensations may also occur in the bladder or the groin area. Pleasurable sensations may be experienced following the caress of the nape of the neck, ear, eyelids, or other previously unexplored body areas. Some cord injured patients experience pain when stimulation is applied to skin areas bordering on the level of the lesion.

Sexual Response with Incomplete Lesions

The effects of incomplete lesions on the genital, extragenital, and mental components of the sexual response depend on the damage to the required pathways and cellular structures. For example, in some central cord lesions the sexual response might not be disturbed. If the lesion is a hemisection of the cord (Brown-Sequard's syndrome), some responses may remain intact while others may be disturbed. If the partial lesion involves the dorsolateral or ventrolateral sides of the cord, sensory or motor sparing may occur and some aspects of the response may be possible.

Time After Injury

When the reflexes begin to return after the initial period of spinal shock, some of the sexual responses may be exaggerated. For example, in a person with a complete, high lesion, strong and lasting erections may occur in response to even the gentlest genital irritation. This response may last for days and must be differentiated from priapism, which is an erection due to clotting of the blood in the penis. If the erect penis becomes even more erect with touch or if erection subsides when touch is removed, the condition is not likely to be priapism.

Erection in response to mental stimulation may not appear for several months after the injury. It is not known why this time delay occurs. Improvements in sexual responses may be possible in the long run. Once the neurological and hormonal status (37, 38) is settled, however, the sexual responses are not significantly affected by the passage of years.

Other Factors

Observations and research on the sexual response have been almost exclusively on males, and many subjects have been drawn from rehabilitation centers. Perhaps these persons do not represent the total spinal cord injured population. Mention has been made already of the difficulties in identifying complete versus incomplete lesions. Some responses should not be there according to clinical diagnosis. Some individuals are on medications (19). Others might be engaged in severe physical exercises related to wheelchair sports. The effect of these on sexual physiology is unclear. The availability of a partner may make some difference. Perhaps the partner's attitude is also important.

Consequences Related to Sexual Activities

Sex acts may be classified as solitary (masturbation) and partner-related acts. The latter might be subdivided into caressing, kissing, genital fondling, oral sex activities, and vaginal and anal intercourse. Many of the activities require coordinated musculoskeletal activities. Undressing, assuming desirable positions, holding, touching, stimulation with hands, and moving in rhythm with the partner may not be possible for a spinal cord injured person.

In considering sexual responses, the important cord levels were the sacral, T11 and above, and the T12-S1 areas. In sex-related motor functions, the significant dividing line is between those with and without adequate hand and arm function.

Acute spasms may be disturbing but may also have acceptable effects when these occur in response to the partner's stimulation. Severe spontaneous spasms may interfere with the able-bodied partner's attempts at genital caressing, may prevent the act of intercourse, and may even result in a fall from a wheelchair or a bed. Chronic spasticity may be associated with contractures and further loss of functional ability. Similarly, chronic pain or irritating tingling or burning sensations might lead to a cycle of irritability, moodiness, depression, and loss of sexual motivation.

Some acts may require vigorous participation by the partner to achieve desired sensation. This may be the case in some incomplete lesions, such as Brown-Sequard's, in which there might be good sensation available on only one side of the genitalia.

Consequences Related to Sexual Interest

One index of sexual interest is participation in "attempted" or "successful" sexual acts. Another is the mental preoccupation with sex activities. From a clinical point of view, it is difficult to define whether thoughts reflect the genuine sexual desire or not. In a sense, sex activities are playful pursuits. Players may lose their zest when the play turns into a chore.

Spinal cord injured persons with fond memories of a satisfying sexual life-style tend to have a strong motivation to reestablish their former practices. Those who in their preinjury sexual practices have been able to utilize the acts of intercourse, and manual, oral, or mechanical stimulation as desirable options, seem to hold more flexible attitudes about the appropriateness of various alternatives to sexual intercourse. For these persons, experimentation with different acts, different body positions, or altered sensations may now become an extension of their former approach to sex practices. Or if their preinjury sexual experiences had been limited, now they may be motivated to explore the available options.

Sexual disinterest can be caused by chronic pain, discomfort, malaise, and fatigue related to the complications of spinal cord injury. Sedatives, antispasmodic medications, and psychotherapeutic drugs may temporarily depress interest level (17). Drab living quarters or the physical environment of hospitals or institutional settings may also turn off sexual interest.

Still other negative factors include preoccupation and worry about finances, the job situation, housing, relationship discord, depression, feelings of hopelessness, and sexual dysfunctions that existed before the injury. To many, the norm is having the erect penis inside the vagina and coming to climax. Manual or oral stimulation is often thought of as a "preliminary act" that leads to the "real thing." To some anything other than intercourse is "perverse." Among able-bodied people, this focus on intercourse, rather than on enjoyment, is a major cause of erection dysfunction and loss of interest. Among people with spinal cord injuries, this belief may inhibit any experimentation with sex acts other than intercourse.

Two other factors may contribute to loss of sexual interest. One relates to the busy life of the spinal cord injured person. Getting up in the morning, getting dressed, getting to work, looking after urinary and bowel care, all take a great deal of time. Priorities have to be set and less important or less rewarding aspects of life may be the first ones to be dropped from the list of daily activities. When sexual practices were spontaneous in the preinjury days, scheduling them will not be easy now. As days pass by without acting on sexual opportunities, the premium on "making it good" increases. The situation, when it arises, may become awkward, more and more difficult to initiate, and suddenly the couple realizes that they have lost the usual signals and intimate moments that led to former spontaneous sex practices.

The other difficulty with interest arises out of the partner's burnout. Women partners are particularly stressed because suddenly they have to carry the burden of medical, financial, educational, child-rearing, and family management decisions. Fatigue, chronic tension, depression, life-style changes, anger, or resentment may rob the person of zest in general and sexual zest in particular.

Consequences Related to Sexual Behavior

In courting activities the focus is on establishing or maintaining a relationship that includes sex activities. These behaviors may vary in different cultures, and within the cultural context individuals have their own customs. Strong social norms dictate what is right and wrong. Many people with spinal cord injuries feel that they cannot compete with others under the existing rules; some feel totally unattractive and a burden to the partner.

Able-bodied people enjoying the company of friends with spinal cord injuries may be concerned about points of etiquette, caused by a feeling of responsibility for their welfare. Again the injured person is perceived as ill, and people who are ill need looking after.

The limitations in functional living skills, such as eating, dressing, and grooming independently may significantly interfere with the personal independence necessary for getting to the market place.

A 31-year-old woman with a C5–6 complete injury said, "I'm on the shelf. It's too hard for anyone to reach me. Even if someone came along, how would we find privacy? How could I be sure of being clean? What would happen if I fell out of my chair? How would I face the staff here at the hospital. . . . ?"

There is, however, immense variety to human sexual relationships, and there are many ways to overcome seemingly impossible barriers.

A 28-year-old man suffered a C2–C3 complete injury and was on a respirator. Eighteen months later he married a 25-year-old woman he had known for several years. While she is working, he spends 4 days in an extended care setting. On Fridays, he is transferred to their apartment. She says, "We spend much of the weekend in bed: talking, reading, making love. He likes me to have pleasure, and I get great satisfaction out of seeing his eyes light up. It has not been a chore. I feel happy and our families help a lot. The only thing that's missing is that I would like to have a child. . . ."

Even if mobility were not a major issue, courting may be negatively influenced by either the injured person's concerns over appearance or the partner's worries about showing interest and, thereby, making the spinal cord injured feel inadequate (10, 13, 14, 15, 39).

Consequences Related to Urinary and Bowel Problems

Both men and women tend to worry about offensive genital odors and "accidents," and the unsightly nature of catheters and conducting devices. Bladder and bowel accidents may occur more commonly when sex acts occur spontaneously. If there is time for planning, most people restrict their fluid intake and empty their bladder. Bowel accidents are more difficult to avoid, particularly if the routine calls for bowel care only every second or third day. Women may have more problems with this than men, presumably because the penis inside the vagina activates bowel reflexes.

A recurrent concern for some cord injured males is that the penis may have become smaller. They notice that when applying the condom drainage device, the shaft of the penis appears to be shorter than before. The reason for this is not clear. Perhaps the weakness of the pelvic floor is responsible for this change. In any case, when pressure is applied to the perineum, the penis becomes longer again.

A legitimate concern of males is that genitourinary surgery, such as prostatic resection or external sphincterotomy, may interfere with erectile ability. Injury may occur to some of the nerves required for erection when the external sphincter is divided. Using appropriate techniques, the current estimates suggest postsurgical erection problems in 5% to 20% of the patients (27, 44).

Consequences Related to Fertility and Contraception

Many people with spinal cord injuries have urgent concerns about fertility and contraception. An early concern of women is a missed period. Clinical experience suggests that in many instances menstrual periods are delayed until 2 to 4 months after the injuries. Thereafter the periods resume a predictable regularity. Regular menstrual periods are presumptive evidence of female fertility potential (23).

Women in their childbearing years are able to get pregnant in spite of their injury, although it is not known whether they are as fertile as able-bodied women of comparable age (20, 40). The fertility of men with spinal injuries is very much subject to dysfunctions. However, even a small volume of seminal fluid, a very low sperm count, and the presence of nonmotile or deformed spermatozoa show some capability for fertilization. Lack of erection ability or inability to experience penile sensations or orgasm is not a reliable indicator of infertility. Careful application of a vibrator to the tip of the penis may cause muscular spasms and ejaculation in some cord injured men.

The motor deficits and propensity for circulatory problems in the extremities complicate selection of the most suitable method of contraception. One way to get an idea about the possible limitations imposed by cord injury is to view birth control methods as "you-do-it" or "done-to-you" procedures.

You-do-it methods necessitate some motor and intellectual performance. When these are lacking, the done-to-you methods are useful. Condoms and withdrawal are the you-do-it methods used by men. Both methods require a certain level of motor coordination for correct application. The you-do-it methods used by women include barrier creams and foams, the diaphragm, oral contraceptives, and rhythm methods. Appropriate insertion of anything into the vagina requires specific physical abilities. Few people think that oral contraceptives have complex requirements. Yet appropriate use of oral contraceptives includes a series of motor acts that may be beyond the abilities of some quadriplegic women. The done-to-you methods available to women include intrauterine devices, tubal ligation, hysterectomy, abortion, and depot hormone injection. Vasectomy is the only done-to-you method currently available to men.

Virtually every birth control method is reputed to have some hazards. Some of these side effects are accentuated in the spinal cord injured because of the nature of the disability. For example, the thromboembolic hazard in the use of oral contraceptives containing estrogen may make this method inappropriate for a woman with a spinal cord injury who spends a large part of the day in a wheelchair. Progesterone-based oral contraceptives may cause weight gain and contribute to depression. Intrauterine devices may be inadvisable when a woman cannot feel discomfort indicating possible uterine perforation or pelvic inflammatory disease, or when increased menstrual flow would be difficult to cope with. Tubal ligation has few if any contraindications specific to physically disabled people. Hysterectomy has the added attraction of reducing the hygienic problems associated with menstrual flow. Postcoital contraceptive medication and even abortion might be considered for a person who has been sexually assaulted (48).

Consequences Related to Sexual Self-View

The significance of "doing well" in the doing, courting, and marketing continuum varies tremendously with individuals and perhaps even in one person over a long period of time (4, 5, 9). Comments like, "I'm not a man," "What else is there to life," "If I can't be a father, what else matters" are frequently heard. A pessimistic or distressed opinion about oneself as a sexual partner should not be mistaken for or labelled as loss of body image or loss of self-esteem. It is more valuable to find out, for example, in what specific way the person is "not a man" now than to dwell on the abstract concept of identity. The partner's opinion is also required to corroborate the complaint. Specific management approaches might be available to correct what appears to be overwhelming difficulty.

A 52-year-old man suffered a conus lesion. His main concern was over his sexual difficulties. He was able to perceive some sensation over his genitalia, experienced a modest increase in sexual tension on strong stimulation, and had a weak release sensation. While able to have penile swelling, it disappeared in a matter of seconds. He was distraught. This became the focus of his complaints, almost forgetting all other disabilities. He ignored his wife's reassurances regarding her satisfaction. The man visited several neurologists, neurosurgeons, psychologists, and family therapists. He was labelled as "unstable," "insecure in male identity," having "sexual envy." By accident, he read about a ring that could be applied to the base of the penis to retard outflow of blood. This appliance indeed helped him to retain his erection, to his tremendous relief. His wife also admitted that this was more satisfactory for her. His penis-oriented complaints disappeared.

SEXUAL ASSESSMENT

Sexual assessment is a way of adding up where a person is on the "marketing–courting–doing" continuum, and includes evaluation of past and present sexual functioning status, discovery of available potential, and detection of problems and their significance to the person and the partner. The process is also a vehicle for helping the person acquire a framework within which his concerns may be presented, considered and, in the long run, measured against a baseline.

The assessment has three interrelated parts: history, physical examinations, and investigations. In practice these would flow together. For example, some historical questions are best asked during a physical examination. In what follows, a more structured approach is presented to portray the content and the method of the assessment process.

The History

The objective is to let the patient and the partner explain what they have observed and experienced in the various sexual function areas and how these differ from the accustomed state before the injury. Assessment begins with a biography. Age is important because, of all variables, age influences sexual practices most. Marital and partnership status explains the context in which the patient lives and identifies the "significant other." Children give an idea of reproductive accomplishments in the past. Having children may also interfere with privacy. Occupation and education level sometimes predict the patient's way of handling explanations. Religious beliefs might indicate perspectives to be aware of. Medical condition gives information about health status and medications taken concurrently. Mood level exposes mental state. Current litigation may explain why the patient wishes to have an assessment now.

An important part of assessment is the detection of beliefs that may influence the patient's acceptance of a range of norms in sexual functioning. Expressions of these beliefs may often surface spontaneously. There are several give-away comments that reveal the patient's stance about "what should be." For example, the patient may use the word sex synonymous with intercourse, as in "We played around but did not have sex." The notion that sex equals intercourse implies that other forms of physical contacts are preliminary to the main act, or childish, or even, perhaps, perverse preoccupations. Sometimes, this idea is just a manifestation of not knowing; at other times, it is a deeply rooted conviction.

Another expression with similar tone is, "He should know what I want." In this instance, the partner implies that a man is born to know what a woman wants and when she wants it. "There is no spontaneity" is yet another expression revealing the need for communication. Human "doing" activities are far from ever being totally spontaneous. Anything from arranging the bedroom to washing hands or combing the hair, arranging pillows or applying perfume and deodorant to the body, or using contraceptives is, to some degree, contrived. "I am over the hill" or "I am too old to learn new things" are expressions revealing deeply held beliefs about waning sexual powers with advancing age. More significant is the fact that many persons at any age say, "It's ridiculous at my age," even though, inside themselves, they know that it is not.

These expressions serve as warning signals to the assessor that the sexual objectives of the person or couple may be very limited and focused. The reasons for asking intimate sexual questions must be explained in detail, and sexual alternatives that might be obvious to the interviewer should be introduced with great care.

Assessment of Sexual Response Status

Knowing the level of injury does not necessarily lead to the right conclusions about a person's sexual response status. Many lesions are called "complete" for all practical purposes, yet vague sensations and visceral reactions may still be perceived. The patient's and the partner's observations are important clues to what potential is available. Physical examination, trial stimulation, and investigations are at times needed to define the extent of the available responses. The information one wants to obtain has to do with erection, ejaculation, orgasm, and genital sensation in men, and lubrication, orgasmic experiences, and genital sensation in women.

Assessment of Penile and Vaginal Responses. The extent of penile responses may be judged from drawings made by the patient or from his estimate, based on a 0 to 10 scale. Zero to 2 is an unresponsive, flaccid penis; 3 to 4 is a soft, swollen, and bendable penis, the glans of the penis able to touch the base of the shaft; 5 to 6 is a swollen penis, still bendable but the glans penis could not be touched to the shaft; 7 to 8 is a firm but not completely rigid penis; and 9 to 10 is a strong erection. It is important to inquire about what happens before the swelling starts, how long it lasts, and what may have caused the loss of the swelling.

Inquiry about lubrication response in spinal cord injured women will not shed much light on sexual responsivity because, for reasons not clear, the vagina of these women tends to retain its moistness even in the resting state. The paraplegic woman may use her finger to test for lubrication; the quadriplegic may need to ask her partner to look or feel.

Assessment of Orgasmic Experiences and Ejaculation. Inquiry about orgasmic experiences of men and women can be done in a similar way. A curve is drawn, as illustrated below. The horizontal axis represents time elapsed in the sexual play; the vertical axis is the increasing intensity of the responses. The curve represents a hypothetical norm: beginning with mounting interest, greater and greater sensations of genital involvement are noted; involuntary muscle contractions occur, and hip movements are noticed; a high level of sexual interest is reached and a tension is building that requires release. The orgasmic sensations, and in men, ejaculation, are experienced, and relaxation flows over the body. The question is: Does this illustration reflect the spinal cord injured person's past experiences? If yes, what does this "sexual mountain" look like now? If the preinjury picture was different, what was it like and how does it compare with events now?

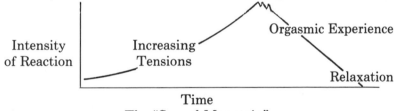

Time
The "Sexual Mountain"

Questions regarding ejaculation should clarify whether or not there is seminal emission. If there is, is it "squirting" or "dripping" and if not but there is orgasm, what happens if the perineal area is massaged? In some instances following prostatic surgery or when the perineal muscles are paralyzed, massaging the area behind the scrotum helps to milk the seminal fluid out of the urethra.

Questions regarding an inability to reach an orgasm may require clarification of the experience. For example, some people may say, "I just don't get any higher, I kind of level off and then the feelings and sensations just settle down slowly." Others might say, "I am quite high, and then suddenly I plummet down into an abyss. That makes me frustrated; sometimes I cry."

Assessment of Sexual Practices

Sexual Interest. There are several ways to estimate sexual interest/disinterest levels. One is to inquire about the individual's personal interest level or interest level with the partner. Indicators of personal interest level may include reports ranging from the frequency of masturbation attempts to the time spent on daydreaming about sexual situations. Interest level indicators regarding partner-involved sex activities include reports of the frequency of attempted and successful activities—for example, in the last 2 to 3 weeks and how that compared with past activity levels.

Reports of the present situation need to be compared with information about past interest levels since characteristically, persons belong to low, mid, or high activity level groups, and tend to remain in these groups as they grow older. Again using a scale representing a continuum from disdain/disgust through indifference to a high positive response is useful in quantifying interest.

In some instances, the interest is present but it turns off at a certain point, or conversely, there is general indifference, but a "turn on" may occur during such activities. Disinterest sometimes begins when one partner does not get "anything" out of sex activities. This, of course, might affect the other partner. While some people really do not get "anything" out of, for example, intercourse, most persons enjoy some part of physical caress and the attendant intimacy. The assessor will want to broaden the customary narrow definition of sex activities to include all activities that provide even a semblance of feelings associated with sexual sensations.

Motor Abilities. Here the assessment is a checking out of the motor function requirements for preparation toward sex activity, engaging in the activity, and disengaging from the activity. The intimate nature of sexual activities usually precludes observation but descriptive reports from the patient and partner often suffice. These activities may include hygienic preparations and transfers to bed, touching, holding, grasping and caressing with hands, moving, inserting, and removing the penis, applying the mouth to various parts of the partner's body, breathing at an increased rate, dealing with spasms, transferring back to wheelchair, and looking after clean-up procedures. The assessor should be able to formulate a mental image of what the patient can do and come up with alternative motor actions when requested.

Genitourinary, Bowel, and Menstrual Hygiene. Much of this assessment will be done during the physical exam. However, patients have so much anxiety about accidental bladder and bowel incontinence that a review of diet and fluid intake is essential to see if prevention of accidents, by planning ahead, is possible. Other questions may relate to the most successful urinary conduction methods and the length of time it is safe to be without a condom drainage device. Can the patient take it off/put it back himself? In women, can the catheter be left in? If so, can it be tied off or does it need to be connected to drainage? Women often have more problems with involuntary bowel movements because the penis inside the vagina may inadvertently trigger the bowel reflexes. Are there positions in intercourse that are better or safer? With regard to menstrual hygiene, is there the motor ability to insert/remove tampons?

Fertility and Birth Control. Here assessment is largely dependent upon the physical examination. However, the patient and the partner may be able to report on observations. For example, secretion seen welling up from the cord-injured man's penis may have been seminal fluid, or an increased vaginal discharge may indicate problems with an intrauterine device.

A very difficult aspect of the assessment is the evaluation of the desire to become a parent. At times the social and personal significance of parenting or of being perceived as a potential father or mother is more important than actually having children. Sometimes there is an enormous preoccupation and concern with the issue of parenthood and the appropriateness of artificial insemination by donor. Questions may need to be aimed at discovering how the couple visualize themselves during the period of pregnancy, birth, postnatal period, and in the first few years of child-raising. Their concerns about public knowledge of the child's genetic heritage need to be explored. Family attitudes about the alternate ways of acquiring a child should be elicited. The intention of these questions is not to dissuade but to clarify feelings and purposes. In this area assessment and treatment clearly overlap.

Sexual Behavior. Sexual behavior refers to the etiquette of entering into and maintaining relationships and includes sex acts as one component. Questions about sexual interest levels and motor abilities do in a way search for answers relating to sexual behavior. Courting is an interpersonal skill usually acquired in the teenage years. A review of the past is therefore relevant. Past expertise can be reactivated, and conversely, inexperience may cause reticence to begin a new relationship. The intent is to identify and explore capabilities and opportunities unique to the person.

Sexual Self-View. The two areas of interest to the assessor are: (a) the patient's evaluation of his or her competence in all the various sexual areas discussed above; and (b) what beliefs might determine the meaning of some of the sexual losses or gains? For example, how significant is it to the patient that intercourse might not be possible? How significant is it to the partner that the cord injured person may not respond as obviously as able-bodied persons? Does the spinal cord injured person feel that he is "over the hill?" To what extent is the injured person's "manhood" or "womanhood" threatened by job changes, income level changes, partner reactions, or parenting difficulties?

The Physical Examination: Three Parts

The examiner first wants to get a good idea about the physical capabilities of the patient (49). Watching a person move out of the wheelchair onto an examining bed and how he/she undresses (or cannot undress without help) give an estimate of the person's potential for various sex acts. In women particularly, the flexibility of the hips has to be checked and the significance of spasms estimated.

Next the examination focuses on general hygiene and on cleanliness in the genital area. The examiner would look at the condom drainage device, and check the tubing and leg bag. Is it clean? Are there offensive odors? If there is underwear worn (many cord injured males prefer not to wear underclothing), is it clean?

In women, the catheter would be examined for cleanliness. Given the physical structures of the woman, would the catheter be in the way in face to face intercourse? Can this person use tampons? If not, what are the manageable alternatives?

In the third part of the examination, the neurology of the genitalia is checked. This is useful for estimation of orgasmic capability and, in men, may serve to sort out whether tactile or psychogenic erections will be available.

This part of the physical examination may also offer an etiological explanation for physiological problems. For example, in an incomplete injury, all the relevant sensations and reflexes may be present but the man may not have the desired penile erection or the woman experience orgasms. In such situations, further history and examinations are required to explain the reason(s) for the situation.

Two tests are of value to determine the potential for orgasmic reactions in response to genital stimulation:

1. Testing pain or heat/cold sensation in the genitalia checks sensory pathways between the genitalia and the brain. These tests give information about the lateral spinothalamic tracts that are considered intact if a pinprick on the penis or the woman's genital area is immediately perceived as sharp and painful, or if hot and cold stimuli are immediately and correctly identified.

2. Contraction of the anal opening on command provides information about the motor fibers going to the genitalia from the brain along the fibers of the pyramidal tract systems. If in addition to correctly perceiving pain, heat, or cold, a patient is voluntarily able to contract the anus the basic tracts are open for genital sensation and for male and female orgasmic reaction.

If one of these tests is negative, the patient will not be able to experience orgasm or, in the male, ejaculation. The male patient may still be able to have reflex touch or psychic erection, depending on the level at which the injury has occurred. Three reflexes are tested to clarify the situation:

1. Sensory fibers of the testicle enter the spinal cord at T9. Absence of sensation when the testicles are squeezed indicates a lesion above T9 and there is no possibility for "mental" erections. If the patient experiences acute testicular discomfort, the lesion is likely below

T10–T12, and the chances are strong that psychic erections may occur (3).

2. Squeezing the tip of the penis normally elicits the bulbocavernosus reflex, indicating the sacral segments of the spinal cord are open and tactile erection is likely to occur.

3. The examiner's finger is placed in the patient's anus to test for the anal tone reflex. Contraction of the internal muscles over the examiner's finger confirms that both the sacral and lumbar segments of the cord are intact. When both the bulbocavernosus and the anal tone reflexes are present tactile erection is usually strong, because the level of the injury is higher up in the cord.

In women the bulbocavernosus reflex can be tested by pressing the clitoris to elicit anal contraction. Anal tone is tested in the same manner as for men, but the significance of these is not understood.

On the rare occasion when an injury occurs at the L2-S1 level, the bulbocavernosus reflex and testicular pain reaction can be elicited, but there is no perception of pain in the genitalia, no anal tone, and no voluntary ability to contract the anus. In this situation, both mental and tactile erection may be expected, although of poor quality. Orgasm and ejaculation will still not be possible with ordinary stimulation.

Investigations

Investigations aimed at delineating remaining physiological potential or sexual interest are few and disappointing in their lack of precision. The simplest form of investigation is to ask people to experiment privately, with or without a partner, and collect their reports. Other investigations include:

1. Nocturnal penile tumescence measurement is based on the observation that, with normal neurological systems, continuous erections occur during the REM cycle of sleep. This test is of uncertain value in persons with incomplete injuries and of no value in a complete injury (29).

2. Laboratory tests may include serum testosterone levels, sex hormone binding globulin ratios, and LH, FSH, and prolactin levels. The norms are not yet understood in spinal cord injury, so occasional tests are of dubious value. More important is to check urinary and blood sugar levels, and estimate thyroid function in persons whose sexual symptoms do not make sense in relation to the physical findings.

3. A series of urological tests have been developed in the last few years to estimate the dynamics of bladder function. These are indirectly useful in estimating integrity of the genital system (43).

4. Fertility studies in men and women are available. The reader may wish to consult specific descriptions in relevant texts.

MANAGEMENT

Flexibility of Norms

Problems in marketing, courting, and doing have three sources:
1. Physiological impairments caused by the lesion or as side effects of medical or surgical treatment.
2. Physical disabilities secondary to the impairments.
3. Handicaps brought on partly by the impairments and disabilities, and partly by the individual's past and present perceptions of what is normal, right, acceptable, or desirable.

As management of sexual problems in the spinal cord injured person often means reaching for alternatives, flexibility about norms in the sexual areas is a key determinant in satisfactory sexual rehabilitation.

Most people consider alternative sexual practices on a continuum from "good" or "highly desirable," to "bad," "inappropriate," "immoral," or "childish." The norms are derived from isolated personal experiences, hearsay about other persons' experiences, or from religious edicts, legal precedents, and poorly informed authoritarian medical opinions. One's own opinions are often reinforced by those of others. Many able-bodied think of people in wheelchairs as unmarketable as husbands, wives, or parents. Some parents try to dissuade their able-bodied daughter from marrying a spinal cord injured man. Some physicians suggest abortion in spinal cord injured women. Unfortunately, these suggestions are based upon unsubstantiated beliefs. Interestingly, recent achievements of wheelchair athletes and the portrayal of spinal cord injured lovers in movies has begun to alter this image. Most newly injured persons, however, still feel that their whole world has just collapsed. It is at this point that the consideration of alternatives has to move away from the "good"–"bad" continuum toward a "first among equals" image.

Some persons hold on to their beliefs about good or bad with such tenacity that the belief has to be looked upon as malignant. The management dilemma here is not that the patient or partner have substantial sexual problems related to the impairments and disabilities, but rather that they are handicapped by preexisting beliefs that more or less extinguish their motivation to look for options. Either partner may believe the type of sex they can offer is of no value anymore in achieving closeness. They feel there is no point in talking about sexual rehabilitation or exploring the larger meaning of human closeness and the role of sexual practices in it.

On other occasions, however, similar sounding beliefs may be relatively easy to change because they were based upon misunderstanding or ignorance about physiological, anatomical, or behavioral possibilities. A fundamental aspect of management is, therefore, the assessment of all aspects of sexual knowledge and practice, contrasting the past with the present.

In some situations the injury represents a turning point in the person's (and the partner's) life. An existing or new partner might be able to provide the required sensitivity, tolerance, and patience. Each might make attempts to have oneself better understood. In this regard, individuals and their partners need to know early in the hospital stay that sexual concerns are common, and that the staff will accept their expression. Early information is particularly useful to those cord injured who had a variety of favorable past sexual experiences. While also devastated by the situation, they soon begin to sense that their valuable interpersonal skills have not been damaged. Having experienced a flexible life-style before, they now seem able to capitalize on past experiences.

Management Approaches

Treatment methods for the sexual consequences of spinal cord injuries may be psychological (talk and guidance oriented), physical (focusing on positioning, environmental arrangements, using external devices, appliances), pharmaceutical, or surgical (using internal devices) (2, 9, 11, 18, 22, 26, 31–33, 36, 41, 52).

Psychological Methods

The goals of the psychological approach are to dispel myth, increase freedom of choice, and support the patient's right to feelings and their expression. These goals are formulated on the notions that knowing about a situation is essential to coping with it, and specific beliefs such as "intercourse is the only acceptable sex act" tend to get in the way of experimentation. Psychological methods may include education to increase biological and self-knowledge, reassurance about adequacy, diminishing of hesitation toward alternative sex activities, and increasing acceptance of viewing and touching one's own and the partner's body.

Education about sexual functioning in the spinal cord injured may be provided in various ways, including pamphlets, books, videotaped informational packages, or lectures. A wide spectrum educational approach allows the individuals to choose the appropriate method for themselves and get involved at the level that is most comfortable for them. The disadvantages are that most of these methods are too general in their approach and may allow one to opt out of these methods at the slightest apprehension about the content.

Education and reassurance can be offered in a low-key manner. For example, a 24-year-old single woman said to the intensive care nurse days after her injury, "I guess I will never have a child now."

Nurse: Why do you say that?

Patient: I am paralyzed. Finished from below the belly button. How could I become pregnant or carry a baby?

Nurse: I am not sure of your specific situation, but in general, women with spinal cord injuries can become pregnant, carry, and have the baby even if they are paralyzed.

Patient: I never knew that! I heard somewhere that men with spinal cord injuries cannot become fathers!

Nurse: This is not always so either. It depends on the type of injury, and they also have methods to help some of the men. But if a spinal cord injured woman is in her childbearing years, is healthy, and does not use birth control, she can have a baby.

Patient: Hm . . . that kind of changes the picture . . . So then . . . sex is also possible?

Nurse: By sex you mean intercourse? Yes! It would be quite possible . . . the sensations might be different in the genital area. . . .

Patient: How about my breasts?

Nurse: Your lesion is low so that your breast sensations are not expected to change.

Patient: I have to tell this to my boyfriend! I thought I was finished. . . .

The nurse provided reassuring information that was new to the patient and limited to her immediate needs. Because it was personal, factual, and delivered at the instant required, it made a deep impression.

An in-depth educational approach is needed when certain deeply held beliefs surface during the interview.

For example, a 28-year-old man with an incomplete sacral lesion said,

Patient: I just feel that I am not a man. What can I offer to a woman? There is no purpose left.

Nurse: It looks to me like you are saying that the woman does not look at you beyond your penis.

Patient: Well, maybe when I become old sex won't mean much, but let's face it, there are a million other guys out there. Why should she put up with me?

Expressions of beliefs like these may indicate deep-seated opinions and perspectives about life. An assessment of recent and past sexual experiences, sexual growth and development, current sex physiological knowledge, and perceptions of behavioral norms would be needed here. The need is not to define when or how such beliefs become set but to provide the therapist opportunities to correct misconceptions, offer new information, and force the patient to examine his beliefs, which until now, were based on what he considered clear evidence. Repeated use of this approach often weakens firmly held beliefs and provides the opportunity to look at sexual issues from other perspectives.

The techniques of low-key and in-depth educational approaches are the same: one would clarify questions before giving information, ask "open-ended" rather than "closed" questions, ask for permission to proceed to unexplored areas, and explain why the question is asked.

Techniques for diminishing hesitation toward alternative sex activities and increasing acceptance of viewing and touching one's own and the partner's body are borrowed from "sex therapy" methods (28). These differ from other psychological treatment methods in two respects:

1. The goals are limited to the relief of the patient's sexual symptoms.
2. Its methods include prescribed sexual experiences.

Originally devised for able-bodied persons suffering sexual dysfunctions, these methods shift attention from intercourse and orgasm to giving and receiving pleasure. The couple learns that apprehensions about any sex act may cause erection, ejaculation, orgasmic difficulties, and eventually sexual disinterest. An expectation of the therapy outcome is that as various nonintercourse sex acts are accepted by the couple as pleasurable, they will be approached with less apprehension. As performance anxiety lessens, the sexual response is more likely to unfold.

In spinal cord injured persons, the sexual response physiology is usually impaired, so the full benefits of sex therapy cannot be realized. However, the components, namely education, reassurance, and sexual skills practice, can be used in various combinations and appropriate levels of intensity just about any time after the injury.

Prescribed sexual skill practices serve to introduce or rekindle intimate activities when a person or couple is too apprehensive to attempt them, or when those activities are not part of a couple's past sexual experiences. Practical sexual prescriptions should usually be made only by qualified therapists who will take a detailed sexual history before deciding where to start in the experimentation. Offhand suggestions, like "Well, try it with the mouth," may be harmful if considered offensive to the couple. An equally important reason for reserving this approach to qualified therapists is that the results of experimentation need appropriate follow-up.

When it was suggested to a 29-year-old male with a complete T4 lesion and his 27-year-old wife that, as a first step, they attempt to caress each other just to find out which areas of the body would still feel "good" when touched, they came back quite disappointed. She said nothing happened, and he agreed. It turned out that she was still so worried that he would feel like a failure that they did not even try the exercise. In this instance, perhaps the therapist did not explain the purpose of the practice clearly enough. More likely, however, the couple required further explanations and reassurances before they could experiment.

These psychological approaches are short-term treatments to deal with current problems. They best suit the psychologically well-functioning who have clear-cut, well-defined sexual concerns. Noncompliance with these methods may signal the presence of other preoccupations or stresses, or may indicate the need for longer term treatment of personality disorders, depressions, or psychoses. Psychotherapy, marital therapy, assertiveness training, or other behavioral modalities may be of value in enhancing the cord injured person's life and indirectly solve sex-related problems.

Pharmaceutical Methods

The goals of this method are limited because no known medications directly increase sexual interest or restore erection, ejaculation, or orgasmic experiences.

Drugs are used for two purposes:

1. To foster a healthy and pain-free existence in the face of a crippling condition.
2. To limit the patient to medications that are the least likely to interfere with the physiological process of sexual functioning.

Medications used to reduce anxiety, relax spasms, or provide rest or pain-free periods may help indirectly, presumably because the patient feels more zestful. Many medications, however, interfere with interest and function. These include sedatives, analgesics, anticholinergic and antiadrenergic drugs, muscle relaxants, estrogens, and the major tranquilizers (40).

The therapist must remember the sexual side effects of illness and medications, and must inquire systematically about changes in interest, erection, lubrication, and the orgasmic and ejaculation process. This may lead to recommending alternate medications when untoward changes do occur.

Physical Methods

Here the goal is to give technical assistance in the physical aspects of sex activities. Promotion of independent movement, dressing and undressing, cleanliness, and secure bowel and bladder management are part of this approach. Occupational and physical therapists may wish to conceptualize a "bedroom scene" and apply the principles of activities of daily living toward the requirements of sexual interaction. On a more specific level, the patient may need technical advice about positions, the use of a water bed, or extra pillows under the hips. Unfortunately, no specific information is available about the relative value of these, but using common sense in dialogue with the couple, one can identify guidelines to problems that may otherwise baffle the patient.

Sexual practices include preparation for, engaging in, and disengaging from sexual activities. Consideration may have to be given also to assistive devices, family planning, or birth control management.

Preparation. The spinal cord injured person may have to plan for and rehearse many of the activities that others take for granted. Preparations may include bladder and bowel check, disconnecting urinary and drainage devices, oral hygiene, moving to a bed or other suitable place, transfers, positioning, and undressing.

The skills for independent management of these activities are described in other chapters. Many however, prefer a degree of continuity in sexual activities, and the partner may elect to help the quadriplegic disrobe, lift the partner into bed, or elect to conduct their activity in the wheelchair. New partners may first need guidance as to the complexities of wheelchair management, undressing, and catheter or hygiene routines. A recent partner may be surprised at the skills required and energy expenditure needed for activities that come easily to most persons. Many couples find it useful to keep towels, pehaps a dish, close by, in case of urinary or bowel accidents, or to clean off perspiration or genital fluids.

The Setting. Preparations may have to be made to find an appropriate place for sex activities. Privacy is an important consideration, particularly in group living situations. However, the concept of privacy may have to be enlarged to include an attendant if two disabled persons want to get together.

Adequate space is another consideration in selecting a place for sex activities. If a bedroom is used, space should be available for wheelchair movement and transfer to bed.

Some spinal cord injured persons prefer a waterbed to add to the rhythmic movement of sex acts. When a hard surface or cramped quarters are the case, the quadriplegic may wish to use supporting pillows and change positions every few minutes to avoid pressures or abrasions to the skin.

Bowel and Bladder Hygiene. Individuals may wish to plan ahead and reduce fluid intake in the 2 or 3 hours preceding sex activities. When fluid intake is restricted and the bladder emptied just before sex, urinary accidents are unlikely. Men using condom drainage may disconnect their apparatus. Some men prefer to use a fresh condom to catch small amounts of leakage during sexual play.

Spinal cord injured women with indwelling catheters may disconnect the catheter and tap the end to the lower abdomen or groin area. Men with indwelling catheters may first disconnect their catheter then close off the end of the tube. After producing a reflex erection, they bend the free portion of the catheter back on the erect penis. Finally, they may apply a condom to cover the erect penis and the catheter. Lubricant on the condom may facilitate easier entry into the vagina.

Stomas. Some quadriplegics with high spinal cord lesions may have a tracheostomy, with or without a breathing apparatus. They may need to learn the best positioning for easy breathing and the continuous ventilating action of the respirator.

Ileostomies, colostomies, and urinary bags should not produce undue complications to sexual practices. Preparation may include emptying the bags and assuring that the adhesive holding the appliance binds well. Some persons may wish to wear an apron-like garment to cover the bags.

Engaging in Sexual Activities

Manual Stimulation. The quadriplegic may wish to use the fingers, hands, arms, nose, lips, ears, and hair to rhythmically caress the partner. Some of the activities are best accomplished if the able-bodied partner is positioned within reach or if the partner moves against, for example, the immobile hand. Other activities may be managed with the movements a quadriplegic has learned to manipulate various objects. For example the penis may be held between the heels of the quadriplegic's hands or an overhead sling may be adapted to permit rubbing of the vulva or clitoral area of the well-positioned female partner. Principles of tenodesis may be adapted to breast or genital stimulation. The back or side of the hand may prove to be softer than the fingers in caressing the face, breasts, or other desired areas. Aids and splints may be employed in several ways. For example, caressing may be accomplished using a hand splint covered with sheepskin or other soft material.

Caressing the spinal cord injured person may require considerable guidance. The cord injured person may need to indicate both the areas still sensitive to touch and those that might be hypersensitive or even painful to caressing. The nondisabled partner may need to prepare for longer periods of stimulation.

The method devised for caressing or the time spent on touching each other is not, perhaps, as important as knowing what the partner requires at that particular time. Directions to each other therefore may lead to exploration of a wide variety of high quality experiences.

Oral-Genital Sex Acts. These acts may require body positioning by the able-bodied partner. Adequate hygienic preparation would reduce concerns over the degree of cleanliness of urinary or bowel openings. When the act is applied to the quadriplegic, urinary flow may occur in spite of normally adequate bladder management. Spasms in the adductor muscles of the hips and thighs may temporarily trap the head of the partner. If stopping the activity for a few moments does not reduce the spasm, the gentle, steady pressure on, for example, the knee, may reduce the muscle tension. Sometimes medication may be required to prevent spasms. However, some cord injured with higher lesions may enjoy the rhythmic contraction of the hip and leg muscles in response to active genital stimulation.

Gagging, choking, or not getting enough breath may be a problem for the quadriplegic engaged in oral sex. Experimentation with these acts and becoming proficient in giving clear signals to the partner to move, are the ways to manage these situations.

Intercourse. For many, sexual intercourse provides both emotional closeness and physical pleasure. Suitable positioning may require assistance by the partner or application of techniques of self-positioning in bed. The various methods of turning, moving down the bed and the use of an overhead bar for bed mobility can be well applied here.

Sitting on top of the cord injured male may provide for the comfort, mobility, and stimulation required by the female partner. This position also provides for a face to face view which may offer additional stimulation to each.

Women with low cord lesions may prefer to lie on their back with their legs separated. Spasms in women with higher lesions may make this position impractical. On occasion, pillow support under the knees helps to open the legs. Other women may wish to lie on their side, with one or both knees pulled up. In the man-on-top position, the quadriplegic woman may have to pay attention to her freedom of breathing. She may have to tell her partner to avoid pressing on her chest. Leg spasms may allow for holding the partner.

Intercourse in the wheelchair may be an alternative to lying down. The quadriplegic man would ease forward in the chair so that his partner is able to straddle him. Similarly, the injured woman can slip forward in the chair and the partner kneel between her legs.

The mechanics of intercourse require thrusting the penis in the vagina in a rhythmic manner. The quadriplegic lying on his partner may contribute to this action by using his skills to roll from side to side. On his back, he may wish to use his overhead strap to produce a bouncing motion in rhythm with his partner's movements. Lubricating jelly applied to the penis may reduce chafing the vaginal opening and the vaginal wall.

Spasms occurring during intercourse may add to the rhythmic movement, but in men with high lesions, severe leg spasm may make intercourse difficult. Gentle, steady pressure on the legs may release the spasms. Occasionally medication may be required to control extreme sensitivity to touch.

The soft penis of the cord injured male can be "stuffed" into the vagina. This technique is easier to accomplish with the man on top and the partner's legs drawn up. The partner moves her seat so that she can guide the well-lubricated soft penis into her vaginal opening. She can then contract her vaginal opening in a rhythmic manner and gently move her hips to expose herself to the desired stimulation.

Disengaging from Sex Activities. The technical aspects of disengaging include bathing or washing the genitalia, getting dressed and transferring back into the chair, and may take as much energy and organization as preparation for the activity.

For some the period after sex activity may be characterized by elated feelings and strong energy. Others find they have become quite tired. Some couples find they can go only so far, and then have to rest or stop. Yet others might feel frustrated and angry that they cannot achieve their objectives.

The psychological aspect of disengaging is clearly of importance. This time period may be of value to "debrief" each other about the preparations, the positions, the preferred ways of stimulation, the nature of the responses, the newly-discovered potentials, and the plans for next time.

Assistive Devices. Some couples may wish to enhance their sexual experiences through technical means. Penile rings and dildos are external methods to assist with erection. Rings may capture blood in the penis and thereby produce and maintain erection. They come in several forms, some flexible, others more rigid. Any of them may be effective sometimes, if applied to a partially swollen penis. Placing the ring on the penis requires a degee of manual dexterity, which may not be available to the spinal cord injured. The risks of using rings are poorly documented, but medical concerns include causing skin damage to the penis, damage to the erectile tissue inside the penis, and even bruising of the urinary passage in the penis.

Dildos are rubbery or hard casings that fit over the soft or semierect penis. The casings may be held on with suction devices, adhesives, or straps. The purpose in using dildoes is to provide stimulation inside the vagina.

Some couples may enjoy using these implements; others may find them strange or repulsive. Common sense must rule. If the applicance is of value and acceptable to the couple, then it might have a place in the management of their sexual problem.

Stimulation may be enhanced by vibrators used by either partner for several purposes. An abled-bodied partner may enjoy the sensation of vibration on the body as well as on the genitalia. To provide this stimulation, the quadriplegic may need to use a wrist-driven flexor hinge to assure a good grasp on the vibrating appliance. The cord injured man or woman may enjoy the vibration sensation on the neurologically intact areas of the body. Application of the vibrator to the tip of the penis or the clitoral area may produce abdominal and leg spasms. These spasms may become rhythmic and in some instances be accompanied by internal feelings of tension even though the genitalia itself may be insensitive to touch. In persons with high lesions, the prolonged application of the vibrator to the genitalia may also cause extragenital responses, including elevation of pulse, respiratory rates, and blood pressure. Some quadriplegics may experience headaches in such situations. The vibrator may cause skin abrasions or burns on the skin (40, 50).

Birth Control and Male Fertility. Advice may be required for the selection of the safest and most protective birth control method. This area has been discussed earlier and as noted must take into consideration both medical indications and contraindications, and the person's physical capabilities. Vibratory stimulation of the penis and electroejaculation techniques show promise for management of infertility in men with certain lesions (6, 19, 51, 52).

Surgical Method

The only surgical approach to the management of sexual problems is insertion of an internal penile prosthesis, making possible a reliable firmness of the penis. These devices are either firm or flexible rods or fluid-filled cylinder-like structures inserted into the erectile tissues of the penis. Some need to be pumped up when erection is desired. The pump is located inside the scrotum and activating it requires strong finger power. The quadriplegic may require assistance from the partner. Similarly, manual dexterity and strength are required to press the release button.

A secondary benefit of prosthetic devices is that the rods or the casings for the cylinder provide for a degree of firmness of the penis even in the resting state. Some men find it easier to apply their condom drainage device over this semifirm penis.

The prosthesis neither promotes ejaculation nor does it restore sensation to the penis. It seems to be of greatest value to patients who have no touch-reflex erections. Designed to assist both able-bodied and spinal injured men, these devices require substantial surgical procedures that may not be in the best interest of the individual. A concern with any internal prosthetic device is that pressure sores may develop in the shaft or perineum (30, 42).

Choosing the Treatment Approach

The choice of treatment depends on many factors. One should rarely reach out for a surgical solution in the first 2 years following injury since return of function may well occur in that time. An educational or talk-oriented approach would be appropriate at any time. The approach might be less directive if an unpartnered person is asking for help than when an interested couple comes to inquire about specific sexual issues. A "marital" rather than "sexual" approach might be indicated if not only the couple's "bedroom" but their "living room" is in turmoil.

Administrative decisions about the inclusion of sexual rehabilitation in the institutional setting is another determinant of treatment approaches. Availability of trained personnel, specialist backup, and payment schedules for professional treatment programs are yet other variables.

Selecting a treatment approach can be visualized in six steps:
1. Clarify the problem.
2. Compare and contrast pre- and postinjury sexual functioning status.
3. Define physical and physiological capabilities (through examination and investigations).
4. Explore realistic sexual goals.
5. Define psychological capabilities and resources available in moving toward the patients' goals.
6. Explore other alternatives, if necessary.

Treatment Approaches With Children

Little is known about the sexual concerns of young spinal cord injured children. Parents, however, might have grave concerns about the sexual future of the injured child. Some parents prefer to withhold information from their child about the likely losses, particularly in the fatherhood area. Other parents encourage an outgoing life-style for their injured child. Both hope for ultimate adjustment, but the first believes there is a specific time in the growing person's life when sexual issues should be dealt with, while the second hopes that adjustment will come through daily experiences, in school, sports, and friendships, over a long period of time.

There is some evidence that exposing the injured child to the tumults of daily experiences is better in the long run than saving him from uncertainties, until he is "more mature." Formal sexual assessment and management efforts are probably out of place for very young children. However, sexual assessment seems to be appropriate, with parental permission, for the pubescent boy and girl. Preliminary discussions with parents are important because they need to know what the sexual counselor will present to the child. If the parents prefer to withhold sexual information, even after discussion with the counselor, then, at least under current social arrangements, this is their right.

The situation is different if a teenager has had preinjury sexual experiences that represent adult behavior. While the parents' approval should still be sought, if it is not forthcoming, a second professional opinion should be requested. If it is in agreement, sexual assessment and management should be carried out when requested by the youngster. In the prescription of contraceptives, the same safeguards may be applied.

One dilemma is in the use of a prosthetic device for young persons. For example, a 16-year-old boy suffered a L1-S4 injury. He had no erectile response to physical touch or to mental stimulation. He was sexually active before his injury and gravely concerned about his sexual life now. There was no change in his situation 2 years later. A decision was made to proceed with an implant. In the short run, this has worked out well. However, presumably he will live another 40 to 50 years. Will medical and technical advances be available in the next few years that will make the surgical approach look like a mistake?

Parents of cord injured youngsters may develop sexual problems of their own. The reasons for this are not clear, but several factors seem to be operational. Adult couples who see sexual practices as "stolen pleasures" rather than as means of closeness often break off sex activities when they feel depressed and guilty about, or preoccupied with, the gravity of their child's situation. One parent is often in the hospital for days at a time, inadvertently neglecting other members of the family or preventing them from offering support to the injured child. This distancing may lead to a break in sexual routines and difficulty picking them up later. Couples often stop talking to each other because they are so sad and they do not wish to cause each other more distress. These circumstances may lead to sexual disinterest, and erection or orgasmic problem. It is clearly the professional's role and responsibility to mention to parents that interpersonal conflicts, including sexual ones, are not unusual features in the life of the injured person's family (8).

Institutional Approaches to Management

Over the last 40 years there have been three administrative approaches to the sexual concerns of patients and partners:

1. To deny or repress sexual expressions. The philosophy behind this approach is partly that sex is an inappropriate area for professional exploration, that the patient's whole attention should be focused on return to work, and that it may be a further strain on the patient to learn about sexual disabilities on top of other problems.

2. To tolerate expressions of sexual needs and even offer some answers or suggestions when this appears to be appropriate or when one or two interested health professionals are willing to get involved. This approach is usually haphazard and often undertaken with only token support from the medical staff. It is characterized by a well-meaning surge of interest in the plight of some patients, exclusion from consideration of the needs of the young and the old, dependence on a few interested staff members, and a "wait and see" attitude in most of the nursing and medical staff. If an untoward incident occurs, such as a phone call from a wife who is upset that "someone talked sex with my husband," the staff member involved may be reprimanded and memos may fly!

3. To organize a program of sexual rehabilitation. An organized program needs clearly defined goals acceptable to the staff members. There must also be a clearly stated outline of the specific services required, the type of personnel who will be responsible for offering various aspects of this patient-partner care service, and their relationship to other team members. The relationship has to be spelled out in terms of the referral methods and the role of staff members "before the specialist arrives," the methods of reporting back to staff members, and the inclusion of reports in the agenda of team meetings. A protocol must be drawn up for both introducing the service to the patient and the family, and communicating with staff of the next institution assuming care of the patient. The plan must provide ongoing staff education and introductory education for new staff members, coordination with other programs, means of supervision, consultations, backup services, and in-service training programs, materials, supplies, and physical space for various required procedures. In addition, there may be the need for a protocol to manage areas of conflict for staff.

A Model of the Organized Approach

There are few models of the organized approach. One example is the Sexual Health Care Service located in the Acute Spinal Cord Injury Unit of Shaughnessy Hospital, the G.F. Strong Rehabilitation Centre and Pearson Extended Care Hospital, Vancouver, B.C. The service is offered by sexual health care clinicians (with a background in one of the health care professions) working with a physician specializing in sexual medicine. The service includes staff education and research in addition to patient, partner, and family care (34).

Services consist of assessment, education, and sexual skill training. These are extended to the patient, his or her present or intended sexual partner, and the patient's family (parents of adolescents, for example). The services can be followed through the following steps:

1. Soon after admission the patient's primary care nurse takes a history, and in the course of obtaining data from the patient, inquires about any concerns the patient may have about sexual functioning. The nurse offers reassurance that such concerns are common, tells the patient there is a specialized care service on the ward, and that the sexual health clinician will introduce herself later. The existence of the service is brought to the attention of the partner and family as well. This first step legitimizes the early ventilation of sex-related concerns and establishes sexual rehabilitation as a routine part of the unit's medical program.

2. Introductory visits. The sexual health clinician visits the patient frequently. During the first few brief meetings with the patient and family, the clinician tries to elicit any sex-related concerns, helps the patient organize these concerns, obtains preliminary evidence of physical dysfunctions, and outlines future steps in the rehabilitation process. The physical examination, the brief diagnostic procedures, the clear questions, and the direct approach all tend to legitimize the patient' inquiries and give an air of openness and competence to the program.

3. Assessment. By the second month, most of the patients are over the acute phase of their injury and are usually ready for a major assessment of their sexual potential.

   If a partner is available, a private assessment is made of the partner's experiences, present sexual tensions, and methods of resolution. The partner is then invited to participate in the patient's assessment, which includes a physical examination. The assessment deals with each of the categories of the patient's sexual functioning status. Specific alternatives are then explored and on occasion demonstrated. For example, the partner may want to see how to bring on a reflex erection, or both may want to know what position in intercourse is most feasible. Some patients may want to know about sexual aids. A private room is made available to the couple for unobserved use at their convenience.

   A record of the assessment is summarized under the various headings of the sexual functioning status list. After review with the patient and partner, the summary is placed in the chart. No final diagnosis is made because the patient's physical and social circumstances may change in the future. Follow-up, therefore, becomes very important (21).

4. Follow-up visits. Follow-up visits are carried out to correct areas of confusion and misinformation, to monitor changes in the patient's sexual functioning pattern and marital and social relationships, and to encourage experimentation with alternative sex activities. The follow-up includes preparation for discharge and periodic progress visits thereafter. Some patients do not wish to have follow-up visits. Other patients wish to delay experimentation until they are in their home environment. Patients who have no partners may be encouraged to experiment by themselves.

Outcome evaluations of this program are inadequate. The objective of patient care services is to provide treatment on the basis of assessment. This requires a highly individual approach to each patient and a range of goals that can be very broad, from reassurance and relief gained through accurate information to a reorientation of the patient's perspectives about the acceptable range of sexual expression.

Immediate and retrospective reviews indicate that in nearly all instances the clinician's interaction with patients and partners leads to a clear definition of the patient's functioning in sex response, sexual activity capabilities, interest level, fertility status, and urinary-bowel hygiene relevant to sex activities. About two-thirds of the patients and partners are able to refocus their sexual expectations on goals consistent with their physical disabilities. This process may take several months or several years. It is not yet possible to assess the relative significance of factors such as the clinician's input, the behavior of the existing partner (or the appearance of a new partner), the success of vocational reorientation, or the financial status of the family.

One recurrent observation is that the nature and severity of the injury is not the important determinant of the outcome. Two factors that seem to help the patient refocus and work toward realistic sex-related goals are: (a) active, varied, and satisfying sex relationships before the injury, and (b) an interested and adventurous partner. If these factors are missing, or if one or both partners are consumed by anger related to the catastrophic injury, it is more difficult for the clinician to help the couple achieve significant goals in the short-term.

Less Formal Approaches to Management

Although an organized sexual rehabilitation program may be the ideal, it is not always possible. Patients will, however, still approach nurses, therapists, psychologists, social workers, and even housekeepers with their sex-related concerns. If there is specialist backup, both patients and team members feel more at ease discussing sex issues. But even without a specialist around, patients want to explore their sexual situation.

Should the nurse, social worker, physiotherapist, or occupational therapist be involved in sexual care? If so, should this involvement be limited to informal and private discussions with the patient or should it be a formally assigned task? In either case, should the interaction be reported at the team meetings? Should the patient's physician be informed about the patient's concerns? Should these staff members give advice? If so, what guiding principles should be followed? Who should set these? For example, to whom should the nurse be accountable if something goes wrong, and who should reward the nurse for excellence in the practice of sexual health care? The answers to these questions are not always clear-cut. An important role can however be identified for the nonsex specialist health and social care worker.

Sexual First Aid. As the name implies, this approach is a form of brief intervention applied at the time the need for aid is perceived. It might include defusing anxiety by providing acceptance and limited information, and finding more qualified helpers. The intensity of this type of first aid varies with the perceived need, the professional's preparedness to clarify the type and nature of complaints and provide limited information, the physical environment, and the ease of access to specialists in the sexual field.

The four components of sexual first aid are:
1. Accepting sexual concerns (which may be expressed directly, indirectly, or obtained in the course of specific enquiries).
2. Clarifying the concerns.
3. Giving information.
4. Applying professional knowledge to sexual areas.

Accepting Directly Expressed Sexual Concerns. The early introduction of the idea that "sex is spoken here" lowers the patient's anxiety about the topic being ignored. It also helps the staff. Sexual concerns will be part of the problem list now, and it will be relatively easy to approach the patient again at some appropriate moment in the future.

Other ways of letting the patient know about acceptance of sexual questions or concerns would be in a pamphlet describing the services offered in the treatment unit. Some patients prefer to read about sexual alternatives rather than discuss them. For example, the 45-year-old wife of a doctor suffered a T12-L1 fracture with complete paraplegia. She thought sexual health care was a "wonderful idea," but she preferred to "read about it rather than talk." She studied the few pamphlets the nurse gave her but did not ask any questions. She was seen, however, introducing other female patients to her reading material.

Acceptance of Indirectly Expressed Sexual Concerns. Examples of indirect expressions of sexual concerns include repetitive references to one's past sexual prowess, repeated compliments about the nurses' desirable physical attributes, jokes with sexual connotations, hypothetical questions like, "If you were my wife, would you care to go to bed with me?", or statements like, "Maybe my husband should find another woman." Patients may also make inappropriate sexual propositions or gestures to staff members.

Sometimes what the patient does or says is not an indirect expression of sexual concerns or desires but behavior representing indirect complaints about the treatment program or concerns over not making good progress in recovery. The staff person's task here is to find out what these expressions really mean. Where they are truly sexual concerns the task is to project acceptance and encourage the patient to express them.

Doug, a 28-year-old man, married 6 weeks, suffered a C6–7 injury. Two months after his injury, he was being prepared for his first weekend home visit. Although usually a cooperative and well-motivated patient, he became abusive to the staff, yelled at his wife, and refused to participate in physiotherapy. When the physiotherapist suggested to him that the exercise would help him transfer into bed, he said, "You'd think I'm training for my second honeymoon."

Doug's nurse picked up on this and attempted to clarify.

Nurse: Is that the way you feel?

Patient: What way?

Nurse: Like you're going on your honeymoon?

Patient: Are you kidding?

Nurse: Well, no, but I can imagine that you might feel some pressures. (This is acceptance of feeling.)

Patient: What the hell are you talking about?

Nurse: Well, we somehow haven't talked about you and Jane being in the same bed. (This directs the interview toward the sexual area.)

Patient: Maybe we didn't talk because it's none of your business.

Nurse: Perhaps not. Have you talked with Jane about this? (This is further directing.)

Patient No. What's there to talk about?

Nurse: Well, this first visit home is kind of an experiment. (This focuses the discussion.)

Patient: There you are. Sex raises its ugly head.

Nurse: I did not say sex, or intercourse, or erection, or orgasm. Maybe the two of you want to try something, maybe not. What I am saying is that you and Jane may want to agree before the weekend what your plans are. She might just want to know how the two of you can be side by side. (This gives options and responsibilities to the patient.)

Patient: Yeah. Hm . . . Is this written down somewhere?

Nurse: Well, no, but when Jane comes in today, we could make a list together.

Patient: I wouldn't mind it.

This brief illustration shows how the nurse disarmed the patient's angry outburst, clarified the main concern, and helped the patient acknowledge his hurt and fear. The patient could now explore alternatives with dignity. The nurse accepted sexual issues as part of the person's daily life, and used common sense and interviewing skills to handle the situation.

Barbara, an 18-year-old woman (partial C6–7 cord injury), was engaged in a light-hearted conversation with a male nurse about fashions and clothing styles while doing her exercises in the physiotherapy room. Discussion focused on the differences between "sexy" and "sensuous" clothing, and she turned to him for an opinion.

One would not immediately identify this conversation as a cry for help, yet Barbara recalled the incident several months after her discharge from the unit. She said, "I desperately wanted to know, am I attractive enough for a man to have interest in? Do I still come across as a sensuous person in a wheelchair? But nobody heard my questions!"

Clarification of Concerns. Once a patient's complaint or concern is out in the open, it has to be clarified. To which of the categories listed earlier does the patient's complaint belong? Is it worry about erections and orgasms, loss of interest, loss of the partner's interest, new relationships, active participation in sex acts, or managing urinary and bowel control during a sex act? Is it a concern about becoming a father or mother, or about contraception? Clarification translates the patient's diffuse worries into manageable bits. It also reassures patients that their concerns are not unique.

A 52-year-old woman, married for 28 years and the mother of three sons, suffered an incomplete injury to the C6–7 segments in a car accident. Two months after her injury and just after her husband had visited, she turned to the nurse and said "I think I want to talk to somebody about our sexual life. This was very important to my husband . . . to me, too. You know . . . not that we are like kids, but we enjoy each other. I guess I can live without it, but it was so much a part of our life."

Nurse: I'm glad you're feeling comfortable enough to talk about sex with me (acknowledgment). I guess you know I don't have special training in sexual counseling, but I would be glad to listen. Would I do? (This indicates limitation and invites further information.)

Patient: I'd like it if you would listen.

Nurse: I might have to ask you a few questions, too. (This is asking for permission to explore when appropriate.)

Patient: I could talk to you.

Nurse: Should we arrange a time then? Like around 2 p.m., just after your treatment? (This gives an official seal of approval to the discussion, lowering the anxiety level.)

Around 2 p.m.:

Nurse: We have some time now.

Patient: I hope I'm not holding you up. I don't even know where I should start! I've never known anybody with my type of injury before. Does it cause any sex problems?

Nurse: Well, you know, just the other day one of the other patients said exactly the same thing and asked the same question (This reassures the patient.)

Patient: You mean other people ask about sex too? That makes me feel better. I thought I might get reprimanded or something.

Nurse: More and more people want to get proper information now. But sex means so many things. How would you feel if I asked you a few questions?

Information Giving. Information giving is the third level of "sexual first aid." It is most appropriate when the patient expresses a specific concern about sex. Giving specific information is an organized approach to the patient's distress. Once the main complaint is isolated and the reason for its timing understood, the staff member has a good opportunity to clarify misinformation and provide relevant new information. Equally important is a closure to the brief discussion. This may consist of a promise for more information, a check with someone more expert in the situation, or a discussion with the partner.

Staff must accept the patient's statements without cover-up or offers of false hope, clarify specific complaints and misinformation, and if it appears to be in the best interest of the patient, arrange for a visit with someone more knowledgeable.

A special aspect of information giving is to introduce the patient to self-monitoring of visceral sensations relating to the genital area or accompanying sexual activities. Spasms, nasal congestion, or headaches are some of the many indirect body expressions that may occur in response to genital touch or body caress. Recognizing these early may help the patient to realize that he or she is not "dead." Partners also benefit from knowing about such reactions, because, however minimal, these are responses!

Applying Professional Knowledge To Sexual Areas. In certain situations, professionals may focus their expertise on a specific sex-related problem. The nurse, physiotherapist, occupational therapist, social worker, psychologist, or other professional may become a temporary "sex consultant" to other staff members, the patient, the family, or the sex specialist (1, 2, 25, 47).

Physiotherapists may be helpful in considering alternative positions. The possibility for using adaptive equipment should not be overlooked and the occupational therapists expertise utilized. The skills of the social worker or psychologist may be beneficial in managing problems related to sexual communication.

The following is a summary of some of the techniques that may help staff in giving sexual first aid:

1. Ask for permission. Whenever a new sexual area is about to be discussed, a good approach is to ask: "Can I ask you a question about your relationship?" or "I would need to know if you have experienced an erection in the last few days. May I ask you about this?" If the patient says, "No, I don't want to talk about it," the staff member can safely reply, "I'm glad I asked you first. I wouldn't want to invade your privacy." While the nurse should stop this line of questioning, the reason for the patient's somewhat frightened reply may need to be investigated.

2. Be specific. Most patients find it easier to deal with well-stated questions than generalities. For example, "What sort of erection did you notice this morning?" is a question that can be answered with some specificity. "What was going on down below this morning?" is such an unclear way of asking that the answer might not be trustworthy.

3. Avoid irrelevant questions. A useful rule is to ask oneself, "Why did I ask this? Could I explain the reason for my question if the patient challenged me?" If the answer is "yes," the question was not irrelevant.

4. Start with reassurance. "Many women with spinal injury go through periods of loss of interest, but tell me . . . this loss of sexual interest that's concerning you now . . . have you ever experienced it before your injury?"

5. Proceed from least sensitive to more sensitive areas. "I wonder . . . in your conversations with your friends, have you heard about self-stimulation? Have you read about it? What sort of feelings have you had about it? Many young children stimulate themselves—what was your experience as a child? What has your experience been in the last few years?"

6. Use language that is clear to the patient. The language can be medical, slangy, or earthy, depending on the patient's needs and the nurse's comfort. Patients sometimes say "organism" meaning orgasm, "pee-nuts" instead of penis, or "clidoris" instead clitoris. In these instances, correction may be embarrassing, but letting the patient know that "not that it makes any difference, but here we usually say orgasm" may be helpful (46).

Practicing to Provide Care

Staff members need to practice fulfilling a role in sexual health care. Even if they have a great deal of knowledge about the sexual consequences of spinal cord injury and the best of intentions, they may feel so awkward, vulnerable, and concerned about causing hurt to the patient that a sexual conversation is impossible. One way to acquire the necessary confidence is to practice various conversations. By role-playing staff members can rehearse various ways of detecting concerns or giving sexual first aid. Audiotape or videotape equipment is useful because it is possible to review style, sound level, points of hesitation, methods of reassurance, clarity, and so on.

In some institutions, staff members participate in "desensitization" programs that include viewing explicit sexual films, discussing reactions to sex-related words, and describing sex acts. The value of these programs is not clear (24).

Perhaps a more fundamental approach to acquiring a facility with sexual conversation is to reflect on the fact that health professionals are motivated in their work by their desire to help people. There is plenty of evidence that sex problems are distressing to most patients. Their desire to talk and enthusiasm about receiving information usually motivates health professionals to help. This motivation leads the staff member to seek more knowledge, better communication skills, and sometimes, promoting the creation of an environment where the sexual consequences of the patient's disability are formally considered.

REFERENCES

1. Ambramovitz, N. R. Human sexuality in the social work curriculum. *Family Coordinator*, 20:349–354, 1971.
2. Annon, J. S., and Robinson, G. H. Behavioural treatment of sexual dysfunctions In: *Human Sexuality and Rehabilitation Medicine*. Edited by Sha'ked, A. The Williams & Wilkins Company, Baltimore, 1981.
3. Bermant, G., and Davidson, J. M. *Biological Basis of Sexual Behavior*. Harper & Row, Publishers, Inc., New York, 1974.
4. Bors, E. Perception of gonadal pain in paraplegic patients. *Am. Med. Assoc. Arch. Neurol. Psychiatry*, 63:713–718, 1950.
5. Bors, E., and Comarr, A. E. Neurological disturbances of sexual function with special reference to 529 patients with spinal cord injury. *Urological Survey*, 10:191–222, 1960.
6. Brecher, R., and Brecher, E., editors. *An Analysis of Human Sexual Response*. New American Library, New York, 1966.
7. Bregman, S. *Sexuality and the Spinal Cord Injured Woman*. Sister Kenny Institute, Minneapolis, Minnesota, 1975.
8. Bregman, S., and Hadley, R. G. Sexual adjustment and feminine attractiveness among spinal cord injured women. *Arch. Phys. Med. Rehabil.*, 57:448–450, 1976.
9. Brindley, G. S. Reflex ejaculation under vibratory stimulation in spinal cord injured men. *Parapleia, 19:*299–302, 1981.
10. Brockway, J., Steger, J. C., Berni, R., Ost, V. V., Williamson-Kirkland, T. E., and Peck, C. L. Effectiveness of a sex education and counseling program for spinal cord injured patients. *Sex Dis., 1*(2):127–137, 1978.
11. Cleveland, M. Family adaptation to the traumatic spinal cord injury of a son or daughter. *Soc. Work Health Care, 4*(4):459–471, 1979.
12. Cole, T. M. Sexual problems of paraplegic women. *Med. Asp. Human Sex, 10:*105, 1976.
13. Comarr, A. E. Marriage and divorce among patients with spinal cord injury. *I-V. Proc. 11th Ann. Clin. Spinal Cord Injury Conf.* (VA Hospital, Bronx, New York):163–215, 1972.
14. Comarr, A. E., and Vigue, M. Sexual counseling among male and female spinal cord and/

or cauda equina injury, Parts 1 and 2. *Am. J. Phys. Med.*, *57(6):*107–122, and *57(10):*215–227, 1978.

15. Conine, T. A. Sexual rehabilitation: the roles of allied health professionals. In: *Rehabilitation Psychology-A Comprehensive Textbook.* Edited by Krueger, D. W. Aspen Systems Corporation, Rockville, Maryland, 1984.

16. Crewe, N. M., and Athelstan, G. T. Spinal cord injury—pre and post injury marriages. *Arch. Phys. Med. Rehabil.*, *60(6):*252–256, 1979.

17. David, A., Gur, S., and Rozin, R. Survival in marriage in the paraplegic couple: psychological study. *Paraplegia*, *15:*198–201, 1977–1978.

18. Deyoe, F. S. Marriage and family patterns with long-term spinal cord injury. *Paraplegia*, *10:*219–224, 1972.

19. Diamond, M. Sexuality and the handicapped. *Rehabil. Lit.*, *35:*34–40, 1974.

20. Drugs that Cause Sexual Dysfunction. *Med. Lett.*, *15:*73–76, 1983.

21. Eisenberg, M. G., and Rustad, L. C. Sex education and counseling program on a spinal cord injury service. *Arch. Phys. Med. Rehabil.*, *57:*135–140, 1976.

22. Francois, N., Maury, M., Jouannet, D., David, G., and Vacant, J.: Electro-ejaculation of a complete paraplegic followed by pregnancy. *Paraplegia*, *16:*248–251, 1978–1979.

23. Goller H., and Paeslack, V.: Pregnancy damage and birth complications in the children of paraplegic women. *Paraplegia*, *10:*213–217, 1972.

24. Griffith, E. R., and Trieschman, R. B. Sexual functioning in women with spinal cord injury. *Arch. Phys. Med. Rehabil.*, *56:*18–21, 1975.

25. Griffith, E. R., and Trieschman, R. B. Sexual function restoration in the physically handicapped: use of a private hospital room. *Arch. Phys. Med. Rehabil.*, *58:*368–369, 1977.

26. Griffith, E. R., and Trieschmann, R. B. Sexual training of the spinal cord injured male and his partner. In: *Human Sexuality and Rehabilitation Medicine.* Edited by Sha'ked, A. Williams & Wilkins, Baltimore/London, 1981.

27. Hamilton, E. A., and Nichols, P. J. The problem of period control in disabled women. *Ann. Phys. Med.*, *9:*288–294, 1968.

28. Held, J. P., Cole, T. M., Held, C. A., Anderson, C., and Chilgren, R. Sexual attitude reassessment workshops: effect on spinal cord injured adults, their partners, and rehabilitation professionals. *Arch. Phys. Med. Rehabil.*, *56:*14–18, 1975.

29. Higgins, G. E. Sexual response in spinal cord injured adults: a review of the literature. *Arch. Sex. Behav.*, *8(2):*173–196, 1979.

30. Hodges, L. C. Human sexuality and the spinal cord injured: the role of the clinical nurse specialist. *J. Neurosurg. Nurs.*, *10:*125–129, 1978.

31. Hohmann, G. W. Considerations in management of psychosexual readjustment in the cord injured male. *Rehabil. Psychol.*, *19:*50–58, 1972.

32. Jameson, R. M. Division of the external urethral sphincter and potency in spinal cord injury patients. *J. Urol.*, *130:*86–87, 1983.

33. Kaplan, H. S. *The new sex therapy: active treatment of sexual dysfunctions.* Brunner Mazel Inc., New York, 1974.

34. Karacan, I., Williams, R. L., Thornby, J. L., and Solis, P. J. Sleep related tumescence as a function of age. *Am. J. Psychiatry*, *132:*932–937, 1975.

35. Kolodny, R. C., Masters, W. H., and Johnson, V. E. *Textbook of Sexual Medicine.* Little, Brown & Company, Boston, 1979.

36. Larsen, E., and Hejsaard, N. Sexual dysfunction after spinal cord and cauda equina lesions. *Paraplegia*, *22(2):*66–74, 1984.

37. Light, J. K. and Scott, F. B. Management of neurogenic impotence with inflatable penile prosthesis. *Urology*, *17(4):*341–343, 1981.

38. Martin, D. E., Warner, H., Crenshaw, T. L., Crenshaw, R. T., Shapiro, C. E., and Perkash, I. Initiation of erection and semen release by rectal probe electrostimulation (RPE). *J. Urol.* *129:*637–642, 1983.

39. Masters, W. H., and Johnson, V. E. *Human Sexual Response*. Little, Brown and Comany, 1966.
40. Melnyk, R., Montgomery, R., and Over, R. Attitude changes following a sexual counseling program for spinal cord injured persons. *Arch. Phys. Med. Rehabil.*, *60:*601–605, 1979.
41. Miller, D. K. Sexual counseling with spinal cord injured clients. *J Sex Marital Ther.*, *1:*312–318, 1975.
42. Miller, S., Szasz, G., and Anderson, L. Sexual Health care clinician in an acute spinal cord injury unit. *Arch. Phys. Med. Rehabil.*, *62:*315–320, 1981.
43. Money, J. Phantom orgasm in the dreams of paraplegic men and women. *Arch. Gen. Psychiatry*, *3:*373–382, 1960.
44. Mooney, T. O., and Cole, T. M. *Sexual Options for Paraplegics and Quadriplegics*. Little, Brown & Company, 1975.
45. Naftachi, N. E., Viau, A. T., Sell, G. H., and Lowman, E. W. Pituitary testicular axis dysfunction in spinal cord injury. *Arch. Phys. Med. Rehabil.*, *61:*402–405, 1980.
46. Phelps, G., Brown, M., Chen, J., Dunn, M., Lloyd, E., Stefanick, M. L., Davidson, J. M., and Perkash, I. Sexual experience and plasma testosterone levels in male veterans after spinal cord injury. *Arch Phys. Med. Rehabil.*, *64:*47–52, 1983.
47. Ray, C., and West, J. Coping with spinal cord injury. *Paraplegia*, *22(4):*249–259, 1984.
48. Robertson, D. N. S. Pregnancy and labour in the paraplegic. *Paraplegia*, *10:*209–212, 1972.
49. Romano, M. D., and Lassiter, R. E. Sexual counseling with the spinal cord injured. *Arch. Phys. Med. Rehabil.*, *53:*27–33, 1973.
50. Rossier, A. B., and Fam, B. A. Indication and results of semirigid penile prostheses in spinal cord injury patients: long term follow-up. *J. Urol.*, *131(1):*59–62, 1984.
51. Rydin, E., Lundberg, P. O., and Brattberg, A. Cystometry and mictometry as tools in diagnosing neurogenic impotence. *Acta Neurol.*, *63:*181–188, 1981.
52. Schoenfeld, L. Carrion, H. M., and Politano, V. A. Erectile impotence: complications of external sphincterotomy. *Urol.*, *4(6):*681–685, 1974.
53. Sha'ked, A., editor. *Human Sexuality and Rehabilitation Medicine: Sexual Functioning Following Spinal Cord Injury*. The Williams & Wilkins Company, Baltimore, London, 1981.
54. Stevenson, R. W. D., Szasz, G., Maurice, W. L., and Miles, J. E. How to become comfortable talking about sex to your patients. *Can. Med. Assoc. J.*, *128:*797–800, 1983.
55. Szasz, G. Sexuality curriculum for physiatrist, physiotherapist and occupational therapist. In: *Sex Education for the Health Professional: A Curricuum Guide*. Edited by Rosenzweig, N., and Pearsall, F. P. Stratton, New York, 1978.
56. Szasz, G., Miller, S., and Anderson, L. Guidelines to birth control counselling of physically handicapped. *Can. Med. Assoc. J.*, *120:*1353–1358, 1979.
57. Szasz, G. Sexual health care. In: *Management of Spinal Cord Injury*. Edited by Zejdlik, C. P. Wadsworth Health Sciences Division, California, 1983.
58. Szasz, G. Vibrator-induced ejaculation in spinal cord injured men. Personal communication.
59. Szasz, G. Vibratory stimulation of the penis in spinal cord injured men. Paper presented at the Canadian Congress of Rehabilitation, Vancouver, 1985.
60. Van Arsdalen, K. N., Klein, F. A., Hackler, R. H., and Brady, S. M. Penile implants in spinal cord injury patients for maintaining external applicances. *J. Urol.*, *126:*331–332, 1981.

Index